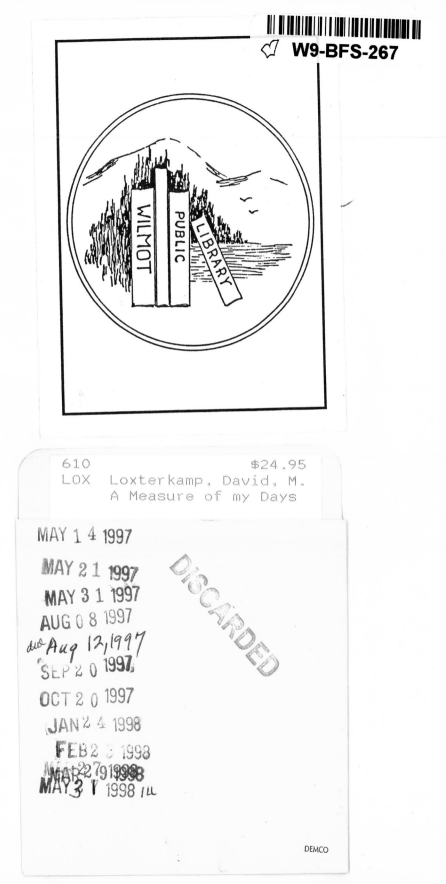

A MEASURE OF MY DAYS

A MEASURE OF MY DAYS

The Journal of a Country Doctor

DAVID LOXTERKAMP, M.D.

University Press of New England

Hanover and London

University Press of New England, Hanover, NH 03755
© 1997 by David Loxterkamp
All rights reserved
Printed in the United States of America

5 4 3 2 1

CIP data appear at the end of the book

Acknowledgment is made for permission to reprint the following previously published chapters:

"A Good Death Is Hard to Find," *Journal of the American Board of Family Practice* 6, no. 4 (July–August 1993).

"The Watch," *Journal of the American Board of Family Practice* 6, no. 1 (January–February 1993).

"In the Midst of Death," *Commonweal* 122, no. 15 (September 8, 1995).

"Taking the Gravel," *Journal of Family Practice* 39, no. 6 (November 1994). Reprinted by permission of Appleton & Lange, Inc.

For those with whom I share this place and time,

especially my beloved Lindsay,

and our children,

Clare and John, whose blessing is immeasurable.

Contents

Preface

The journal chronicles a year in the life of a rural family practitioner. The year is 1992. The place is Belfast, Maine. The value of such a testament may lie in its plain description, its breadth of focus (on a community rather than a single inhabitant), its writing in the pitch of a prolific life, and my earnest attempt to look honestly at my labors. The reader is permitted to follow me behind the closed doors of the examining room and operating suite, down a path to a trailer in the woods or home for supper, and inside the doubts and fears and self-deceptions that I see as plaguing the human condition, particularly my own.

I hope to practice medicine in Belfast for many years to come. To succeed at this means that I must measure up to, and keep, the confidence of those patients who come to me for their care. Therefore, all of their names have been changed or omitted. Many of the patients described in the journal have died, but, where he or she is still alive, I have also altered the description of the illness. Names of colleagues are left largely unmentioned except where the mentioning is of little consequence or I doubt their disapproval.

I would like to thank a number of people whose love, support, and guidance have made this book possible. First of all, I would not be a doctor were it not for my parents, Edward and Rosemary Loxterkamp, a general practitioner and charge nurse cast from the old mold. Dr. G. Gayle Stephens has been a lifelong inspiration, correspondent, mentor, and friend, and sustains my vain attempt to record what we see similarly in medicine. My office staff has made Searsport Family Practice a home to write about. We now number sixteen, including Tim Hughes M.D., Cathy Heberer, Trudy Norman, Scott Bailly P.A.C., Bonnie Allard R.N., Nancy Rivers R.N., Debbie Dakin, Mary Beth Leone L.C.S.W., Donna O'Leary R.N., Lisa Nielsen M.D., Kim Ashey, Keirstin Wyman, Amy Barden R.N., Theresa Dyer, and Becky Helm. I cannot thank all of my patients by name, or thank them enough. But it is for them—their suffering, courage, gratitude, and understanding—that I labor. I am indebted to my agent, Faith Hamlin of Sanford J. Greenburger Associates, who never lost hope that she would find a suitable home for my manuscript, and to the many people at University Press of New England who worked hard to bring it to press, especially my editor, Phil Pochoda, and copy editor, Carol Sheehan.

Lastly, I must thank my family: Lindsay McGuire, who inscribed on my wedding ring *toi et nul autre* and made good on her word; and our lovely daughter, Clare, and long-awaited son, John, who waited for me, too, while I typed and revised "just another line." They have always been the hardest test and the best of all possible rewards.

Belfast, Maine   D.A.L.
September 1996

A MEASURE OF MY DAYS

Introduction

VIGILS

A monotone pulse penetrates my unconscious, wiggles between the sheets, and rouses me from my bed. I hobble toward the window where the alarm clock rests. With a flick it is silenced, and I gaze out to a billowing gray mist, the cool breath of Belfast Bay as it blows past my window on an early midsummer morning. It is 4:30 A.M., light enough to convince me that day has begun. Cats scampering underfoot, I creak downstairs and begin the morning chores.

I grind the coffee and set it dripping, blend the crunchy cat food into raw scrambled egg for the felines, Kitty and Dinky, and choose the morning chants, which today are the *Carmelite Vespers* of George Frederick Handel, scored in sacred choral polyphony. There is an easy, unfettered satisfaction in these mechanical motions that gently wake me, and peel the sleep from my eyes. I smell the vapors of coffee dripping, hear the faint coughs of my wife and daughter stirring overhead in their gentle dreams, feel the vibration of wooden legs squeaking across the floor beneath me as I slide to my desk and create a time and place for the world opening to my imagination.

What I see in my practice shapes my life. And through my writing I return to see it better: bits and strands of everyday medicine woven into one's conscience like a robin nesting, in a place where earaches and bellyaches, "bunches" and "risin's," or some unutterable sorrow provide the day's take in "accomplishment" or "insight" or, not uncommonly, a niggling sense of defeat. It is a world that seems light-years from the glamour, drama, or cutting edge of the university medical center, one where the rewards for your labor are found in the bargain bins and dumpsters of a general practice.

The morning vigil to the computer has become my bread and butter, especially when I realize that in two brief hours I will lose control, sacrifice my calm to the chaos and appetites of a busy practice. So I tread here in search of happiness—

I

happiness in the form of order, peace, and solitude. These only do I need, because in love (from my family and friends) I am secure.

For my patients, too, I wish this happiness. Do we share the goal if we should call it, say, "the desire to avert misery"? For what reason would they otherwise come? "Take your pills," I urge them, "quit the booze, lose weight if you hope to escape your father's stroke or his emphysema or his violent end." But these threats are toothless. Every prescription is written with a statistical faith; my orders draw from a tradition that is blind to the doubters and the disinclined, and to those who comply under the pain of death and die anyway.

I cannot dispense happiness any more than a parent can hand it down. But I give to my patients a replenished heart and ears that will listen. I can hold up their fears and doubts and dispirited dreams as we strive toward that mutual goal, happiness. This does not deny medical science its death-defying feats. But physicians realize that the hardest work begins when the cure is evasive and "the plan" is our only defense—plans fabricated countless times over countless days, by doctors and patients who infuse a diagnosis with different meanings in order to disperse the unknown and light the trail to their recovery; plans to create order; plans to sustain hope.

Good planners do not bury those delicate moments. One time in ten, or one in ten million, a patient stumbles, the doors of stubborn pride swing ajar, and raw feelings are exposed. Who is this man if not my neighbor, vulnerable yet deserving of God's grace? Only when I embrace him as my brother can I offer him something more than pills, more than companionship, but mercy also, and every intercession against despair.

Through the journal, I have come to appreciate what doctors bring to the bedside. Not only skills and training, but also our very lives and needs. The challenge, we suddenly realize, is to give back to our patients more than we receive. And we know that we can succeed only by fostering in ourselves a deep sense of purpose, and by sharing whatever blessings we find along the way. Luke makes this clear in his Gospel, "Give, and it shall be given to you. Good measure pressed down, shaken together, running over, will they pour into the fold of your garment. For the measure you measure with will be measured back to you" (Lk 6:37–38).

Like the Medieval memento mori, the doctor's work, more than anything else, reminds us that our days are numbered. We are given in abundance what the psalmists craved: a chance to glimpse "the measure of my days, what it is, that I may know how frail I am" (Ps 39:4). The journal, more than anything else, is a compendium of stories that tell of the irrepressible human spirit, refined by adversity and renewed by love.

We often hear that God is in the details. But why should He cling to so cluttered a plane? It is rather here—in the empty pages of a journal, and along the backwaters of our big-notioned society—that I seek my Maker. I have come on the counsel of Father Henri Nouwen, who finds "God dwelling where man steps back to give Him room."

Of course, we are the ones stuck in the details; they dot our disjointed lives. This journal records the particulars of a life lived on the coast of Maine. Of Belfast and its seven thousand inhabitants, including my wife, Lindsay, and daughter, Clare. It is a story about my work and those who share it: my partner, Tim Hughes; my associates Scott and Mary Beth and Cathy; the countless nurses and office staff and patients who constitute the sublime pleasures of a medical practice. Through my practice I have discovered what Sir William Osler, father of American medicine, once observed: "Nothing will sustain you more potently than the power to recognise in your humdrum routine, as perhaps it may be thought, the true poetry of life—the poetry of the commonplace, of the ordinary man, of the plain, toil-worn woman, with their loves and their joys, their sorrows and griefs."

The journal entries are merely bookmarks in a bountiful life. They are sketches from a year in medical practice, a string of facts and circumstances that have moved beyond the mere documentary. It has demanded of me—like the very act of writing—a stepping back, a giving over, a letting go. It has provided me with an awareness that one often reaches in the fifth mile of a run or the tenth year of a medical practice or when infatuation peels from the person you love. In finding my stride, I have found the reasons to run.

The vigil is my daily comfort. But rarely do I appreciate it except in its absence, when I grumble at the interruptions or feel the knot of deprivation. It happens all too often, what with the exigencies of a hospital practice, the cries of a patient in labor, or a second glass of wine that follows the evening meal, all of which lie in ambush at the sound of the morning alarm. Then, not even the hunger sirens buried in the bellies of our felines (who expect to be fed by 5:00 A.M.) can rouse me from slumber or settle the cloud that hovers in my brain.

Until I can return to my desk, I carry these memories inside me: an aftertaste of strong coffee, etched impressions of a flaming sunrise, the flicker of the computer screen, the touch of varnished butcher block, the click of plastic computer keys beneath my fingertips. They are the accouterments of my sacramental time . . . time enough to snatch a handful of pages from a book, jot a letter to a long-neglected friend, or log an entry into my journal. Two hours of silence and solitude, when distractions dissolve, words weld themselves to the page, reminiscences are savored, and the heart heaves with joy and gratitude. Two hours that fold into the morning bustle, as twilight dissipates into the radiance of day, and the mists and fog burn off yet linger in the recesses of the mind.

3

JULY

What good will it do us to know merely that such things were
said? The important thing is that they were lived. That they
flow from an experience of the deeper levels of life.

THOMAS MERTON

The Wisdom of the Desert

On a ridge of Route 1, in the orange globe of the rising sun, two ungainly crea-
tures mounted the pavement and ambled to the opposite wood. They were altogether too large for stray dogs, too clumsy for deer, too fearless for the coyotes
that roam our rural coastline. Still squinting, and now barely pressing the accel-
erator, I realized that these beasts were a moose cow and her calf. The cow bent
her head toward me, shook it whimsically, then nudged her calf down the opposite bank and disappeared into a stand of pine.

I had needed a sign, longed for an apparition—some divine confirmation that
I had come to the right place at the appointed time, that my journey was in some
way sanctioned and secured and readied in advance. You see, I am a young physician of an older school, one who feels called to his practice and destined to be
here. Yet, only a decade into my work, I am riding in the rut of despair. Now
these early mornings I will curse less loudly at my inconvenience and offer the
road to Elena.

Almost six months ago, at the close of my sabbatical year, Elena Moulton was
diagnosed with amyotrophic lateral sclerosis (better known as Lou Gehrig's Disease). This was not the first adversity she had faced in life. Elena was born an

4

achondroplastic dwarf and raised by a rigid, overly protective mother. After college and her elopement with Harry, they adopted a son whom they later discovered was mentally retarded and emotionally impaired. But ALS is altogether different. It is a rare and invariably fatal neurologic disorder that whittles away at the body's functional capacities, rendering useless, first the limbs, then the larynx, and finally the muscles of swallowing and breathing. Elena had come to the second stage of her illness when I paid her that first call.

I remember watching her struggle, nodding and grunting at a plexiglass message board as she tried to express herself with the remnants of a language. Two letters constructed, then three; a word, then another, until they strung together in a simple phrase. From my vantage I noticed the panic in Elena's eyes, saw the desperation in the wave of her head. Finally she could go no further, her efforts washed away by a flood of tears. The palpable tension between husband and sister (who had been hovering behind Elena) now ignited into petty bickering.

At that moment I vowed to get Elena a computer and find a way to make it work. After several phone calls and a long talk with a local computer aficionado, a plan was hatched: we would need a Macintosh computer, software that displayed a keyboard on the screen, and a pointing device that responded to head movement and a puff on a straw. How long could Elena maintain the necessary strength and head control, or have the lung capacity for puffing? I didn't know. When the materials finally arrived, I brought my computer to her home *temporarily* while I hunted for a loaner, just to get her started. And so began my early morning junket to the office in search of a computer from my personal use.

Despite telephone calls and a personal visit to the Kodak Center for Creative Imaging in nearby Camden, I could not secure a computer for Elena. A week went by without leads. I lost patience, sunk into despair, imagined myself "The Writer" who had sacrificed his principal means of self-expression for his patient. It was a lovely, romantic, ennobling thought until the reality struck home: my computer was allowing a dying patient, with no use of her limbs or voice, to peck a bare-bones message—nothing but the basics of need and desire—to family and home health aides, who waited with Job-like patience at the computer's side.

In a few days, Elena developed a head cold. The abundance of mucous and saliva, difficult to clear or suction from the throat under the best of circumstances, was now audibly gurgling in her chest, and causing her, and those around her, untold mental anguish. Elena once confessed to me, while speaking of her prognosis, her two greatest fears: choking to death and dying alone. Before I could return a telephone call to the family, they had summoned the ambulance and whisked Elena to the hospital, where I would care for her over the next five days. It was a trial run, working out the kinks for the more urgent journey they saw looming ahead; Elena's X-ray, blood counts, vital signs were all normal, and she happily discovered the security and attention that a hospital could offer. The oxygen and IV antibiotics had done little more than justify the necessity of her admission.

In the meantime, I seized the opportunity to take my computer back and puttered happily on it for the few days that Elena recuperated in the hospital. As the discharge date neared, I explained to her that I was looking for a *larger* screen, something easier to work with. True, I admitted to myself, but far-fetched. Three days passed and still no computer in Elena's home. My great pleasure—my mornings at the computer—was now guilt-ridden by the injustice: I had stolen Elena's computer for my own use, solely for the recreation of it. I must give it up. Five days after Elena's return from the hospital, I brought back her Macintosh with apology and regret.

"Sorry, but I struck out, Elena; I have no larger screen for you, just this homely little Classic." Elena's eyes gleamed as I set up the computer, and she motioned for me to mount the headset. I watched intently as she marched the first eleven letters onto the screen: n i c e   m a c h i n e . Red-faced, I now felt redeemed by the Elena's quick, accepting smile.

For whatever the reason, after the computer, after that trip to the hospital, Elena changed. For the first time in months, she asked to leave her home in order to visit her mother in a nursing home. She typed messages to her nurses, a moving account of which was reported to me yesterday. When asked about the most difficult part of having ALS, she listed, first, her inability to speak; second, her struggle to get an itch properly scratched. Now the computer sings sonnets for Elena. And in the past two weeks, there has been new movement, rediscovered strength in those stubby fingers, in her limp and dangling legs, and a growing stamina for holding herself erect, a posture essential for puffing at the computer. But recovery is virtually unknown in ALS.

Elena attributes her improvement to the oxygen she received in the hospital, reading somewhere that patients with multiple sclerosis benefit from hyperbaric oxygen. If not from that, then from the antibiotics. What Elena has "recovered" from, at the very least, is the hopelessness of her condition. She has reclaimed a life and the possibility of living, perhaps more fully and for however long, in the good fight against her relentless slide toward that moment when at last she will be stripped clean of all her capacities. In her trip to the hospital, Elena had faced death and flown home again. And she continues to live, ever so convincingly, with the love and attention of her husband, son, and caregivers—and with that homely little box that has given her a voice.

After returning from three days of vacation, mounds of charts towered above my desk and clamored for attention: abnormal laboratory tests; requests for disability reports; phone messages from visiting nurses and referring physicians;

phone messages from patients needing a clarification of their prescriptions, their diet, their progress, all begging for "only a minute of your time, doctor."

Before breakfast with Lindsay and Clare at 7:30 A.M., I must hospitalize a patient with *hyperemesis gravidarum* who has come here more for the indoor plumbing than a magic cure. No doubt I will disappoint her; my role is peripheral, just a twelve-hour plug in the hospital dike.

It promises to be quite a year: I am the reputed age of Jack Benny and will engage my fortieth year in a few fleeting months. But more ominous is the failing health of my mother. She convalesces now in a nursing home, following surgery at University Hospitals to evacuate a blood clot beneath her skull. She had fallen at home, a victim of her drinking and memory loss and poor balance, all of which will continue to plague her after the surgery. She will never return home. Her apartment, in my hometown of Rolfe, Iowa, lies waiting, furnished and heated and hauntingly empty. But Mom is growing accustomed to the security of her new surroundings, the reliability of three square meals and the companionship of her nurses and neighbors. Fortunately, with her poor memory, she does not press the issue of going home. And the chances diminish with each passing day. As *her* life crumbles, I in turn lose that Maginot Line that separates youth from old age. Is this not the cause of the midlife crisis, rather than what they would have you believe: the slip-sliding away of your youthful dreams, or the discovery that the promise of material success was an empty one?

Another momentous decision faces Lindsay and me: will we add to our family, give Clare a sibling, or call it quits in our advancing years? Our four-year-old has raced beyond infancy. Could we recapture it with the life of another, toss the dice once more for a package of healthy genes, brace ourselves for the sleepless nights and endless interruptions, scramble our plans again for God knows how long?

I am covering the Fourth of July weekend for family practice. At a moment's notice I could be summoned for a hospital admission, emergency room consultation, obstetrical delivery, medical examiner's case, telephone call from a worried patient, or a surgical assist. The beeper at my waist is the devil's plaything.

On most occasions I suffer the "on-call" role gladly. Patients appreciate you more on weekends, especially the tourists passing through. The work is considered "extra," something above and beyond the call of duty, and sets the doctor apart, marks his devotion, elevates his cause, and earns his place at the banquet where the chronically overworked and underpaid are said to feast.

A beeper, moreover, provides a convenient excuse for a late arrival or early departure at the Hospital Aide Potluck Dinner. But it cuts both ways; it may equally deprive me of a moment's peace, a quiet run, a warm supper with my family, or an uninterrupted night's sleep.

I have, over these last eight years, made peace with the beeper. I now try to erase every expectation from the on-call weekend, and accept whatever morsel of free time falls my way. Before, I resented the burden, hated the patients who abused me, who got sick "stupidly" or at the most inopportune time, or who waited too long and by rights should be forced to wait a day or two longer. The illusion of freedom, the wisp of hope that I could *enjoy* such a weekend, became my curse and suffering.

Cursing and suffrage brought me to the crux of the matter: After choosing this career, could I swallow the responsibility? But only after doing so could I enjoy a life in medicine. The idea sounds saintly—perhaps even dysfunctional, in the way martyrdom has been revisioned—but it is key to a country doctor's survival.

One patient of mine is in labor; six others rest comfortably in their hospital beds. I have only a few clinical quandaries left hanging from the workweek: a child, feverish and fussy and eating poorly for three days, whose illness I am calling viral; an emphysematous man with chest pain, right-sided and knifelike. A chest X-ray would be useless in the diagnosis of pneumonia or bronchitis, so I will treat the pain only. I am reassured by the absence of cough, fever, or shortness of breath and suggest that he take ibuprofen. A young woman with abdominal pain has defied my testing; her thick chart suggests an hysterical personality, but she rejects any suggestion that stress or anxiety may be contributing to her pain. And she flaunts the episode when—after eleven days of hospital testing—a surgeon opened her belly and found the adhesions that were responsible for her pain. Now the family is outraged that "these doctors" cannot fix her. I am temporizing, playing for time, hoping to find my patient an honorable out when the tests return negative. She does not *need* any more surgery, which has already cost her several dispensable organs. But the more tests we perform, the longer the hospital stay, the more inflated the bill, the higher the stakes. And, as I am frequently reminded, tests can be wrong.

Maybe this weekend I can turn the compost, mow the lawn, go for a long run, fly a kite with my daughter, treat her to lunch in the hospital cafeteria, or play long enough for my wife to make a hospice visit. But, as is often the case, maybe I can't.

It was a dismal showing, yesterday's log. A long and arduous labor ended in cesarean section at 6:00 P.M., and that was the crown jewel of my accomplishments. She had consumed most of the day's worry. She had been laboring for two days, stop and go, when I finally ruptured her bag of waters. There was every good reason to get on with it: she was five days overdue, had a ripened cervix, and was running low on energy and optimism. When a strong contraction pattern did not ensue, I gave her a sedative. She woke up often during the night with irregular pains, and by morning the contractions were still five to eight minutes apart. So Pitocin was started to intensify the pains and narrow their frequency. It worked well enough; the cervix reluctantly widened, and by 2:00 P.M. she was pushing. The deep decelerations that had plagued her earlier continued into the second stage, so I remained close by. Finally, after three hours of pushing in every conceivable position and with no descent of the head, I called for a C-section.

These are the worst of labors: hours of intense pain that come to naught under the quick and anesthetized slice of the surgeon's scalpel; fretting over falling fetal heart rates, suffering the cries and moans of the labor bed, hesitating to call for the section despite the mounting need, and finally summoning the OR crew on a sunny holiday afternoon. A doctor learns most about himself in the face of adversity. Coming to the correct diagnosis, initiating appropriate treatment, assuring the cure of a patient through the glorious exercise of science . . . a rare outcome, indeed. Most of the time, the patient gets better regardless of what we know or do. After a few years in the trenches, doctors face this truth and adjust accordingly.

The more basic need is for companionship in the patient's struggle. Our patients ask us to help them bear the pain, quiet their fears, face the certain diagnosis of cancer or an incurable condition. Often our own bellies tighten as we see ourselves, or our families, in the frantic eyes of the patient, and we shudder at that reality. I cannot sit with a laboring mom without reliving, in some small way, my wife's three hours of pushing before the birth of our daughter. I cannot erase the anger of patients or their families who felt I hesitated too long in ordering a C-section; cannot forget the limp and ghostly babies I have pulled from between their mothers' legs after a series of deep decelerations in the fetal heart rate, or the embarrassment of calling in the surgical cavalry only to have the mother deliver in the wings of the OR.

Any doctor can make the right diagnosis and do the right thing; our regimented training secures that claim. But how do we, individually, connect with our patients, knowing when and in what ways they will need our support, our frankness, our heavy-handed opinions? At best, I serve as their guide. Doctors have grown familiar with the terrain of pain and fear. Patients trust us to stare without blinking at their base instincts and unguarded moods, having seen them all, having grown accustomed to our own. We are expected to recognize the truth of their lives without messy revelations. Surprisingly, we sometimes do. But these understandings cannot be taught in the way a skill or technique can be taught. They are not a shamanic gift. They rather emerge slowly over time to those who outlast a million complaints in a thousand stuffy exam rooms, over the wail of toddlers, in the instant before the patient permits your escape. It is a waiting game out there along the parade route of cures and declines.

Of the many chores I had hoped to accomplish yesterday, I succeeded in

9

finding only fifteen minutes for the compost. It is now a dense, rich, aromatic mixture of grass clippings, leaves, kitchen scraps, and other organic debris. How satisfying to watch nature digest itself. I enjoy the outdoor, backbreaking work, the steamy stench of it all, the smell of silage wafting from my Iowa boyhood, this tiny token for the environment. Now, if only our manure man would deliver, our compost could attract even fatter worms, which are the gardener's benchmark of good soil.

Of course I lay no claim to the title "gardener." It properly belongs to my wife, Lindsay. I am here for the spading, the lugging, the sheer *progress* of it all. You cannot take the farm out of the Iowa-born boy.

The most depressing part of the long weekend was yesterday's endless showers. Lindsay played Leonard Cohen and we ran the furnace to lift the damp and chill; at noon it was fifty degrees out of doors. Last night we celebrated an Olde-Fashioned Fourth by racing around the backyard with jumbo sparklers. Afterward, we hunted for night crawlers. Clare is unabashed about grabbing almost any slithery thing (except slugs, which she prefers to skewer with a stick) and is apprenticing in the art of hunting crawlers. The key, of course, is to search on the eve of a steady rain, shortly after dusk, skimming the beam of a flashlight over the bare earth. First identify the tip of the crawler, then swoop toward the end nearest the hole. Crawlers escape at lightning speed and exert a tremendous pull once they have gained a toehold. A soft approach and quick wrist are the essentials of the art.

Yesterday morning I toured the hospital, visiting my convalescing patients in the ICU, OB department, and medical-surgical floor. In the afternoon, I admitted a patient with severe bullous emphysema, saw another with lobar pneumonia (a dwarf known as Yoda in the nursing home*) in the emergency room, and consulted on an orthopedic patient with delirium.

The hardest part of the weekend was OB. When obstetrics is good, it is very, very good, but when it is bad it is horrid. My patient presented to OB at 7:00 Sunday evening, with a recurrent, irregular backache that had deprived her of sleep the night before. Now her cervix was seven centimeters dilated, membranes bulged with each contraction, and we conspired to rupture them, thus calling labor's bluff. Active labor ensued. By 11:15 P.M. she was bone-tired but fully dilated and ready to push; I watched her nod between the pains. Almost the same history, I recalled, as the patient we sectioned two days ago.

We prodded her into a squatting crouch next to the bed, then onto her hands and knees, and finally into an upright sitting position supported by a horizontal

---

* Yoda died two days later, as she thought she would.

bar. She simply could not budge the head beyond the narrows of her pelvis. Stuck, frustrated, exhausted. I stayed with her throughout most of her gymnastics, coached and supported her in labor, tried not to show my concern when two hours had elapsed, then another half hour, then another. Finally I approached her with the options, waited for her nod of approval, met the eyes of that wide gentle face now drained of all vitality and dotted red from pushing. Labor wound down to this moment of truth, when the patient and her doctor abandoned hopes for a "natural" birth. It had been a good, hard, well-managed campaign. Why a baby cannot pass is almost never known, hence the vague alibi "failure to progress." The patient and the operation cry for a more satisfying explanation. Questions gnaw in the minds of the doctor, the mother, her family: why did we fail; should we have persevered longer, intervened sooner, tried one more maneuver or an aliquot of Pitocin?

I return to the medical-surgical floor at 4:00 A.M. after the section, only to learn of another admission waiting for me down the hall, moaning quietly beyond the darkened doorway.

I owe my mother a telephone call. It has been put aside for two weeks as one day's duties have spilled into the next. But her forwarded mail—volumes of Medicare and Blue Cross "explanations of health care benefits"—jogs my memory.

As Mom's power-of-attorney, I also collect her interest earnings and dividend checks, money that offsets the high cost of convalescence. On my last visit to Rolfe I finally looked squarely into her finances. She had been after me to do it for years, wedging her requests into the first fifteen minutes of every visit home. "When I die," she would insist, "everything is in the safety deposit box at the bank. Marv and Rosella (my aunt and uncle, our closest relatives) will take care of the funeral arrangements, pick out the dress, see to the obituary. Just don't you kids fight."

I spent two hours in a stuffy cubicle at the Rolfe State Bank sorting through legal documents from the family estate. It was, in ways I could not have imagined, a nostalgic time. Here was material proof of my father's hard work and devotion, the evidence to support his claims. I was twelve years old the year before he died. How clearly I can remember the five of us seated around the supper table, listening to my father's declaration, while his hand hit the table like a gavel, "I just want you kids to know that, when I die, you will be well taken care of." How ridiculous to imagine! When I die! We might as well worry, as my mother once did, about being nailed by falling Skylab debris.

But there it was, irrefutable proof. After his death, our material lives marched on: we still vacationed at Lake Okoboji, bought a new Chevrolet every third year, pursued our college interviews, received help with mortgage down payments and the much-needed checks at Christmas time and after the arrival of our first child,

Clare. And still there was an estate, built by my father during a scant fifteen years in general practice, and preserved by my mother with the motto "Never go into principle."

It was, to an older generation, proof of parental love, of family values, of duty and devotion, of a responsibility fulfilled. It sustained my sense of importance, the feeling that I was set apart, endowed, heir to something beyond a tiny farming community and the glory of high school success. I am sure that love and attention and sacrifice were the active agents in the creation of what is now popularly called self-esteem, but accomplished with an impressive sleight of hand. I never knew it then. And what remains is my parents' estate.

So now, as I handle my mother's retirement checks, earned on the house calls and home deliveries that took my father from us, I have a greater sense of their love. These are not a substitute for horsey rides on my father's knee, or whisker rubs, or home movies in which I was the star, but they are love just the same, in a different package.

Today is electric with anticipation. At 5:00 A.M. the air is sweet and warm, and the yolk of a sun is cracking through an absolutely clear eastern sky. My desks at home and office are symmetrically tidy and unfettered by obligation. This morning I will meet with Cathy, our office manager, for the weekly business report, visit briefly with a patient, mow the lawn, buy a birthday gift, and pen a letter to a friend. I will return a dulcimer to Bob Ranney, along with the book he loaned me, and a copy of a reference letter I have prepared for him. Bob grew up across the street from me in Rolfe, Iowa, on a wide and shady thoroughfare lined by elms. The Ranneys and the Loxterkamps, 807 West Elm Street and 808, local dentist and doctor, respectively. Bob, ten years my senior, took an early interest in me, looked me up on Christmas breaks for basketball in the school gym, then invited me to his Walden Pond when I turned college age, a place called Bull Creek in the Missouri Ozarks. It sealed our friendship, those sweet nights of Harry Carey baseball on the St. Louis Cardinals sports channel, unlimited watermelon, sumac lemonade (our marketing strategy would pitch the name *Sumade),* and stories of my father, dead these half-dozen years, whom Bob knew in a way I hungered for, at Dad's heels on many a home visit.

The birthday gift is for my partner, Tim Hughes, who always appreciates a good book or gag gift but not the social obligation that birthdays sometimes impose. We will gather tonight, husbands and wives, for a celebration six days in advance. The ostensible reason will be to report on recent travels: Tim's trip to Disney World and his wife (Cris) and daughter's (Rozy) sojourn to a Friends retreat.

I know now that Cris's hopes were not fulfilled. Will we broach the question, raised in recent conversations, of why bright, talented, likable doctors' wives lose their way in search of self or career? Are they attracted to the doctor's iron-clad identity and sense of purpose? Do they take as their own his displaced doubts and uncertainties? Of course, there's the rub, because our roles become polarized and fixed through the daily grind. Lindsay has commented on what a relief it is—almost a pleasure—when I become downcast, when my boundless energy slackens and I lose my competitive edge. Such moments come rarely. I witnessed this once in my partner, during my sabbatical year, when the doubled work load dampened his spirits. But it is far more difficult to detect, or to acknowledge, in myself.

Yet here we are in marriage, making do. It does no good to say "girls, buck up, deal with your problems," even if the roots lie in the social or biochemical circuitry of their brains. Mary Beth Leone, the therapist who works our office, has two doctors' wives for clients and knows Lindsay and Cris well. She sees in all of us that peculiar and intriguing equation. But how to understand it, reshuffle it, right the balance that elevates the doctor and subordinates his wife? More on that tonight over dessert and presents.

We had a very robust evening together, Tim and Cris, Lindsay and I, in honor of Tim's forty-first birthday. Questions of mood did not arise. Instead we talked of travel. Ever since moving to town eight years ago, we have cultivated a tradition of celebrating birthdays together. Last night we gave Tim an astrologically appropriate pet (a hermit crab whom he dubbed "Hermes"), a worry stone, and a fake rubber hand. He especially liked the package illustration of a hand emerging from a vest pocket, a cargo trunk, and the fly of a pair of trousers. Our final gift was a book on death and spirituality, wrapped in the cover of John Berger's *A Fortunate Man*. Berger's 1967 account of the life of a country doctor in rural England is still, a decade since I discovered it, my favorite doctor story. Last year I gave Tim a copy for the second time, a gaffe he did not let pass unnoticed. So I created the appearance of giving it a third time.

Yesterday, after celebrating Mary Beth's birthday at noon, the room began to spiral with loud chatter and wild gesticulations; suddenly I felt compelled to remove myself to the doctor's room and sit silently with my thoughts and creeping mood.

Patients would arrive in a few minutes. If I began late, I would run late and finish even later with each successive patient. So it was imperative that I rock myself out of the rut and begin on time. The tension in my upper back and neck, the heaviness of my eyes, the dullness of my thoughts had suggested to me all morning that something physical was wrong. Then, at the noon staff meeting, I could say nothing that, once beyond my lips, did not twist itself into dark humor, a supercilious statement, or a belabored point. Why not shut up and let the meeting pass as painlessly as possible?

The afternoon drained me. I seemed forever on the verge of a yawn. I gazed helplessly out the window, hoping for simple patients with simple needs who would ask nothing more of me than a prescription refill, who would not judge my lackluster performance unkindly. There was nothing in it for me, not an ounce of pleasure. No pull into the lives of my patients, no tolerance or pity for their problems. It was as if the electromagnetic current had been severed. My eyeballs felt like lead shot, the inside of my head was a washing machine. Comments from my partner—innocent on the surface—seemed terse and critical and cutting. The nurses chattered incessantly, aimlessly, hurtfully. I did not trust the advice I was giving my patients, so I ventured nothing beyond the simple, safe, and automatic. Lindsay was working in the office that day. Had she been ignoring my gaze? Had all the affection between us gone? Did I notice a perky employee too conspicuously? Why was everything an annoyance and a distraction?

By midafternoon the tide was ebbing, and I recognized depression for what it was. Yet it never *feels* like depression. It will leave for a week, perhaps a month, and then sweep back in a tempest. Thank God it is brief, lasting a day or two at the most. I can ignore it—even, at times, convince myself that it is the full moon conspiring, or a virus replicating, or pure exhaustion taking its toll. But today I have no clear answer. It is, in some ways, a blessing. It is a peephole into depression, one day's share in what others—my patients, my family, my wife included—battle daily. Will they find happiness or optimism or energy? Or will they travel their whole lives with the sorrowful mysteries strapped to their backs?

I feel better today. I am typing, enjoying a flaming-orange sunrise, and listening to chirping birds and Handel's *Carmelite Vespers*. I hope to enjoy a part of the day with Lindsay. Perhaps I will run this afternoon, or return a letter to Gayle Stephens, who has been my writing mentor for the last fourteen years. We are not friends, I readily admit. If you pushed us onto the open floor at a medical convention, our talk would turn stiff and formal. We are constrained, I suppose, by our manhood, our doctorhood, and differences of a generation. But there is an affection between us, a bond and an abiding respect.

Gayle is one of the most admired essayists in family medicine, a moral being whose vitality over the years—I am now convinced—has been maintained by a proximity to his patients, and to their sorrows and ills. Recently he sent me two pieces awaiting publication. Both are very good and a pleasure to read in their raw form, before the publisher has edited them. In his letter he mentions his new role as a retired physician, "an informal consultant to friends, neighbors and former patients." He speaks of his patients, a black women with ALS, a lady in his church whose husband is alcoholic. Gayle is the associate editor of the *Journal of the American Board of Family Practice* and has, most ardently and patiently over the years, encouraged me to write. Because of him, I have sent a few stories to the *JABFP*, which, with his editorial help, were accepted. He now tells me that the journal has created a new column called "Reflections in Family Practice" that is ideally suited to the stories I spawn. So I'll enjoy returning Gayle's letter, reporting on my life in Maine, and unveiling my plans for this diary.

Standing on the back stoop, I face a cool southerly breeze and its threat of rain, smell the heavenly valerian standing shoulder-height beside me, hear the caw of distant crows and the *wheeip, wheeip, chir chir chir chir* of our cardinal-in-residence, and ready myself for a run. I look forward to the long stream of purple and pink lupines along the backstretch of Route 1, where the goldfinches nest and scatter from me as I churn past.

Today is the Feast of St. Benedict, abbot, father of Western Monasticism, writer of The Rule to which all Roman Catholic monks adhere in one form or another. I will make a special point of going to 7:30 Mass. There is much to be thankful for in the fruits of Benedict's labor. I have come inexplicably to his monastic tradition: the Gregorian chant, simple Cistercian architecture, the writings of Thomas Merton, retreats to the Trappist abbeys at New Mellary near Dubuque, Iowa, and St. Joseph's in Spencer, Massachusetts, and New Clairvaux near Vina, California.

I love the order of their day: work and contemplation punctuated by common prayer. The *offices*, as they are called, gather the monks seven times a day to sing the psalms, listen to the Word of God, and celebrate Mass. It is precisely this order that I rebel against in my own chaotic life. Yet chaos is no better. I long for structure that is freely chosen, that strengthens my work and focuses my energy, that liberates me from the zillion dispensable decisions of daily living, that creates a space for the All and helps me sift for the essential and come to terms with my fears and insecurities and loneliness. It is tempting to discard such structure and let life be manipulated, distracted, and deluged by the cornucopia of choices in the Land of the Free.

Yesterday Lindsay and I shared a lovely drive to Rockland, where we shopped for shrubs for the front yard. Lindsay's great passion is gardening, the only family trait (other than love of the evening news) that she readily acknowledges. She enjoys nearly all aspects of horticulture—naming the names (for which she has a categorical gift), absorbing sun and wind and dirt, composting and fertilizing the earth, ordering the grounds, picking the wildflower bouquets, and drawing in the fragrance of sweet flowers, only a trace of which can I appreciate. She is forever shouting, on an evening walk or during a tour through a neighbor's garden, "what's that incredible scent?" Then searching wildly for a flowering tree, shrub, or garden row until she has located the source of her delight.

I first met Lindsay in Hyde Park while attending the University of Chicago. I was working on a master's degree in the social sciences, she as a clerk in the catacombs of the basement bookstore called Seminary Coop. And though she was seeing someone else at the time (on a daily basis, actually: they were living together), she agreed to meet me for beer and conversation at the Woodlawn Tap, better known on campus as Jimmy's. That was January 26, 1983, a date more secure in my feeble mind than the day of our wedding.

We quickly became friends, correspondents, travel companions, paramours. Lindsay found me an easy conversationalist, someone who returned her probing questions as fast as she dealt them. She thought my work "interesting," at least in comparison to tales from the polymer chemistry lab, where her old boyfriend worked. I, on the other hand, liked her looks—fresh, petite, brown-eyed, mysterious, and pretty. I enjoyed her interest in books, films, ideas. I shared her passion for diners, Thai food, strange beer, and old bars, like the venerable Berghoff in Chicago's Loop. I loved her peculiar and active curiosity. I loved, too, her precise, clipped manner of speaking, heavy on the consonants; her languages, French and Latin; and the worldly experiences she had amassed at such a tender age: raised in Washington, D.C., she had traveled in England and lived briefly in New York, Paris, and Chicago.

For all the sizzle of courtship, our year and a half together in Chicago had its trials. I felt awkward around Lindsay's friends, with whom she seemed hopelessly entwined. I felt needled by her opinions, which were sharp and plentiful, judging and cajoling, as if she expected me to spar with her, to return them tit for tat. But it was not my nature. I felt it a duty almost to stifle opinion: as a doctor, you are there to support the patient, apprise him of the bare clinical facts only, which often meant overlooking, at least for the moment, his carelessness or stupidity, his inattention to hygiene or good manners.

On the other hand, Lindsay was not enamored with my friends either, and she was forced to ignore the poor taste I displayed in what I wore and what I drove, where I lived and how I "accessorized." Her old boyfriend had been a "stylish, young, urban esthete," while I was an apparition out of Middle America, the acrylic-on-velvet big-eyed boy you could find hanging above any living room sofa. Our move to Maine was as much an escape from my belongings as it was our adventure of a lifetime that we would risk together.

Lindsay, like all of us, is a strange combination of her parents. She grew up in suburban Washington, the last of three daughters born to a Jack-Mormon journalist and a commanding Presbyterian housewife. From Ray she inherited a love of words and their uses; from Helen, a ticket to perform with the Little Singers of Montgomery County, who exposed her to foreign language through a repertoire of twenty-seven different national anthems. From Ray she acquired a love of gardening; from Helen, an aversion to organized religion. From Ray she derived her relaxed, disarming chuckle; from Helen, her sharp opinions that intensified as they descended in a line from sister to sister. From Ray she got skinny, hairless legs; from Helen, the fear of dying young, as Helen had (of ovarian cancer) when Lindsay was fourteen, and as Helen's mother had when Helen was twelve. But it was this early death that liberated Lindsay during her rebellious teenage years, and it gave us, Lindsay and me, that similar excavation of the heart that distinguishes the child who has lost a parent prematurely.

Lindsay also inherited Helen's tortured ambivalence about career and motherhood. When Helen's mother died, Helen assumed the domestic chores of cooking and cleaning for her father and three brothers. But fortune shone when Aunt Emily invited her to come to Philadelphia and attend Girls' High School. She advanced to college, thoroughly enjoyed it, majored in math and physics. After college she took a job with Eastman Kodak in Rochester, New York, where her talents were recognized. Then war broke out, and she was off to the Women's Army Corps as an intelligence officer in charge of aerial photography. During her wartime travels, she met Lindsay's father. When the war ended, they were married and moved to Rochester so that Helen could resume her career with Eastman Kodak.

But conditions had changed: the G.I.s flooded home, Helen's desk was moved into the hall, and she was passed over for promotion. Her spirits sagged. Bowing to the advice of friends and the dictates of society, she had a baby. The baby did not adjust to kindergarten, and it was advised that Helen have a second child to support the first. The young family moved to Bethesda, where Ray became employed as a speechwriter on Capitol Hill. Helen's unhappiness deepened, especially after the birth of their last child, Lindsay. Her dreams of career vanished only to resurface as the hopes and ambitions she would fashion for her daughters.

I am not sure if this helps to explain the quandary we faced as we contemplated having a baby. Lindsay seemed poisoned by a desire for career that had been force-fed to her as a child. She was afraid of losing herself to play groups, burp pads, and the latest notions in *Parent* magazine. She had grave doubts about her abilities or worthiness as a mother, especially given the truncated and distorted example left by her mother. Marriage to a physician only complicated matters. Doctors are afforded an instant prestige, instant identity, instant career. And Lindsay worried, "When you're on call, I'm on call, so that I won't have a life, basically. I'll be as tied to a baby as you are to your practice, which is something I don't think most doctors remember or fully appreciate. I'll wait for you to jump and run out the door."

But we have a child, thanks to our therapist, Mary Beth Leone, and thanks to Lindsay's courage, and thanks be to God who blew that tiny spark into our lives. I am indebted to Lindsay for her steadfast loyalty; for her affections (sometimes distant or spare) that are, at any rate, more generous and spontaneous than I deserve; for her sensitivity and her gentle tears that fall during a sentimental movie or a sappy poem I pen on a birthday card; for her exquisite taste (and sense of smell); and her own opinions, which have softened through the years to sift comfortably through our conversations in the waning moments of a day.

I set out at a trot down the sloping hill toward the Bay, admiring the placid, pale waters before me that stretch toward Blue Hill and Cadillac Mountain. My legs are rubber bands, wound for action, and I feel the firmness of my undercarriage, the sureness of my knees and ankles. There is in me a full-headed, deep-rooted, summer enthusiasm for the call of the road. An offshore breeze billows through my T-shirt and cotton shorts.

Within a half block, I turn left on High Street, the town's major artery. Here the streets take a different name in each direction: Northport Avenue to the right, Condon Street ahead, Salmond to the rear; as always, I proceed left along High Street, holding back the horses, tempering the pace for the long run ahead.

High Street is canopied by towering black locusts, maples, oaks, beach. I run past old mansions and estates that date from Belfast's era of affluence, the period of the American Greek Revival in the mid-nineteenth century, when she built and sailed vessels the world over. At Peach Street and on through Park, my stride lengthens as I lope down the hill. Here the peeling paint and storefront facades begin to mark what has become the commercial district. On the left I pass a nursing home, the group home, the Belfast Free Library, and finally reach the downtown. We cherish this cluster of large, brick buildings, including the Masonic Temple and the Progressive Age Building, whose faded letters boast of "Steam-powered Printing." Most was rebuilt in brick after the devastating fires of 1865 and 1873, and is listed on the National Historic Register. I sneak under the stop light at High and Main, the only one of its kind in Waldo County. On past the McClintock Block and Phoenix Row, whose upper apartments teem with the Welfare crowd, youths raising youths, where I have thrice visited wearing the coroner's badge. On past Colonial Cinema, City Hall, the Courthouse, and a large, weathered frame structure that once housed U Otta Bowl, a candlepin alley that was still operating when we moved to town.

It is an easy run thus far, with time and inclination to let the mind wander and take in the public bustle. But now High Street turns up Primrose Hill, a grouping of eight impressive homes that mirror the historic affluence of Upper High Street. Admiral Pratt's estate is principal among these. This is my first test, the journey's leg that tunes the hamstrings and readies the diaphragm and rectus abdomini for the approaching campaign. In the next mile, I will be leaving Belfast, running past the Gov. Anderson School, the Head Start grounds, the old Waldo Shoe Factory (one of the last to close), and the overpass of Routes 1 and 3, which lead the tourists to Bar Harbor and Acadia National Park.

And then, suddenly (even to a runner), the trail drops away, down, down to become City Point Road. The air chills and dampens in the shaded overgrowth. Dilapidated shacks (what the realtors call "camps") peek timidly out from behind the trees; Budweiser packages, bald tires, plastic motor oil quarts, cigarette wrappers are littered along the route. For the next half mile, the Belfast & Moosehead Railroad parallels my path. These tracks once hauled grain and other products to support a thriving poultry industry; it too has failed, and now tourists travel the twenty-five-mile round-trip excursion to nowhere, to the interior where the real Maine, of trailers and junked up dooryards, is stowed away.

Out on City Point Road and across the Upper Bridge, Belfast village first rose on its toddling legs. Passage there challenges the runner with a series of steep hills along a twisting, narrow ribbon of road that shoulders the Passagassawakeag River. Finally the terrain levels out, and I cross the bridge to Head of Tide. Here, houses are not as grand or well kept as those closer to village center. But they date from Belfast's beginning, a fact established by a plaque on the homestead of Glenview Farm, "Est. 1798." Capes, federals, gambrels, and saltboxes all intermingle, dogs jerk at their chains, the smell of honeysuckle and the brilliant flash of poppies greet the runner as he glides by. The air warms and sweetens in the open sunlight. It can be stagnant and thick with mosquitoes and black flies, but today a light breeze dries the sweat from my brow. On this half mile, my legs finally stretch to relive the wide-open runs of my youth on the Iowa prairie. I spot an Osprey nest atop the utility pole, dodge red-wing blackbirds who defend their marshy nests, and smell the mud baking in the tidal basin below.

Finally I begin the ascent. The next mile is alternately a gradual, then steep, climb away from the sea. I set a pace and cling to it. After a quarter mile, the road turns back toward town, south on the Doak Road, over a gorge where rapids roar and sharp plates of slate jut into the broiling stream. In the spring when the Passy is full, this is the most serene place on earth. But no time to gaze. The road rises menacingly and I focus on survival. Sweat pools in my eye sockets. My legs ache and lungs strain for oxygen. Up past the cemetery where I once paused, rich in sea lore. I remember the captains buried here: F. A. Patterson, Simeon Rider, and Charles Brier, whose son Henry died at sea on October 6th, 1860. Martha J. Mayhew's children honored their mother with poetry etched in stone:

Heaven retaineth now our treasure. Earth the precious casket keeps.
And we often love to linger where our dearest mother sleeps.

As for their father, the Captain Vinal Mayhew, they put it plainly: "To Die Is Gain."

Here lie George U. White and his three wives; Eliza Jane, dead at the tender age of thirty; Katie, gone at thirty-eight, and Sarah, who buried her husband and lived twelve years a widow. Here lie the Soldiers of '61, brothers A. F. and F. A. Patterson, Jr., representing Company H of the Eighth Maine Regiment and Company K of the Fourth Maine Regiment, respectively. The latter survived the war only to perish "On the passage from Africa to New York, AE 35 Years."

I keep climbing, climbing, hoping to catch my breath as the upward grade slackens. I push past the old Doak homestead, appropriated now by the general surgeon, and the Doak Repair Shop, owned and operated by a direct descendant. Still climbing, I pinch the stinging brine from my eyes and fight to hold the pace.

I am always, on this stretch, pierced by the loneliness of the long-distance runner. I speak not of solitude, for that is a welcome companion in my line of work. I have never passed a runner on this route, nor do I nod to cars that rocket by, or wave to the old men mired in their dooryards. I give up intention, all conscious thought. I slip inward to where the question is put in inescapable terms: why do you run? what makes you a runner? It is not for the endorphins or for a longer life, though I would not begrudge a runner these reasons. I, too, am in training. It is the distance that attracts me, the long haul. It is the solitude; it is a challenge in such simplified terms; it is the lure of accomplishment; it is the sense of sole responsibility. I relish, too, the sweat and strain, the responsiveness of muscle and will. I enact, on manageable terms, our lifelong journey through time and space, at a more livable, observable, thinkable speed.

For the seventeen-year-old in Alan Sillitoe's novella, "This long-distance running is the best lark of all . . . [A]s soon as I take that first flying leap out into the frosty grass of an early morning when even birds haven't the heart to whistle, I get to thinking, and that's what I like. I go my rounds in a dream, turning at lane or footpath corners without knowing I'm turning, leaping brooks without knowing they're there, and shouting good morning to the early cow-milker without seeing him. The long-distance run of an early morning makes me think that every run like this is a life—a little life, I know—but a life as full of misery and happiness and things happening as you can ever get really around yourself" (p. 10).

Finally I crest the hill and stare a quarter mile down the wooded valley. I know now that I'll have the lungs to finish, though the steepest climb looms ahead. I clear the summit, recover my wind, straighten my drooping frame, and picture the graceful, undulating, two-mile stretch of road home. The race is over. I accept the accolades, the melodramatic finish, the chance to untangle my knotted legs. I sail past the redemption center, legs rebounding; past the new high school, lungs sucking deeply; arrive at the downtown from Waldo Avenue and slide past the Post Office and Customs House, the First Church and William J. Crosby School, and along picturesque Church Street, with houses boasting their considerable age. At last I draw a bead on the stop sign at the end of the road. Just beyond lies the finish, with home but a short walk up the grassy slope of our neighbor's lawn. Home, what I have been searching for, and have finally found.

This morning I lay in bed a few minutes after the alarm to enjoy Lindsay's legs interfolding with mine, the cotton sheets drawn snugly against the cool breeze, the catbirds cawing and chickadees chattering outside our window, and, intermixed, the whining of our fat felines who were unwittingly locked outside last night. Truth in fact, our doors never lock, nor do most of those in town. The fear of the city has not yet seeped into our insular community. I don't doubt that it will come. But for now we live with one less fear.

Hospital rounds were a breeze: the brushfires in OB and the ER were easily snuffed, and I set off happily for the Belfast Free Library to spend my lunch hour with Joseph Williamson and his double-volume *History of Belfast*. Then the beeper sang, summoning me back to the ER. Two admissions awaited: a seven-week-old infant with fever and an old man with stroke. I was nearly two hours late to the office, and, even with radical surgery on my afternoon schedule, never caught up.

The journal has caused a shift in my thinking, a reordering of priorities. It consumes every free shred of my morning; it occupies my idle thoughts—not in a disturbing way, but constantly and completely. The bookshelf gets fewer glances. My running has slackened to three times a week. I wonder, too, what behavior has changed because of it. I don't want to "freeze" or capture my life over the coming year, nor should I change for the sake of a story. What did Heisenberg say? You cannot simultaneously record the speed and location of a particle in space. You cannot observe without changing. So it is good to paw over my tiresome routines and snap judgments, to extrude doubts and worries and clean out that hog barn . . . I think, hmmm, "this would be good topic," or "better resist that temptation." This imaginary audience, like a guardian angel, has become my conscience and changed my approach to the world.

Yesterday was Tim's birthday, proper. The office celebrated with a traditional potluck feast. Charlotte's incredible spinach lasagne, Lindsay's tuna pâté, Scott's homegrown broccoli with dip, Cathy's tossed green salad, and becandled cakes by Bonnie and Trudy. The staff doesn't miss a trick, laying out a spread for every occasion. The format rarely changes, and is ripe for scrutiny: a birthday card signed by all, the gag "last patient of the morning" (your wife in disguise), a loud chorus of "Happy Birthday" as we pile in close together. But, when *your* turn arrives, suddenly it is a nice surprise and a warm feeling to have the ten of us huddle around the ping-pong table with too little to say and too much to eat in honor of the day of your birth.

Last evening Tim picked me up for a family meeting. After a winding, wooded drive ten miles into the interior, we arrived at a shingled bungalow, the home of Bernitha and Ted Truman. Bernitha is dying of lung cancer that was diagnosed three years ago. Jean Goldfine, the Hospice social worker who lives up the hill from the Trumans, arrived fifteen minutes before us. She's been a regular companion at our recent meetings, and it is comforting to have her along. It is good, too, to be here with Tim. Doctors, especially generalists, operate in relative isolation. What we value most in family practice—dealing in relationships—is often exercised in privacy. The area of obstetrics is a prime example. I have watched only one delivery by a fellow physician since my formal training ended. The family meeting, in contrast, requires a team approach, depends upon it for mutual support, and creates an environment where everyone is a novice, a witness, and a full participant.

The family meeting is simply a glorified home visit, an occasion for the doctor to come calling. Today "the doctor" will be two physicians and a social worker. By prior agreement, Tim will lead the meeting and Jean and I will take a back seat. "Family" becomes whomever the patient has identified. Such a meeting provides an invitation for family members to broach a topic they might otherwise ignore, or subvert, or quarrel over without getting to the crux. In a family meeting, everyone is asked to speak and listen. We take an hour to say, or begin to say, what is most important to communicate before the time runs out.

Bernitha's house is tiny, a single downstairs room divided by lines of furniture. The five of us fit snugly on the sofa and three chairs that are clustered near the door. Tim and Bernitha share the couch, where she has spent nearly every waking hour (and many nights) listening to the traffic, imagining cars careening through her bay window. "I'd be a goner," she announces matter-of-factly. Portraits and religious calendars, posters in biblical verse, knickknacks of every persuasion hang scatterdash along the walls. A portable TV occupies the center stage, like its dooryard counterpart, the satellite dish. A little dog scrambles from lap to lap and finally nestles between Tim and Bernitha, where it will receive the most affection.

Tim's method is uncomplicated, based on the interview style of Michael Murphy, medical director at St. Peter's Hospice in Albany, New York. He will steer back and forth between patient and husband, asking "what is your story, what are your worries. Tell me about when you first learned of your cancer, Bernitha. What were your feelings then, Ted?" Trolling back and forth between them. We learned that Bernitha's doctors had not initially told her of her cancer, and when they finally did, they had said it was treatable. I squirm in my seat because I was one of "those doctors." I remember the tearful visits two years ago when we ordered the chest X-ray for bronchitis and found instead a spot on her lung. I informed Bernitha that it was most likely cancer and packed her off to the specialists. Then I left for sabbatical as Bernitha set out upon her odyssey with the oncologists and radiation therapists. Only months later, after she finally wandered back to Dr. Hughes, did her case move from the back burner. Why the delay? What actually happened then?

Bernitha spoke, too, of her emptiness and loneliness when Ted becomes engrossed in the television or trots off to bed. There are strings of days when no one pays a visit. Yet she is happy for the neighbors who drive her to her appointments and take her out to lunch, who walk down the road three times a week just to say hello, fellow parishioners who pray for her and cook the meals and dote over her. And she spoke of a son in Oklahoma whom she has only rarely heard from since his last visit a dozen years ago.

Bernitha's fears all stem from loneliness. Her greatest fear is that Ted will go first, what with his emphysema and all, and leave her no choice but to sell the house and move into town. Ted spoke sparingly during our visit. I do recall his offer to sing for Bernitha if she wanted, and his mention of the movies (which he thoroughly loves, except, of course, those "of naked women"). But he never acknowledged that Bernitha was dying—because, as he kept saying, "she looks too well."

It is easier to clamber out of bed this morning than I would have imagined last night. After Lindsay returned from a Hospice meeting, we stayed up for the Democratic National Convention. We listened to a speech by Jerry Brown, the grand oration of Mario Cuomo, political commentary by Gergen & Shields, and the roll call of the states through the Maine delegation. I didn't feel sluggish when the alarm beep-beep-beeped out of control (the switch broke yesterday in a fall from the dresser). As I moved through morning chores, I was rewarded by an absolutely blue sky, the hint of rose and melon leaking from the subterranean sunrise, a scent of sweet salt air wafting up the hill, streaks of sunlight running over the ribbons of cut grass, and silhouettes cast by the majestic, towering trees along High Street.

On most days I punch a time clock, settle for the satisfaction of doing an average job on average problems and meeting an average degree of success. Once in a while a patient will come along to whom I can offer something special, make an individual difference, feel the privilege of my post. Such a person came in yesterday, a walk-in (rare as hen's teeth, even in a poultry town) with a swollen ear. He was a regular patient of one of my vacationing colleagues.

"Happened ten years ago, just about the same, and I did well on pills," he offered.

It would be a simple matter, no doubt, of identifying the pills, confirming the diagnosis, and prescribing that medicine again. But the conversation led to the fact of his treatment a week earlier with a cream for psoriasis, aggravated by stress. He owned a business in town and had worked over a hundred hours the week before in preparation for his vacation. He showed me an empty prescription for Valium; wouldn't I refill it?

"Someday the boys will take over. And I just hired a top-notch employee to share in the responsibilities. Another helper is coming back in August, so, Doc, it's getting better."

On examination, his ear was minimally swollen and slightly red, but I could find no hint of a problem in the auditory canal, ear drum, temperomandibular joint, or lymph glands. So why had he come in today? Was he worried about his ear, or seeking a refill of his Valium, or needing to talk, or hoping the doctor would order him to restrict his pace? He had chosen a hard life, like his father, who owned the business before him. He wanted to save it for his sons, who deserved a decent job and a secure future in a county that offered precious little of either. The temptation was to sell and be done with it. But how could he let a life's work and the family tradition slip away?

We talked about his sons, what hard workers they are and how they came by it. He was sixty-two. How much longer did he hope to live? What good was he to his sons or the business if he should die tomorrow? What values other than hard work had he passed along to his kids? In the end, he admitted that stress was the lion's share of his problem, and that pills were no answer. But better times were ahead, he assured me.

So we planted a seed. And I pray that he's right about better times ahead, or that the first heart attack won't kill him.

The cats were sitting on their perch on the front steps this morning, whining as I came down the stairs. More and more they prowl at night, up to no good, engaged in all manner of foul play (or rodent play, judging by the carnage they deposit at the back door for our general inspection).

Today I could not raise myself at the alarm's first beckoning. The switch is still broken, and I had to dismantle it before snuggling back under my sheets. By 5:00 A.M. the elements conspired to awaken me, and I tumbled downstairs for the morning chores. Last evening Lindsay and I listened to speeches by Al Gore and Bill Clinton and absorbed the political commentary about Ross Perot's decision to quit the race. I slept through most of what had been billed as "the speech of Clinton's life," but revived myself at the end. I hope the candidate follows suit. The country has its best chance for a national health plan under the Democrats.

Tim, Mary Beth, and I met yesterday for our customary hour, Thursday mornings at 8:00 A.M. We talked about the competition that arises between partners. Tim, who is becoming more aware of what Carl Jung and Robert Bly call the "shadow side," sees it cast over his glowing orations about marriage, daughter, and work. Tim operates, I believe, closer to the surface than I, not so laden with emotion. But for me to say so sounds like sour grapes, after all the crap I dish up about my own life.

Ours is not an easy association, tagged as it is with the warning labels "male," "doctor," and "partner." Mary Beth once suggested that I represent Tim's brother. "My *big* brother," Tim rejoined. And I certainly see the makings of that dynamic in our friendship. I am an oldest son, thrust to the head of the household during adolescence when my father abruptly died. Tim has a strong, successful, poker-faced father, and an older brother who aspires to the role. He often instinctively rejects what I instinctively offer: advice, assistance, a "helping" hand. But we each know the value of friendship, and have been blessed by it since childhood. I still keep in touch with Bob Ranney, who grew up across the street from me, Jim Jordan from high school, Bill DeMars from college, Pete Kerndt and George Schoephoerster from medical school.

My relationship with Tim is full of expectations laid by these preceding friendships. And I recognize at least one trap: the hope that Tim will look after me, guard my fragile feelings, know intuitively if they are at risk, and rush to their defense. Lindsay has already proven herself, but more often now coaxes me to defend myself.

I have known Tim since 1984, when, on a brilliant day in June, Lindsay and I dropped by the Donald Walker Health Center in Liberty to meet the young physician on duty there. We were in town looking for potential practice sites. It was blistering hot. We were utterly spent, our patience and pluck drained by an endless hospital tour, talk of income projections, and all those panoramic views of the Bay. So we welcomed Tim's outstretched hand and his warm, unassuming invitation to spend the night at his place and stay for the morning meal. Tim is an easy person to meet and, like the rest of us, hard to get to know. We have been working at it ever since.

My partner is a Midwesterner like myself. He grew up in suburban Cleveland, the last of four children in a comfortable home. He attended Dartmouth College, Case-Western Reserve School of Medicine, and family practice residency in California. Both of us landed here in similar ways: neither had any prior knowledge of or connection to Belfast. Both of us set out, two years out of training, to find a place to live. For each of us it was love at first sight. In Belfast it is possible to inhale the history, briny and fresh and intimately tied to the Bay. The brick buildings of the downtown convey a feeling of stability, and the bustle of the commercial district confirms your sense of community and of civic pride. You have ocean at your feet, hills all around, and the most magnificent architecture imaginable, largely in the style of American Greek Revival, which has been "improved" only slightly by the march to modernization.

Tim and Cris drove to Belfast from California, hoping to find a small town near the wilderness. Lindsay and I wanted to live "East," upon her insistence, and "rural," upon mine. Tim was content with a place "as good as any other," but I needed a new start and a place I could call home. Neither of us has been disappointed.

They say that medicine is a mistress, and your practice partner becomes a spouse. But the record shows that these marriages quickly crumble over matters of money or personal difference. I believe that Tim and I have made it over the watershed and will survive together until the chapter closes on our lives here. We earned each other's trust and respect in the early days of long hours and little pay. Tim and I sacrificed for each other (and the practice) when we left for year-long sabbaticals in Costa Rica and San Francisco, respectively. We both enjoy rising early, spending time alone (in a rowing shell or along the back stretch of a country road), sharing gems of stories we acquired in the line of duty. For what it's worth, we both have a wife and child, are left-handed, and were born under water signs.

But we have also learned to live with our differences. I cannot resist the doctorly impulse to offer advice, and Tim cannot help but reject it. He becomes anxious and annoyed when others speak for him, so I write these words with trepidation. But our differences are also complementary. Tim is methodical and patient, and wary of the instinctive or obvious. He trusts my business savvy and I trust his clinical sense.

For Tim, there is much of the boy left in the man. He has a childlike heart, a student's love of books and ideas, a youthful vigor and daring, a sportsman's love of rowing and bicycling, a soft spot for Gary Larsen and gag gifts. He operates from the foundation of a happy childhood. As the youngest of his siblings, he is a man whose approach to life is open and uncomplicated, not burdened by parental expectation, doting, or worry. Nor does he obsess over the deeper meaning of things. I once asked Tim about his preference for partnerships, having, of course, myself in mind but thinking, too, of his wife, Cris, his rowing buddy, David Simmons, and his journalist companion, Jay Davis. With a shrug of the shoulders, he replied, "I'd just rather work with somebody. It's more fun to resonate with somebody. It's the resonating that's fun for me."

And that is my partner through his partner's eyes: often innocent, sometimes gruff, never pretentious or oblique in his ways, and as loyal as the day is long.

This past weekend we went on a family retreat to Baxter State Park. It had been scheduled last January, when four of us in the office mailed away for reservations at the premier campsites of Kidney and Daicy Ponds. We left at suppertime on Friday, and leisurely drove the two-and-a-half hours to the Togue Pond entrance. When we arrived, a young ranger checked our tickets, inspected her clock, and duly informed us we were a few minutes late. "Sorry, go back to Millinocket and find a room there for the night," she flatly instructed us. I had no energy to argue, and wished to spare Lindsay that embarrassment, but fumed during the entire twenty-minute trip back to town. Fortunately, I held my tongue about our late start. Any comment about Lindsay's working late that day would have been a declaration of war. We took a cheap room in Sweet Lillian's B&B (discounted for remodeling) and rose early the next morning for the second assault.

It was a wonderful weekend. As I type I am itching from mosquito bites from elbow to ankle. Our cabin was next to Tim, Cris, and Rozy's on Kidney Pond. The whole entourage (thirteen strong) hiked along mountain streams to cascading waterfalls, below which we swam in the frigid, clear water. Next to Big Niagara Falls, the children slid down smooth boulders into a basin of water for nearly an hour, squealing with glee. Everyone brought extra food just in case the rest of us forgot. We had a campfire that night, ending with ghost stories. I told the tale of the mummy's castle, "reputedly true," for I had the names and dates to prove it. Clare, the youngest camper, hid inside the cabin with Lindsay, though she listened intently through the window and periodically bellowed out her questions ("were they friendly mummies?") and warnings ("it's *still* too scary!") as I spun the yarn. I used Abram's eyes as a fear-o-meter; he would wince whenever I emitted too hideous a laugh or strung out the suspense. Lindsay's weekend was brought to perfection when, as we were leaving the park, we sighted a moose cow and her calf crossing a stream and stopping to munch leaves on the far bank.

We got home in time for laundry, a car wash, a game of bat 'n ball, and a long run (after which Clare went running with me, down the block and around the corner and back up the neighbor's drive). But the weekend ended in disaster when dad forced the issue of tooth-brushing before bed. My cajoling, bargaining, and reasoning failed; I lost my temper and, later, the war. Lindsay bailed me out with her gentle words, and I made amends and read the bedtime stories, but Clare woke up during the night with nightmares sparked by the embers of our quarrel.

Smokey's Greater Shows has come to town for the Belfast Bay Festival. We visited the midway last night along with a swarm of patrons I knew as my patients, my former patients, or my patients-to-be. It was a night of furtive looks and brief clinical updates as we stood in line for cotton candy or the Twister. It was a reunion where I could mark progress in people's lives by their most recent divorce or newest escort or the number of kids that clung to their leg.

What a celebration on the midway! We witnessed it all, Clare riding ringside on my shoulders. There is something about a summer carnival that draws out the county folk in droves, sifts the loose change from their pockets, and gives us back a glimmer of hope and a reason to gussy up. The Carnival is an equal opportunity entertainer. It is democracy in action. And *there* is the beauty of it. It is a mystery all inclusive, open to everyone and his kid.

It is not at all like the laundromat scene. When Lindsay and I first moved to town, we rubbed laundry baskets with many of the poorer patients in my practice. It was depressing. For a few cycles of wash each week, we entered their desperate lives, inhaled their cigarette smoke, suffered their abusive conversations, stepped over their neglected and under-clothed kids. Our very first capital investment after moving to town was a washer and dryer.

But the Bay Festival is different; it draws out *everybody* for the Saturday parade, the fireworks, the beanos and raffles and footraces and the battle-of-the-bands, but most of all for the rides and promenade of Smokey's Greater Shows.

Clare redeemed herself for last year's fiasco on the Jumping Giraffe—after being nearly trampled by the "big kids," she had panicked and froze and had to be rescued by her father. This year, despite some initial temerity, she screwed up her courage and sprang onto those great loaves of air and never looked back. We tried out the Super Slide, the Merry-Go-Round, the Round House Train Ride, the Fun House (thrice), and the Blue Helicopter. Her companion on the slide and copter was her wild buddy Evan, resplendent in a Batman costume. Clare struggled to remain conscious until 9:00 P.M., but collapsed on my shoulders somewhere along the four blocks of our homeward journey.

The air had already warmed to forty-eight degrees when I opened the back door to let in the cats this morning. Hues of rose and salmon returned to the eastern sky, and nary the wisp of a cloud. What a perfect day for the parade, an afternoon tea at Jennie Baker's, and fireworks tonight! And *possibly* a foot race this morning, the annual Bay Festival 10K. Once a year I race against time to see how I stack up. I declare myself a runner; rejoin the racers' communion. It will take on more meaning today if Clare comes to watch, which is likely given our location directly along the race route.

Yesterday was a wonderful day off. The only things on my docket were malleable goals: turn the compost, mow the lawn, lunch with my partner, nap in the library, and read (at Lindsay's request) a chapter on "Hospice as Community" in Sheila Cassidy's *Sharing the Darkness*. Sheila talked of the natural edges that abrade any professional community that is drawn together by a common cause instead of the love of the group. She eventually learned to find her support outside, and to wait for the "natural" circles of support to form inside. We are feeling the abrasion in our little hospice team, and will be addressing "process" issues next meeting in a longer session. I doubt that it will redress, or even *address,* any of the important problems. We are still a group without soul, without a clear mission, without confidence in our individual territories of service. We have had no crisis to bond us. And we are so very young, a hodgepodge group, a pick-up team. Give us a year or two, I am thinking. Let things sort themselves out. Most importantly, let our patients teach us.

I met Tim and another colleague for lunch. The "agenda" was to discuss the conflicts created by the new obstetrician in town. She has decreed that only *one* of the family doctors (along with the general surgeons) will assist with C-sections; the purpose, ostensibly, is to become well acquainted with one assistant so as to be able to rely upon his skills. But the policy was formulated after the fact, after another family doctor assisted with surgery on one of our patients without our foreknowledge. Tim and I felt the policy to be unfair and divisive, and, practically speaking, untenable in a small community where we constantly rely upon each other's assistance. If the obstetrician needed more able assistance at her C-sections, why not choose the general surgeons exclusively? But not *one* of the family doctors. Or give us all a chance to prove ourselves. We got together at lunch to air our grievances and plot the next step toward settling the misunderstanding. But the next step was taken last night when a patient of ours, needing a C-section, went into labor. She *demanded* that Tim be the assistant. Tim invited the general surgeon to perform the C-section, which he rightly refused, as that only would have expanded the field of conflict. So the obstetrician came, Tim assisted, and mother and baby were—naturally—healthy. Now the dust must settle.

So begins a new week. It is Monday morning, and in three hours I will be strapping on the beeper at the watchman's post. Since returning from sabbatical, Tim and I alternate each week between "office duty" and "hospital duty." The hospital doctor handles all of the clinical responsibilities outside the office: hospital admissions and rounds, deliveries, emergency room visits, trips to nursing homes and patients' homes. He will be scheduled lightly in the office: afternoons only and Monday night. On calm stretches, the hospital doctor is gifted with flexibility, a few degrees of freedom in the morning to drop by the cleaners, the post office, or to attend a hospital meeting or lunch date with a friend. Subject to change without notice. When he carries the beeper, he carries the practice on his hip.

The following week of office duty is our just desert. Duties end at 5:00 P.M., or whenever the office lights go out. Monday and Wednesday afternoons are taken off, and all day Friday. The office doctor must cosign charts for our physician assistant, Scott Bailly, but he has no additional demands. He can plan forays to the library, the bookstore, down the coast, or go out for a run or sit under a tree with a favorite book. What a pleasure this life has become.

Shifting our duties in this seesaw fashion still leaves us with a fifty-hour workweek on the average, excluding the unexpected telephone calls, emergencies, and labor pains. And meetings. The Monday morning "changing of the guard,"

Tuesday hospital committee meetings, Wednesday breakfasts with our office manager, Thursday morning sessions with Mary Beth, followed by a hospice team meeting. And we have made our own bed, choosing these meetings beyond those the hospital requires.

Tim and I established our partnership shortly after we met and began working in the same building. Our office is now halfway between Searsport and Belfast, near Moose Point State Park on the hill-side of Route 1, where we are the beneficiaries of water views and the natural air-conditioning of the offshore breezes. On an average day, each of us sees about twenty patients, from earaches to emphysema, warts to wens. Between patients, and before and after our office hours, we also attend to telephone messages, laboratory reports, drug representatives, disability forms, specialty referrals, the charts of our physician assistant, and the niggling details of running an office.

This is our fiefdom: the Searsport Family Practice, P.A. It is our corporate family, having burgeoned now to a dozen employees. In 1985, the year Tim and I drew up the partnership papers, we were responsible for a single employee each. Tim hired the nurse; I recruited Lindsay to be our receptionist. But a doctor now needs a nurse to assist him, another employee to assist the patient, and an office manager to tie it all together. Scott Bailly, the physician assistant, joined our practice in 1987, and Mary Beth Leone, a social worker from Camden, recently began to see clients in our office on Thursdays of each week. Tim and I are learning, sometimes the hard way, that a social body needs regular attention: monthly staff meetings, annual evaluations, a set of office policies and procedures, and a few kind words to carry us through. It also demands strong leadership, which, more than any clinical challenge, has forced Tim and me to dig deeply into ourselves and our relationship.

Since moving to town I have learned two other invaluable lessons about the practice of medicine: one must swallow his duties, and one must become a team player. Initially, I balked at the endless demands, which seemed needless, unfair, and a great bore. The beeper was a ball and chain. Not infrequently on weekend afternoons, I would discard it on the sofa while I went shopping for groceries or darted out for a leisurely run. I tried to convince myself that emergencies don't arise that quickly. Anyway, I live only four minutes from the hospital. And besides, what is the emergency staff for? And though I'd borne the wrath of nurses who couldn't reach me, and missed a few precipitous deliveries, my rationalization did not waiver.

Until the day Eva soured in the ICU. That Saturday morning, too sunny and warm and expansively free to be inconvenienced by a nagging beeper, I returned from the grocery store to hear my beeper screaming from a fold in the sofa. "Call 114," the message bar flashed. Call the ICU. Minutes later I was at Eva's bedside. We—the nurses and I—all recognized that she was in crisis. She pleaded for me to help her, to ease her labored breathing, to stay by her side. With great effort we hoisted her up in bed, pushed morphine and diuretics through her intravenous line, strapped an oxygen mask to her face, and watched her slip irretrievably to oblivion. I signaled for a Code 99. Eva, white as her mitred sheets, was gone without another gasp or twitch or electrical impulse from her body. I thanked the team for their prompt and professional efforts. Thirty minutes into the code, I pulled a sheet over Eva's hazy stare and went to face her husband.

What I found in that waiting room was not anger or accusal, but rather a family's acceptance, and their genuine appreciation for our efforts. I know now that my coming earlier would not have saved Eva. But it would have allowed me to save face. As hard as it is to lose a patient, it is harder still when you feel you have failed in your duty.

Teamwork, too, is essential. We rely utterly upon our consultants, our cross-coverage, and the nurses whose touch and clinical judgment and attention to oversight are our saving grace. The notion of team, once very much in the medical vogue, has lost its lustre now that the health care pie is slivered into so many technical roles. Maintenance of a team requires a busy meeting schedule, a large payroll, and attention to territorial concerns. The movement now seems to be toward bureaucracy, subspecialization, and a redefinition of the "professional." He has become someone who does something for money, and does it better for more money. We have drifted away from old-fashioned notions of vocation, and from the value of experience.

Perhaps Robert Coles's aphorism, borrowed from his father, has it right: character is how you behave around the company you keep (p. 198). Two years ago I began writing, by which I mean scribbling on paper a few stories about my patients. These were often my favorite tales, the ones that had survived the most retellings: a bizarre medical examiner's case, a troubling moral dilemma, a curious fate. Now that a few have been published in the "personal essay" sections of the professional journals, writing has become my companion. It is an invisible audience, my silent conscience, the filter through which I see the world, an ambassadorship to the hinterlands. It connects me, inside and out.

Smokey's Greater Shows has moved down the coast, and City Park slumbers again in the leisurely lap of the Bay. The summer is slipping by, warm and fragrant.

After ten years on the job, I am growing comfortable in my role as a family doctor. Politics, diplomacy, and conflict resolution are not my forte. But, in the last month, Tim and I have diplomatically transferred a patient from one home health agency to another, helped a colleague achieve better pain control for a hospice inpatient, and successfully pressed for hospice family meetings under *all* circumstances, even in the absence of crisis. As a form of "treatment," such meetings cannot guarantee a better outcome, and Tim and I are not "experts" in the "technique." We bring only ourselves. We offer to sit with the family in their pain, grief, confusion, and isolation, to love them and share in the responsibilities. If they use the occasion to explore hidden conflicts or unspoken fears, so much the better. If we gain insight and direction for implementing care, it is a bonus. We exploit the doctor's privilege to come a-calling, spend an hour, share a cup of coffee. We do it for sacred ends.

AUGUST

It is not a bad place, much as any other, but the secret of our love for it lies in what I have just said—we know it intimately. This is the lesson I got from Thoreau: love your own pond. All are beautiful. Be content where you are.

✷

LINCOLN COLCORD

Sea Stories from Searsport to Singapore

It has been raining all night, a drenching, garden-soaking, eaves-dripping rain. The intensity of the downpour now waxes and wanes outside my window as the day catches on. Our little plants have been singing hallelujahs.

I love coming back from my morning run along the Route 1 bypass around town, often to find Lindsay in the garden pinching the basil tips or inspecting the new blossoms of foxglove and marigold or shading herself beneath the towering sunflower stalks. Clare came running down the drive to announce that our pet hermit crab had died. Hermie had seemed indestructible, having bounced countless times off the hardwood floors and pavement still secure in his shell. He thoroughly enjoyed dips in the wading pool or a crawl in the grass. But we knew something was up; we never saw him eat the "crab cakes" or the minuscule shavings of lettuce and carrot that we cut for him. When two of his claws fell off, it was a signal to summon the priest. Yesterday morning he gave up the ghost, and his poor withered body, falling limp from the shell, was laid in a pillbox coffin and buried between the blueberry bushes out back. Each of us delivered a eulogy fashioned from the fond memories we shared with Hermie.

I am dismayed to consider how long it's been since Lindsay and I entertained dinner guests, or set aside a night for ourselves, or prepared a meal that was the least bit interesting, or discussed our upcoming vacation. Lindsay may ovulate today; will we take advantage of it or allow moods and hospital call or the demands of our child defeat us? We are living day to day, emotionally and financially. How will we pay the October taxes? When will we start saving for Clare's college or our retirement? How did my father, entering practice at age thirty-three and dying just sixteen years later, provide so well? These are my worries as I hunch over the computer beneath the serene image of Saint Dominic, whose cares he commends to an all-knowing God.

The eastern sky, which wore a faint band of silver at 4:45 A.M., is already rosy-cheeked at 5:00 A.M. At this latitude, the seasons shift on a daily basis.

It was a good weekend, owing to the hospital's unexpectedly light demands. I touched all the major bases: running (including the long run yesterday), Sunday Mass, lawn mowing, family barbecues, a badminton spree, and even a little solitude at the Belfast Museum, where I studied an 1855 map of Belfast. I delivered Baby Brittany, hospitalized an old man with prostate cancer and renal failure, and treated an assortment of ills in the emergency room. I'm ready for a lighter week, perhaps to spend writing, or perhaps to organize a visit by our California friends, the Moores, who will be vacationing in Maine this weekend just across Penobscot Bay. Plan A calls for hosting them here on Thursday night, and then joining them Saturday at their summer cabin after they are settled.

The fogs of August have returned. Yesterday they hugged us the whole day, except for a few hours around noon. Quite the opposite of the San Francisco fog, which, during our sabbatical summers of '90–91, blew in every afternoon around teatime, then politely drifted through. The noticeable effect of San Francisco's fog was its chill; natives and tourists alike prepared for that sudden drop in temperature as the banks blew in. But along the coast of Maine, our breathy fog threatens to dampen, to saturate, to mildew every porous surface in the house. The screen is beaded with water droplets, the refrigerator top glows an iridescent green, papers and soft book covers curl whenever they are left the least bit exposed. I rather like the fog, our morning shroud, because it is so like Maine and unlike Iowa or San Francisco. It is a reminder of place, as much as the lobster boats or road kill or thick Down-Eastern accents. Every morning during tourist season, the fog curtains our lives until 10:00 A.M. It is drawn tightly over Lower Main Street, the sail and lobster boats of Belfast harbor, the monument at the mouth of the Bay, the supply ships beyond, and all points east. This I inspect daily as I pass over Memorial Bridge on my way to work. The Bay remains our little secret, the fog an insider's joke played on the cars that strain for a view of quaint, authentic Maine in their gaper's crawl toward Bar Harbor.

Yesterday my first patient upset me for the entire day. She moved here a few months ago with her crippled husband to take up residence in her daughter's home. Leona found me, singled me out, asked me—on that first visit—if I would treat her high blood pressure, monitor her recovery from stroke, listen to her arthritic complaints, and sign her disability papers. Paperwork is a thorn in any relationship, for doctor and patient alike. But it is a necessity of her life and a reality in any medical practice. These papers will recertify her disability and authorize one insurance policy to pay for another and permit state services to flow without interruption and take more of my time than does the patient herself. It has been a year since the stroke, and she walks unaided and without an impediment of speech. "So you're getting along fine without assistance? Able to do most of your housework? Controlling the pain, getting a good night sleep?" She becomes suspicious of my questions and tactfully evades them. I push harder: "Are you involved in a rehabilitation program? If not, why? If your leg is bothered more by arthritis than stroke, if you cannot hold down a job because of your nerves and poor memory, then why don't we work on these?" I am incredulous that she was granted permanent disability by the state. And so I bully her now, fluster her. Her blank stare and helpless stammer make it clear that all she wants, all she is angling for, is The Benefit. She will choose pain if it brings security to her miserable circumstance. So why have I became the Grand Inquisitor, defender of the state's dwindling coffers? Disability determination is the bureaucrats' job, and they ask nothing of me here.

We back up. "So Leona, is there anything that I can do to make your life more comfortable?" I have so intimidated her that she cannot think of one thing, fearful of what she might lose if she "recovers," worried about what improvements I might report. Slowly, I retrace my steps, put the questions back in their most favorable light. This is deception, partly; I want her trust. But mostly I want what all doctors strive for: common ground, shared goals, and half the responsibility for achieving it.

"Leona," I retreated, "you are too preoccupied with your husband. Why not think of yourself? How much more ably you could care for him if you walked well, if you could steady his tottering gait, change his dirty linens, wipe the egg from his face and bib. Why not try another rehabilitation program, or get a second opinion from a bone doctor?" She doesn't buy the argument but agrees to think about it after Russell's MRI in a few weeks. "Maybe then, doctor," she offers. "But I'm too nervous, to stoved up, to ever work again. I just couldn't do it."

Leona scheduled a follow-up appointment in a month. So we will have time to pursue our relationship and forge a mutual plan. Next time I will be ready for the papers.

The California Moores arrived yesterday. They (God bless them) enjoy a certain sanity, generosity, sense of humor, and degree of strife that makes them rare and whole. Add to that an itch for travel, and it is easy to understand why we like them so much. They have made a commitment to return to New England every year so that their children might get to know "family"—the cousins and grandparents, aunts and uncles they left behind. Charlie and Becky are the longest-married couple we know. They grew up in the same Vermont town, became high school sweethearts, married young, became parents late. Their youngest of three, Mika, is Clare's age, and the two of them became instant buddies and constant quarrelers at the Haight-Ashbury Cooperative Nursery School in San Francisco during our sabbatical year. Through Mika, we came to know and appreciate her parents.

But it's not just their visit that I will enjoy, it's the *idea* of their visit. A sense of connection. A sense of enlargement in our lives through this transcontinental bridge. People there know us here! So far only a few people here know us, and scarcely at that. Having the Moores's friendship gives me hope that others will follow.

Visitors are a blessing. I appreciate the sacrifices that go along with travel, especially with three small potatoes, and I know the disruption it brings to a well-ordered life. This makes more precious the balm it brings to the severed ends of a relationship. And it reminds me also why we feel at home here, happy and secure—for reasons, invisible to the guest, that have appeared to us, like objects of the night, over time and with increasing clarity. Much of what we like about Belfast is simply the habit and the routine, and our sense of belonging, at long last. We know this town and its psychological terrain. We have experienced the frustration of caring for kids, the boredom and strain of repetitive work, the lean, long winter and the muddy spring, the busted budget, the empty waiting room, and coming home for another night of pasta or a chicken pot pie.

We have seen this tourist town without its makeup, at the end of summer when the romance wanes and the welcome and for-sale signs are covered and the leaves blown down for another season. We are accustomed to the shortcuts across town, the bargain bins at Reny's, the smalltalk you talk before you commence to deal. We know our neighbors and they know us. And when friends come to visit, I am reminded of all this, and how much water has passed beneath Little River Dam since we first crossed it.

The Feast of St. Dominic. His image looms above me, in the form of a print we bought in Florence five years ago. He sits in perfect repose, absorbed in *Lectio Divina,* his sacred reading. Dominic is slightly bent before the Bible, one hand marking the page, the other supporting his chin, with an emblematic red star floating above his halo. He is portrayed so by the Dominican monk Fra Angelico, who painted this detail within a larger fresco, *Christ on the Cross Adored by St. Dominic*, in the fifteenth century. It is to be found near Cell 46, on the northeast corner of the first floor in the Convent of San Marco in Florence. The print captured me in part because of the piety, devotion, and humility of the artist. I know little of this saint, and would choose to know still less of his followers: Savonarola, and the other *domini-canes* (hounds of God) who played such a dominant role in the excesses of the Inquisition. Yet this Order of Preachers also gave us Thomas Aquinas, the celebrated medieval doctor of the Church. The legend of Fra Angelico supplies a romance: He "never took up a brush without first making a prayer. He never made a crucifix when the tears did not course down his cheeks, while the goodness of his great and sincere soul can be seen in the attitude of his figures." One might believe, more temperately, that "there is no painter whose images are more exactly calculated to encourage meditation and to foster those moral values which lie at the center of spiritual life."*

I am attracted to the romance, to the reflection and calm that we conflate with the contemplative life. I know that I am too restless, too much in fear of loneliness, too needy of others' approval and the products of hard labor. I need tangible results by the end of the day, some *thing* to show for my miserable life. We wish for solitude, those of us who lack it or run from its bidding. But I know this about Dominic: "he travelled tirelessly to superintend his nascent order,"† which had taken root in Toulouse and Bologna, at the University of Paris, at Oxford, and in Spain. And earlier, in his campaign against the Albigensian heresy, he lived earnestly but simply and poorly with Bishop Diego.

What rest did Fra Angelico find in his busy workshop, surrounded by his assistants and pressured by the commissions and papal summons? Did these saints, Fra Angelico and St. Dominic, not find nourishment in their *lectio divina* or their daily toil? Is this not available to me, too, as I tear about on my morning rounds, or at the exam table and beside the bed, or on serpentine roads that lead to patients dying in distant homes? Quiet attention, an observant repose, sitting without doing in the context of an exam, for a few precious minutes before restless action carries me away.

I am thankful for my two morning hours and for the occasional long run or drive in the country. These snatches of calm, spliced into a relentless schedule, are my bread and wine. They require only a space where I sit and listen and let the possibilities come. They take but a moment. And bringing solace to the doctor, they solace the patient too, who seeks quiet attention in the midst of the storm.

---

* John Pope-Hennessy, p. 4.
† Donald Attwater, p. 105.

I slept an hour later this Saturday morning, after Lindsay and I spent much of the night tossing and turning. Yesterday was not overly stressful. But I have noticed that when one of us passes an anxious night, the other suffers it too. It has less to do with emotional sympathy than with the physical constraints of a queen-sized bed.

I have enjoyed the week with my wife. Monday night, Lindsay attended her monthly Hospice board meeting while Clare and I slurped pasta and watched the Summer Olympics. The following morning, Lindsay rose early to "catch up at her desk," but instead we spent the time talking about hospice. Politics, personality, intrigue are a part of every social endeavor, no matter how noble the cause or relaxed the operation. And Lindsay thrives on that, though she keeps a sensible head and her nose to the grindstone of client visitations and volunteer training. This year she will leave her post as coordinator of the training sessions and help facilitate the bereavement support group. It is a step away from large headaches and commitments of time, and toward something I sense she needs personally. Her current hospice patient is dying of ovarian cancer, as her mother did two decades ago.

We visited Peggy together on Tuesday: my house call and Lindsay's visit accidentally overlapped. It was nice company, and I enjoyed talking to Peg in Lindsay's presence. Our patient struggles with every breath; she is suffering from end-stage emphysema in addition to her cancer. But her greatest battle is with personal guilt, and for her daughter's love. She sent Shelly away to a home for disturbed children when she was only twelve years old. The teachers at public school had insisted that Shelly was "mean-spirited and rude," and recommended a corrective action. Peg's fatal mistake—one that she will carry to her grave—was telling Shelly that she was going to summer camp. "Camp" lasted a year and a half. Now Peg desperately seeks her daughter's forgiveness and craves her companionship. But Shelly has constructed a life of her own and cannot drop everything for Mother. Facing again the pain of Peg's desertion, she also knows she cannot heal her mother's wound—the sorrow and shame of having exiled and deceived her daughter. I encouraged Peg to begin talking about this with her social worker and minister when they visited next.

Last evening, we shared a picnic with friends at Moose Point State Park; Laurie is carrying their second child, and Bill lost his job as a boat builder. After arriving home, Lindsay got a telephone call from her good friend in Boston, Anne Eaton. Anne just delivered her second child, and her husband, John, just lost *his* job within the state mental health system. All of this tension, real and imagined, may have precipitated last night's fitful sleep.

All of this is to say that balance and limits are the key to Lindsay's happiness and, as a consequence, mine. She mirrors a reality that I cannot see in myself: too many days of child care, or too long a time without creative expression, or too busy or bare a social calendar as our lives become more strained. The week saw little in the way of romance but was full of affection and connection and good will. And I can go great distances on that alone.

We threw the mother of all birthday parties last night. Cathy Heberer, our office manager, turned forty-nine, so we gathered in her honor for the traditional coffee and cake crumble—on a Sunday evening, with supper thrown in. It was *very* nice; so why do I dread these affairs? Kids raced, conversations flowed, and all thoughts of social obligation vanished into the misty night air.

Yesterday the Stewarts popped over for afternoon tea. We have not seen them for weeks, which, since our return from San Francisco, has been more the routine. But prior to that, in the year Tim and Cris were in Costa Rica, they were our constant companions and confidants. I am not altogether sure what has changed. A distancing at a critical time? Marc's trouble with the church? Or just, as they say, a growing apart?

Marc and Cheryl, both ordained Congregational ministers, moved to town almost five years ago. When the First Church had asked Marc to take the helm, Cheryl stepped aside. She was pregnant with her first son then and anxious to begin a family. This was the second assignment for the young pastors after a rocky start in Virginia.

Then trouble brewed anew. Marc took an interest in the "recovery community"; he rented church space to an organization called Turnabout for their various functions and workshops, joined their board of directors, even directed it himself for a year. He took the Twelve Steps and applied them afresh to his new family, the First Church. Trouble is, Marc (like so many in Turnabout) was "from away," and the First Church stood proudly as the oldest house of worship in Belfast. It was built in 1818 in grand Federal style and represented all that was Belfast, all that is immutable, safe, unyielding, proper, and spoken without words. But Marc doesn't excel in the social graces. Nor does he cater to powers-that-be or to their agendas. He has failed to restore the parish to its glory days of the 1920s to '60s. He has made his mistakes and won his enemies. And his friends—nearly all outside the faith community—have been powerless to help him.

I am one of those friends. I have found Marc to be thoughtful, kind-hearted, and endearing. He is also young and sometimes naive. But what always mattered most was our mutual goal of living our faith authentically within the community. I saw parallels between his ministry and mine, between the suffering and hopelessness of his congregation and that of my patients. We talked long and passionately about the "angels of the church," those traditions that command the helm of the two most powerful institutions in town, the church and hospital.

And, because of our young families, idealistic dreams, and imperfect beliefs, we formed a solid bond in the early years of the struggle.

The Feast of St. Clare, friend of Francis and foundress of the Poor Clares. It was after her that we named our daughter. I will attend morning mass today in her honor.

Yesterday I dragged myself to the hospital, not charmed in the least by the start of the hospital week. My disenchantment is due partly to the added responsibility, partly to the personalities. It is an alien world. It is nevertheless the landscape through which we guide our patients. I am beginning to feel more like St. Jude, patron of hopeless causes, minister to the destitute and dying. Of the five patients I inherited on Monday morning, the first is a nonagenarian who lives alone, deaf as a board, and totally obstructed by prostate cancer encroaching upon his urethra. A Foley catheter temporarily restored the flow, but how much longer can he live by himself, even with a cadre of visiting nurses? The second has head and neck cancer that has mocked every round of radiation and chemotherapy. He is dying but cannot face it, literally, cannot imagine leaving his wife, who is crippled with MS, cannot conceive of giving up the fight. The third should have been dead years ago from emphysema, heart failure, and a car accident that demolished the cupola of the Frost House. He puffed his way back to the ER, mostly now in heart failure and urinary obstruction.

Yesterday exhausted me. It began at 4:30 A.M. with a call to the hospital for a delivery, and ended at 10:00 P.M. with a call from a residency classmate, David Strassler, announcing the birth of their third child and first daughter. Both deliveries went well. I have not spoken to David and Beth in a long time. It was he who initially interested me in a Maine practice, nine years ago, after we shared a Passover feast in his home. I had become a regular guest at Seder, made a commitment to come even when it involved travel from Chicago—not out of love or fascination with Judaism (though as a Catholic I have some, undeniably) but for the sake of friendship.

Then I forgot to come, forgot Passover during our first hectic, poverty-stricken spring in Maine. Beth was deeply hurt. "Forgetting Passover is like forgetting Christmas," she told me. And from her standpoint, it was true. I felt horrible, but what is left to be said after an apology? The invitations to Seder ceased, and the stain of my neglect soiled our interactions ever after.

David and I were "natural" friends; our bond was forged in the combat of residency, out of mutual respect, support, good humor, and (in the words of our deranged director) a shared "siege mentality." But the mixed doubles—Beth and I, Lindsay and David, never sparked. Perhaps the Passover debacle was the pivotal point in a decay that undermines all friendships built on memory, situated in the past. I praise his efforts to keep hope alive, to attend to our lagging friendship, and I vow to make the next move. Why give up on something so rare as friendship, especially between two doctors who live close by and are still sustained by faith?

The day was cluttered with events: a delivery at 5:38 A.M.; a family conference for a dying patient at 9:00; a circumcision at 9:30, and rounds thereafter; two emergency room evaluations, including an eighty-four-year-old out-of-stater who was dragged from death's doorstep and flown here yesterday for the last reunion with his large Maine family;* lunch with Marc Stewart in the hospital cafeteria; attendance at a C-section to "catch the baby"; a telephone call from Tucson inviting my partner and me to be interviewed for a family practice journal; a presentation at the medical staff meeting about a new hospice inpatient wing; a surgical assist for an appendectomy; and, sandwiched between all of that, my regular office load of twenty patients. It is amazing to inventory the working day, and then easier to see why so little time and energy is left for my family and myself. It is Wednesday already; I will get up from my computer and *make* time for the first run of the week.

Last night was one of the summer's coldest, in one of the coolest summers on record. Forty-four degrees when I rose this morning, and cooler temperatures (high thirties) predicted overnight. On this night, the full moon burned torch-like in the winds of a Canadian cold front, flooding the midnight sky. On this day our neighbor's house burned down. We don't have many fires in Belfast; many of the earliest homes and mansions from the town's heyday are still standing. This turn-of-the-century newcomer went up yesterday afternoon around 1:30. It was a grand wooden structure, three houses down from us on Northport Avenue, and known to the community as "the Pitcher House." All the volunteer fire departments from the surrounding townships came; roads were barricaded; Lindsay and Clare and a large share of Belfast watched the blaze for over two hours. Airborne embers landed on the home of our immediate neighbor to the north; fortunately, his roof had already been soaked by the firefighters.

Last evening I stole out of the house around 9:00 P.M. to pay a last visit to Emma Smith. Yesterday the doctors and children agreed that Emma should be given one last try off the ventilator. After the planned extubation that evening, there would be no turning back. By chance I met the cardiologist on the concrete apron outside the hospital's main entrance; he was leaving the ICU as I was going in. I thanked him for his help, his honest opinions, his skill in providing Emma a fighting chance, his willingness to let out line and reel it back in again if

---

* The state medical examiner's office just called; the old man died last night from his widely metastatic, bronchogenic carcinoma of the lung.

the exercise proves futile. I thanked him for his willingness to talk to the family, for being their anchor, and for taking the cautious, negative approach against which the family could balance the more positive outlooks of family doctor and surgeon. We personify the competing emotions that swirl inside the family's minds: give up on their mother? or hope for some small sign of recovery? We agreed to the plan yesterday morning, sat on our decision through the afternoon, and gave the cardiologist permission to turn off the ventilator last evening.

Where was Emma in all of this? Behind a veil of frantic glances, weak grips, and the unintelligible mouthing of words. Knowing that Emma had had a brain stem stroke, two weeks of starvation, and that her aging body was depleted by the effects of surgery and re-intubation did not soften our terrible choice. How can one say no to the positive value of life; how does a patient turn her back on a loved, and loving, family?

When I spoke to Emma, she seemed to recognize me, and her eyes would brighten momentarily. Then I would mention the ventilator—our decision to march on and quit it altogether—and she would avert her gaze and squeeze her lids shut tightly. All the doctors and family had to go by was a living will, drawn up several months ago around the time I began to treat her for depression. But she had often mentioned to me that she would only be happy when she joined her husband in heaven. She had stopped living; she became spontaneously tearful, reclusive, anorexic, silent, and neglectful of her usual habits. I had started her on Prozac a week before we discovered the recurrence of her colon cancer.

When I saw Emma last night, so animated and smiling after the extubation, how could I imagine that, any time soon, she might lose her urge to breathe? What could I tell her of our decision that she would grasp; what could I say without unduly frightening her or extinguishing all hope? I simply spoke of her family's love for her, their sorrow in seeing her suffer, and their acceptance of the fact that someday they would lose her. I told Emma how much I enjoyed caring for her, respected her decisions, always hoped that I might help her but knew that her real pain lay in the absence of her beloved. I asked Emma to trust me and her other doctors, trust that we would make the right decision for her, a difficult decision, carefully weighed, not to reinsert the tube, no matter what. Her bright smile was an unmistakable sign of the old Emma, but what of these words did she understand? I left with a squeeze of the hand and a lump in my throat.

On the way home I stopped by the burned shell of the Pitcher House, so-named for the two brothers who built the duplex (now a four-plex). I immediately found our neighbor (whose roof had been touched by the embers), and he recounted the day's events. In the moonlight, workmen were hauling furniture from a first-floor apartment: chairs and tables and chests of drawers that had been handmade by their owner, Everett Porter. He stood by the waiting pickup, hands in his pockets, a muddled, disbelieving look in his eyes.

A car pulled up. I vaguely recognized the front seat passenger, who greeted me as "Dr. Loxterkamp" and announced that she had made her first Hospice visit today as a volunteer. Now she may have lost everything in the fire. She had made her home above Mr. Porter's apartment for the past three years. She talked of the Pitcher brothers, well known for giving music lessons in their home, who had initially installed a system of pulleys and traps for transporting a piano to the second floor. It was this century-old system, and the Victorian elegance of the apartments, that had drawn her here to live. She had, in fact, used the pulleys to hoist her own pride and joy, a Steinway baby grand, to the second-floor apartment. Now what of anything was left? They would not know until the morning, when she and her husband would receive a sheriff's escort to see.

Fire. The drama of disaster, the licking of the flames, the permanence of its mischief. Thomas Merton once wrote about the summer night his monastery barn burned down. Mark Van Doren spoke of the poem in his preface to *Selected Poems* and recorded Merton's later reflections: "It is for me subjectively an important poem, because when I was a kid in Maryland (yes, even that, for a while) a barn burned down in the middle of the night and it is one of the earliest things I can remember. So burning barns are for me great mysteries that are important. They turn out to be the whole world, and it is the Last Judgement."* The poem is about beauty—the terrible beauty of blazing wood—and destiny.

Among yesterday's many tragedies, I lost my watch. This has happened regularly ever since I owned my first timepiece, owing to my carelessness. But this watch—a plain gold Seiko—is special. It was given to me by an elderly colleague four years ago in appreciation for a favor once granted. The watch symbolizes for me the doctor's ethical duty to stand up for his colleagues, to be aware of their needs and failings, to offer them his services freely, gladly, in the cause of brotherhood. My memories of that old doctor, and of the watch, are warm and fresh and recorded in a short story that is soon to be published.†

I have been expecting to lose this watch for a long time. It is long overdue. But I face the possibility without remorse because I will never lose the lesson it taught me. Tim and I take care of each other, guarding the other's flanks, in the Thursday morning sessions we share with our social worker, Mary Beth Leone. Up until now, the watch had been sticking to my wrist; perhaps there is still more to learn.

As I stretched out in bed last night, I heard the swoosh and clink of a small metal object as it slid from a fold in the covers onto the pine board floor.

Emma Smith died at 3:00 yesterday morning. I called her son last evening to offer my condolences at her passing. Arnie expressed his gratitude for the

---

* *Selected Poems*, p. xi.
† "The Watch," included in this volume.

patience, openness, and kindness shown to him these last, difficult weeks. His only regret was not being present when Emma died. Arnie is an only child. He moved down from Skowhegan some months ago to live with Emma when her depression, forgetfulness, and frailty reached a critical level. He was an immovable rock at Emma's side as she prepared for surgery, underwent the four-hour operation, twice foundered off the ventilator, and drifted further and further from the realm of recovery.

But Arnie was upset that he had not been present when Emma died. Why do we attach such significance to the final breath, the moment of expiration, when the patient swims in a twilight of consciousness where words run loose and emotions high? Arnie had said goodbye the evening before, when his mother's bright eyes took him in and reached back to him with her appreciation and love. Was that the source of the brightness and euphoria that I observed an hour later? Did Emma understand that her last wish had been granted and that she was being sent on the journey with her son's blessing?

When the families of terminal patients call and ask, "Is now the time to come?" I invariably say "Yes, if you can, and if you also understand that you may need to return." Say what is necessary while your parents can hear you, when they still might respond, when reparations are still possible. Come now, and never regret missing the most important moment, which is any of them when honesty and love, hurt and sorrow, and *fear* flow forth like fountains. Come now, and we will help you; we will face your fears together, or stand guard by the door; now, before our tubes and monitors and plunging numbers and streams of providers intrude on your most important of times. Arnie had a moment with his mother before she died, or perhaps many, in degrees. I hope he will cherish those and let go of his regrets about that last flickering moment when Emma was too busy for him, busy with her preparations to embrace her beloved.

We received a surprise visit by way of our friends the Stangrooms. Rob and Cathy, Chris and Caileigh came on Friday and shared supper last night with Lindsay's parents, who were also in town for a visit. Rob and Cathy were among our first friends, the connection made through a kitchen supply store where both of the women worked. They were like us in many ways: they moved to Maine with an abundance of energy and idealism and vision for a fresh start. They were college-educated, liberal-minded, and attached to the modest ambitions of their parents: They strived to pay their bills, provide for their kids' college education, and put something away for retirement. Rob was an entrepreneurial carpenter who owned a mooring business in Camden. He was a dreamer and a jack-of-all-trades, as most men must be who live on the coast of Maine. But three years ago they pulled up stakes and moved to South Carolina, where Cathy has family and a carpenter can earn a decent wage.

Rob says of their move that they still cannot get ahead financially. This, despite long hours at his job with a small construction firm and Cathy's busy days at her mom's gift shop. They have talked of moving back. They miss the people here. The kids are thriving in Hilton Head, though, as kids will do when home is built on a solid foundation.

Lindsay and I felt the same lure to settle in Maine, and the same temptations to leave it. A *New Yorker* cartoon once depicted a man and woman conversing over cocktails. "Maine?" she exclaimed, after discovering his origins, "What an authentic place to come from." There is something about the granite hills, the limitless shore, the thousands of islands that dot the shimmering sea, the ruggedness of the land and the people who inhabit it. The geography has became entwined with our romance. Lindsay and I were married here, nine months after our coming, on the back porch of a rented house. But we were already married to the notion of Maine and rural life and living in a coastal, blue-collar community. So it taunted us, punished us, snubbed us, denied us. For the first several years it took all our strength to hold on and steady a course. We took refuge in our relationship.

Even as a family doctor's family in this small, closely knit community, we had to earn a place here, as all have who came before us and all will who come after. I had to build my practice by word of mouth and to accept a variety of odd jobs just to put food on the table: I became county coroner, worked weekends in a neighboring emergency department, consulted for the Bureau of Vocational Rehabilitation, filled out surveys for the drug companies. I struggled in solidarity with the average Mainer who pounds nails, sells real estate, hauls traps, plows driveways, splits firewood, dabbles in antiques or anything else to improve his odds of survival. In the early years, we took almost no vacation, ate TV dinners or dined at Mc Donald's, and shared stimulating evenings with my patients at the laundromat.

Staying was a matter of pride: we would entertain the thought of leaving only after our survival had been assured. By that time, we had friends enough to stay. True, our poverty was relative to what a "real" doctor should make. But we live in Waldo County, one of the nation's poorest, and feel privileged to have even a small discretionary income. Like most of our neighbors, we have adjusted our expectations to our income, and decided it was worth it to stay. Poverty keeps a certain kind of company; keeps progress at bay; keeps "lesser" values in the running for our time and attention. No doubt, poverty is an identifying feature of this community; it knits us together in a common struggle, like boot camp recruits, and tests the mettle of each newcomer who strives to make his own way.

To a Catholic boy bred on penance and self-sacrifice, suspicious of wealth and good breeding, it all seemed pretty good. I still resent the many—approaching fifty as the recession deepens—green (medicaid) papers that slide across the receptionist's desk. And I compare myself to my more affluent classmates, fellow family doctors who, for reasons of good sense or good luck, settled where the money was. I am trying to abstain from these painful, pointless exercises. I've staked my claim; I'm here to serve, so let the poor come to me, and let me welcome them as if they were angels of God, and surprise me with their grace and dignity and self-revelation.

I still am idealistic, hopeful for family practice that it might close the gap between the lives of practitioners and those of their patients. Tim and I each took sabbaticals at the moment in our careers when matters of productivity, competitive edge, and moral certainty began to lose their grip. Age forty is a watershed, when parents fall from their pedestals, young children emulate their parents' traits, and marriages mature and begin to wear at the edges. We see ourselves in our patients and are exposed daily in the privacy of the exam room, or beside a dying patient's bed, or sometimes, just as assuredly, in a glimpse or a nod or unspoken word in Aisle 5 at Shop 'n Save. We come to learn that there is richness here, *much* to learn, and no shortcuts to the deeper truths. I need, and perhaps all of us need, friendships free of the ethical worry and the power trap of the doctor-patient relationship. I need work that requires of me some creative "solution." But I also need my patients, and am fed by them, in ways that forever amaze me.

Sandwiched in the middle of that abundant weekend was Emma's funeral. En route to other more pressing things, I stopped at the Methodist Church to remember this fine woman. It was the best twenty minutes of my day.

Yesterday, as I trotted down Salmond Street in my sneakers and shorts, I felt in awe of the glory of the morning run. Why do I run? It can be put plainly in these terms: I love the sheer exhilaration. And I love its purgative properties, the drenching satisfaction of a fast pace on a steamy afternoon. I love the freedom it brings, the sense of abandon, and the solitude of the open miles. I love the accomplishment of finishing, and finishing strong. But I also love running—and this is something I have come lately to understand—for the architecture I have discovered along the way.

The pace of a run and the absence of any practical purpose lend themselves to observation. I am struck by sunlight glinting off slate shingles, wet from a recent rain. I compare the squat solidity of a center chimney in a Colonial Cape to the delicate brickwork of a Victorian. I trace the pattern of pilasters and entablatures around the frame of a Greek Revival Home, or ask, "What makes a Cape a Cape?" And I will say to myself, "I love that building," but wonder why. I have many times loped down our gentle hill, rounded the corner beneath the neighbor's towering black locust trees, and covered that quick quarter-mile along Northport Avenue to arrive, finally, at the Y that divides Church Street from

High and discover again, to my utter joy and amazement, the James P. White homestead, our ambassador to the past.

It rises in the lee of a majestic copper beech and stands majestically on the threshold of Belfast's historic district. Like a popular politician or movie star, it stuns you with its poise, charm, and incomparable good looks. You first notice a two-story porch rising on fluted columns to the sleek slated roof, capped in turn by a widow's watch. You admire its perfectly balanced proportions. You are tempted to run your hands across the smooth, white, wooden walls that gleam like marble in the lemon light of the morning sun.

The White house is neither the oldest home in Belfast nor the largest. But it is the crown jewel in a collection of residential architecture that ranks among Maine's finest. It was designed by Calvin Ryder, one of the leading architects of the American Greek Revival, and was completed by master builder Amos Boynton in 1842. It is probably the best example of Greek Revival architecture in the state, along with the Nathaniel Hatch House in Bangor (1833) and the Charles Q. Clapp House in Portland (1833). Yet the building resists airs. It is a neighbor and a friend. It is part of what anchors my sense of place and draws me into Belfast's proud past, engaging me in those deep conversations that architecture often has with a community.

As a physician, I am attuned to human structure. Much can be surmised from a discreet glance at a pill-rolling tremor or a dowager's hump or a barrel chest. An ornamental detail tells a great deal about its owner, from a crusty hairline to fleshy tumors on the trunk to spider-shaped blood vessels branching on the skin. And all of this—body parts missing or neglected or disguised—is worth considering while you wait in the checkout line at Shop 'n Save or Home Supply.

The shell of a person, like the shell of a house, reflects directly upon the architect and the caretaker—their level of affluence, awareness of fashion, and the kind of company they keep. Family doctors notice such things; we probably focus more on appearances than do our colleagues in internal medicine. But it is the soul we really seek; all else is facade, however solidly and handsomely it is constructed.

So it is safe to say that my attraction to the White homestead is not simply about architecture. I too have a taste for history. I wonder how a village or nation (especially my own) becomes what it is. I wonder how people adjust to their bodies, especially when altered by illness. I appreciate that "taking a history" is the most important work that I do. For here diagnoses materialize and rise on their foundations. Here, we consider the patient's prognosis, map out a strategy for change, and size the obstacles that strew our path.

Architecture, no matter how elegant or outlandish or plain, says something about the values of a people at a particular time. To grasp it is to grasp the town—architecture, Belfast, and the Age of the Greek Revival. It is not excessive to say that American Greek Revival became the vehicle for this community's self-image and still drives it today. It gives substance to our civic pride, to our sense of character, to a bold imagination that has finally reawakened after a hundred years' sleep.

That we are Greek is, admittedly, an accident of history. Belfast and the American Greek Revival flourished in the quarter century before the Civil War; then collapsed in an apoplectic state that would seal the association for the next one hundred fifty years. That is often the first lesson of architecture: Towns are adorned in the architectural style of their ascendancy.

Belfast boomed during the rise of the temple design, which historians place between the War of 1812 and the Civil War. In those decades—1810 to 1860—Belfast's census grew by 100 residents a year. Before Lincoln was inaugurated, it was the ninth largest city in Maine with a population of 5,520; now it is thirtieth. The zenith of 1860 would not be surpassed for another century. The shift in the county-wide population is even more striking: In 1860, 47,229 people resided in Waldo County, 50 percent more than today. Shipbuilding became the keel of the local economy, and during the 1840s and '50s the city launched 183 barks, brigs, and schooners, more than half its total production. Again in 1860, Belfast was the fourth most productive shipbuilding district in New England, which, as a region, led the nation.

The first Greek Revival building in America (Virginia's Arlington House) was completed in 1818, but the nation did not awaken to the style until 1829. In that year, Benjamin Latrobe* added a Greek north portico to the White House, and William McNichol designed the Forks of Cypress. Belfast's first Revivalist may have been mayor R. C. Johnson, who reputedly sent six wooden columns down the Penobscot River in the mid-1830s to support a massive new portico. In 1837, Calvin Ryder received his first local commission but was paid to give the First Baptist Church a Gothic look. Not until 1839 did he inaugurate the American Greek Revival in Belfast, with a classic design for the First Universalist Church.[†]

Greek Revival quickly became Belfast's most prolific architectural statement. One hundred thirty-one buildings—nearly 45 percent of Belfast's Historic District—still contain Grecian elements. Temple design would transform every manner of home from connected farms and colonial Capes to cottages and town houses. The Cape Cod style (side gable, single story, shallow pitch of the roof)

---

* William Seale admits to confusion over authorship of the design. Credit belongs to either James Hoban, the original architect, or Benjamin Latrobe, who died in 1820 but left many Greek Revival plans. From *The President's House: A History,* White House Historical Assoc., Washington, D.C., 1986.

† I cannot secure this claim. The Maine Universalist Church has no record, nor does Williamson's *History of Belfast* (which largely neglects architecture), nor do contemporary newspaper accounts.

was often stretched to a story-and-a-half style in order to accommodate a wide band of trim, or rotated ninety degrees to sport a temple front. Even the older, established Federals raced to don a Grecian mantle: aediculas and porticoes rose here, conspicuous cupolas there, and heavy, added entablature came to rest on Doric columns, as in the Johnson-Pratt estate, which wore it over the second-story panes like a droopy sombrero.

Architecture can also show us branch points in a town's evolution. Return for a moment to the James P. White homestead. Here—to paraphrase New England poet Robert Frost—two roads roads diverge at a yellow light. So, too, did the course of local history during the 1840s. High Street, the city's second oldest thoroughfare, was plotted in 1793. It was settled by an original proprietor, James Miller, and his son, Robert. Sea captains Charles Wording and Ephraim McFarland would build adjoining homes here a half century apart. Tradesmen, doctors, lawyers, and ministers chose this prestigious address, as did the important shipbuilding family of Columbia, Horatio, and Thomas Carter, to overlook their shipyards. Gradually High Street would see the full range of nineteenth-century architecture, from Federal to Queen Anne, representing the ebb and flow of British influence across the century.*

Church Street was plotted much later and attracted the growing class of merchants and venture capitalists. They were less interested in building ships (or sailing them, for that matter) than in financing them, insuring them, and marketing their cargo. Church Street pushed onto High in 1826 just in time for the cultural revolution that would become the American Greek Revival. In 1840, Greek Revival exploded on the lower end of Church Street, including the homes of William T. Coburn, John W. White, William H. Burrill, Robert White, Jr., and Hiram O. Alden. Alden's house, along with Sherborne Sleeper's on Congress Street, was designed by Mr. Ryder and these two may be the oldest Greek homes in Belfast. Over half the dwellings on Church Street are Grecian. Even the commercial buildings near city center are Greek-transitional or Neoclassical in style, including the William G. Crosby School and Maine District Court House. These buildings became the high school and hospital, respectively, for the shooting of another classic, the 1957 film *Peyton Place*.

James P. White, son of an early settler, Robert White, matured and prospered during the rise of Greek Revival; it was natural that he should make his second home a temple. By the age of forty-two, he was one of Belfast's leading merchants and financiers. He founded the Belfast Bank, established the Waldo Insurance Company, ran a paper mill, directed the Belfast & Moosehead Lake

---

* The sequence of nineteenth-century American architecture is as follows: Federal 1790–1820; Greek 1825–55; Gothic 1840–80; Italianate 1845–85; Mansard 1855–85; Stick 1860–90; Shingle 1880–1900; Queen Anne 1880–1910.

Railroad, served as mayor and state senator, and reaped a fortune in Belfast's burgeoning shipbuilding industry.

His community, like the rest of the nation, was entering the "modern world of bigness, specialization, administrative coordination, impersonality, and wide-marketing orientation"* that characterized the years before the Rebellion. America was enjoying an unprecedented period of prosperity and self-confidence and needed an architectural style to celebrate it. American Greek Revival broke with tradition; it was an alternative to the Georgian and Federal schools of English architecture; it avoided domes and arches that smacked of Roman (that is, imperialist) pretensions. It sought no communion with nature (as Gothic Revival attempted) but dominion over it. The new national architecture was to convey a sense of power and permanence, yet also individual freedom and simplicity. It found all that, along with versatility for the individual homebuilder, in the Grecian style.

The James P. White homestead is prototypical of the American Greek Revival style. It contains every key element: rectilinear symmetry; a three-bay front featuring a two-story pavilion capped by a pediment; fluted columns with Ionic capitals; elaborate corner boards (pilasters) and under-eve trim (entablature); an octagonal cupola; flush-board siding; ornamental detail in a floral motif (anthemions and wreaths); and the requisite coat of white enamel paint. The design, however, may not be entirely original. Historian Earle Shettleworth sees its suggestion in Plate 43 of Minard Lefever's pattern book, *The Young Builder's General Instructor,* printed in 1829.[†] But the fashion was honed by Ryder, who borrowed much from the Bangor architects Charles Bryant and Charles Pond and later influenced the local architects James A. Thomas and William Winslow.

Architecture teaches us because it lives. *And we live in it*—from the marketplace to our houses of worship to the roofs that rise above our head. Thankfully, the buildings of Belfast's Greek Revival were built to last by skilled carpenters. They survived the great conflagrations of 1865 and 1873, owing partly to luck (the fires mostly consumed the commercial district) and partly to the slate-shingled roofs that repelled the blowing embers. They survived, too, because Belfast stagnated during the better part of the twentieth century, which spared these homes from the wrecking ball of urban renewal and the "home improvements" that quicken the heart every new homeowner.

Architecture draws you into the culture that spawned it. Greek Revival enjoyed a love affair with the American people because it was more than a fashion (as it remained in Scotland) or a form of political propaganda (as it was in Germany).

* Roger Kennedy, *Greek Revival America* (New York: Stewart, Tabori, & Chang, 1989).
[†] J. H. Mundy and E. G. Shettleworth, Jr., *The Flight of the Grand Eagle: Charles Bryant, Maine Architect and Adventurer* (Augusta, Maine: Maine Historic Preservation Commission, 1977), p. 50.

Indeed, its message resonated deeply with average citizens. It touched a growing sense of national pride and self-determination that Andrew Jackson revived with his victory at New Orleans in the War of 1812. It swelled like the aspirations of the common man, whose per capita income surged in the second quarter of the nineteenth century despite governmental ineptitude and corruption. The ideals of ancient Greece were incorporated into the national psyche, and Americans wore the temple on their shirtsleeves (or rather as the facade for their new homes). Every dwelling, no matter how humble or grand, could boast some element of Grecian style and thus keep pace with the push to progress and the rise of material fortune.

The James P. White house and the grand homes that stretch down Balfast's avenues have provided a sense of place for the citizens of the town across seven generations. Architecture is as much in our mind's eye as the pier at Sandy Beach, or the red tugs moored nearby, or the Bay that buoys our fading memories of a sailing past, or the distant elevations—Blue Hill and Cadillac Mountain and Camden Hills—that cradle us and fill our horizon.

Nothing proclaims the past as architecture does. Our founders and first settlers have long since returned to dust. Remains of Belfast's glorious Age of Sail have fared better inside the exhibition halls of the the Penobscot Marine Museum. But architecture is too large to house. Nor can it be sequestered like the slate markers in the East Side Cemetery, where you can still read those chilling words, "In memory of Ruth Brown, wife of John Brown, Junr, who departed this life April 1, 1798, Aged 30 years & 3 months. Also her infant incircled [*sic*] in her arms." In a family plot nearby lies "Thomas Reed and his son, Silas Lee, who died at sea Nov. 19 1842 AE 30." Three miniature markers huddle beside it bearing a single initial each. But heads no longer bow beside these sunken graves, and Route 1 traffic whines by in oblivion.

Traces of Belfast's booming patent medicine industry can still be discovered at low tide. Lindsay and Clare and I often scour the shores for century-old shards of green glass that still bear the letters of Dana's nationally renowned Sarsaparilla. In our bedroom we keep a wooden sarsaparilla case that proclaims what no modern tonic dares suggest: "Absolutely Guaranteed to Cure Disease." Sarsaparilla is gone, but not the building where the formula was concocted.* Gone is the Broiler Festival that celebrated Waldo County's famous poultry industry. When the Bay was finally cleared of chicken waste, organizers sanitized the festival, too. Gone is the municipally owned railroad, the Belfast & Moosehead Lake. Organized in 1867, it survived its twilight years on freight billings for the poultry plants. Now a facsimile hauls tourists instead. The only living history is architecture.

* It later housed "U Otta Bowl" but is now a warehouse for MacLeod's Furniture.

But buildings should not leave us feeling warmly nostalgic about the past. They are here to cajole us, to challenge us, to inspire us as we respond to the circumstances of *our* day and strive to return something to our adopted community. On close inspection, we see the purposes to which architecture was originally put: the taverns of Thomas Whittier and the Black Horse Inn; halls for the Masons, the Oddfellows, and the Tarratine Tribe; houses for government, commerce, and manufacturing, as well as for Wayward Girls and Aged Women; extended homes for extended families, and a place for them to pray, study, and read. Phoenix Row (1874) on Main Street pays tribute to the spirit that resurrected the commercial district after the city's second great fire. Belfast built *community* during its mid-twentieth-century surge, and struggles to preserve it for the twenty-first.

The challenge for our generation may well be to preserve the great halls instead of building new ones. These architectural treasures stud the centers of small towns all across America. But increasingly, they are being replaced by developers who promise jobs and prosperity. Can business be coaxed to invest in older buildings despite their higher costs? Can zoning boards and granting agencies accept modifications that would preserve only the historic shell of a landmark building? Preservation requires vigilance and collaboration and *action* to slow the leveling march of progress. It demands negotiation between competing groups and community values. But without it, a part of our heritage will be lost forever.

Architecture, by its sheer size, expense, and durability, stands for something that Americans need: lasting value. Like our best literature, like our children who bear our highest aspirations, architecture carries the convictions and dreams of one generation into the next. The historian Paul Goldberger put it well: "Architecture is about the long-haul. It is here to say that something that mattered yesterday still matters today, and, more important, will still matter tomorrow. It is still a way that the generations speak to each other. If there is any real architectural goal, it is not to make one kind of building or another, but to make sure that the dialogue continues into the next generation and the generations to follow."*

There survives in Maine a frontier mentality fed by the spirit of Yankee independence. Some men dream of building houses alone; a few actually succeed. But that is not what architecture is about. Like living itself, architecture is meant for a community. It calls on people to conceive it, to appreciate it, to construct it, and—often many people—to afford it. And it demands dialogue between parties, between the physical and social edifices of a community, about what we stand for and are willing to preserve. It forces us to consider what the builders had in mind, each of us, in every successive generation that calls it home.

* Paul Goldberger, "Does Architecture Really Matter?" Convocation address, Lawrence University, January 1, 1994. Reproduced in the alumni magazine.

Without the James P. White house, my life would be the poorer. In the decade since our introduction, it has been a source of beauty, a symbol of permanence, a prod to my historical curiosity. It has drawn me back to the period of the Civil War, when the children of the American Greek Revival were the architects—the generals and politicians—of that great tragedy. I have come to know and respect Mr. White for his civic achievements, and am indebted to the people of his generation for building a community on this rugged coast. Because of James White and Calvin Ryder and the urban habitat they created, I am inspired to face the challenges of our time and keep the ancient conversations alive.

It has been dreary and drizzly these last four days. The ground, wood, and even our clothing is soggy and mildewed. The day is reluctant to begin: my east window is still pitch black at 5:15 A.M. Running has fallen off, and on the last outing I stopped at four miles because of chest wall pain. We haven't been able to recruit a part-time nurse, who is needed desperately to spell Bonnie when her nursing classes begin, and to allow Charlotte an opportunity to scale back her hours.

At the Perinatal Meeting two days ago, the family doctors agreed to the obstetrician's request that only a "surgical team" perform cesarean sections. For the past fifteen years, family doctors have been delivering babies at Waldo County hospital. And when we needed a C-section, we called the obstetrician and assisted him or her in surgery. This arrangement served us well: it was practical (the surgeon needed an assistant, and the family doctor was already there); it was rewarding (the assistant's fee paid us *something* for the long hours of management without a vaginal delivery); and it was safe (no patient ever suffered the lack of a board-certified surgical assistant). But this obstetrician would change all that. C-sections, she says, are major surgery and require the skills of a "full surgical team," which would, by definition, exclude the family doctor.

But it is the surgeon's decision, and we accept that. Patients will be sliced by the most experienced team. And, in this day and age, the medico-legal ramifications must be borne in mind. But, as one of my colleagues moaned, "it's depressing."

It is further evidence, perhaps, of the drift toward increasing specialization. Family medicine, when it emerged two decades ago, was to reverse that trend, if not win back the ground lost by general practice. It boldly assumed that a doctor's knowledge of the patient is as valuable as another's expertise with a given disease. There will *always* be someone better trained or more experienced than the doctor on hand. So when is enough enough? And what else is relevant to the discussion: cost, availability, continuity, trust, or even (at the risk of sounding scientific) the outcome?

The Feast Day of St. Bernard, abbot and theologian, who died on this date in 1153. Soon after joining the new monastery at Citeaux in 1113, he left to establish a house at Clairvaux, where he built a reputation as founder of the Cistercian Order (known now as the Trappists).

I know little of Bernard's life and have read nothing of his letters, sermons *(On the Song of Songs),* or treatises *(On the Love of God).* It is said that he wrote with an "affective quality" that earned him the title *Doctor mellifuus,* the "honey-sweet teacher." But I am familiar with his Trappist tradition and with monastic spirituality through the houses I have visited, the monks I have known, and the writings of the most popular Trappist, Thomas Merton, who was ordained at Gethsemane on the nine hundredth anniversary of Bernard's death.

Yesterday I received a letter from an old friend, Father William, who introduced me to the Trappist life. Thirteen years ago, a medical school classmate, Pete Kerndt, and I drove to New Melleray Abbey near Dubuque, Iowa, to meet the then forty-two-year-old monk. "Willie"—as I uncomfortably agreed to call him—had proposed a forty-day fast in imitation of Christ and to pray for social justice in Latin America. The abbot would grant permission only if he could secure medical supervision. What did two senior medical students know about prolonged acaloric fasting? It turned into a clinical study sponsored by the University of Iowa Department of Family Medicine, and eventually was published in the *Western Journal of Medicine.**

This morning I have nothing thoughtful to say, no anchored perspective. My mind is full of flotsam and jetsam, the wreckage of dreams and unsolicited childhood memories, the smell of brewed coffee, yesterday's nagging argument with a patient, the transfiguring sunrise, and the cheery call of cardinals outside our screen door. I return each morning to the blessed beach, comb it, inspect the findings, and thank the Good God, mover of tides, for an abundant life on this ledge of land.

At Thursday morning conference, Tim again surprised me with his richness of thought. Healer as illness, illness as healer. Hank was on his mind, an elderly man suffering from incurable squamous cell carcinoma of the head and neck. His variety of cancer has been unresponsive to radical surgery, irradiation, and chemotherapy. Now each chemotherapy treatment leaves him nauseated and dehydrated, with nothing to show for it except the dread of the next one. But, in his mind, *he must go on.* "Didn't I buy into the formula," he argues? "Fight until you drop. Cancer is the enemy, and if you can't lick it, at least go out swinging." It's a familiar strategy for Hank; it had worked his whole life. Why should it fail him now when he needs it the most? His wife withdraws, having seen two husbands precede Hank in their failed crusades; she fights her own war against multiple

---

* P. Kerndt, et al., "Fasting: The History, Pathophysiology and Complications," *Western Journal of Medicine* 137, no. 5, pp. 379–99.

sclerosis. She is suspicious of hospice, which seems too much like surrender. Their lives go on, back to back with bitterness and defeat, within their tiny apartment atop Congress Street. Can the doctors help them to acknowledge the inevitable, shift their goals, accept the new terms of surrender? Healers work with *ideas* of illness as much as they do with putrid flesh; we help create and foster these ideas with patients on the front lines. The illness becomes *ours* as much as it is the patients'.

But also, illness can be the healer, bringing tremendous opportunities for renewal, reorientation, and recovery when it knocks you off your high horse, levels you, grounds you in the human condition that touches us all. This transition—through adversity toward spiritual wholeness, through death to new life—is captured in the Latin phrase *ad astra per aspera* (through adversity to the stars). It is one of the phrases I have considered for Searsport Family Practice's next company T-shirt.

It has been a "family weekend," in this campaign year on family values, and a well-deserved one. After spending most of Friday by myself, in the usual round of writing, running, mowing the lawn, and erranding, I retrieved Clare early from day care so we could spend an hour flying kites at Moose Point State Park. I brought along a snack of potato chips and 7-Up, which were devoured in the car. Our afternoon breeze blew backward: instead of receiving steady offshore gusts, we had to contend with a northerly breeze. But we launched the kite anyway and sent it to incredible heights. Clare then left me with the maintenance tasks and devoted herself to gathering wildflowers in the meadow. What a beautiful bouquet she picked! I was worried about poison ivy as she tromped through the tall grass, but so far no sign of a rash.

That evening we pooled the kids, hired a babysitter, and escaped to the minister's for a gathering of grown-ups. It was gentle rain for our parched friendship. Cheryl Stewart made a very respectable blueberry crisp and we nibbled it on lawn chairs in the summery evening. Conversations with Marc and Cheryl are dependably lively, and this one darted from news of a Down East physician who was sued for sexual misconduct, to the need for collegial support among leaders in a small town, to Tim's comments at our last Thursday morning meeting about the illness as the healer. I realize how much I look forward to removing a wart, repairing a laceration, mowing the lawn, or folding the laundry. For here, anyway, the task has a start and finish; its value is beyond reproach; and here you can lose yourself in repetition or banter, or in its precision of the task or the utterly predictability of its outcome.

Medicine seems seldom that way anymore. We see far too many patients on a far too frequent basis who flash their green cards, chat away the time, ignore our advice about diet and exercise and the need for a balanced life. What good is it;

what little recompense? Marc, of course, sees the parallels from the pulpit, but plays the devil's advocate. Why aren't they enrolled in education classes at the hospital, encouraged to volunteer or attend church for their social needs, curtailed in their abuse of public services, or challenged to get their act in order? I agree: this is all possible. But patients choose *me,* not a hospital or a church or a therapist. They are my responsibility, have given *me* the nod; and I give them back a relationship in which they are at least listened to, shown respect, and find affirmation despite their smelly clothes, unruly kids, ignorant ways, and state subsidies. Perhaps, in time, our partnership will pay off and my patients will improve their lives. Perhaps they never will. But for my part, I find the abuses to be painless, and see value in keeping the hope alive. We are not all that different, patient and doctor. We both have goals and dreams, seek life's meaning, and settle for whatever happiness we can find.

There are so many parallels between ministry and medicine that I appreciate Marc's friendship all the more. Doctors are given opportunities that a pastor is denied. Is it the physical intimacy of our work or its clinical authority that buys the token? Is it the kinds of questions we ask? Is it the life and death urgency, or an assumption about our skills and knowledge, or is it society's preoccupation with health? Perhaps one day we will explore these issues in greater depth.

Today Lindsay, Clare, and I head for the Union Fair, where—the poster promises—we will find amusements, animal barns, craft tents, fried dough and baked potato stands, and a million swarming Mainers. I'll slather on the sun block, which I neglected yesterday at the beach—a carelessness for which I have paid the price by tossing and turning all night in the warm glow of a lightly toasted sunburn. We went to the Swan Lake State Park with Clare's friend Evan and his inseparable mother, Megan. As usual, Evan was costumed in full superhero attire, fretting over nylon ears that wouldn't quite stand at attention. Evan is all boy, serious and silent and secure with his arsenal of sticks and guns. But he and Clare have forged a bond that any parent would be gladdened to see.

Last night, as we nestled in bed, Lindsay whispered to me that her breasts were tender. Nothing more followed or needed to be said. We both sensed the implication, harbored the same doubts and hopes, ruminated on all the changes a second child might bring. We have been "trying" for only a short time, marking the ovulatory green light in our minds but not trying very hard, as sex is a troublesome thorn. We pushed ahead, bent on building the family.

Yesterday I admitted Peggy, Lindsay's hospice patient, to the Hospice Wing with a diagnosis of intractable vomiting and diarrhea. She is the unit's first admission. As construction progressed, she had hoped to live long enough to benefit from it. Her current problem is theophylline toxicity, a drug Peg takes for her asthma. She had not been eating or drinking well for days, and became dehydrated. As her kidneys began to falter, the medicine concentrated in her blood stream. If that is the majority of her problem, Peg will enjoy three or four days in her plush surroundings. But theophylline toxicity may be the first sign of the end of the line.

I saw a patient in the office with exactly the same symptoms she had a month ago: headache, fatigue, low back pain, epigastric distress, insomnia. Divorced three years ago, she is involved in a protracted legal settlement. "Doc, I can't let him get to me," she protests, but he already has. Neither the support of her boyfriend nor the reassurance of a good job has made the legalities any easier to bear. Fighting back the tears, she acknowledges that stress *may* be a factor and assures me that she will call our social worker, Mary Beth—but only after I agree to test for sugar diabetes and infection. We further agree to meet next week.

A young college student returned yesterday. I have tended her minor ailments over the years, mostly during her summer breaks from study abroad. Last year she met a Norwegian boy in Edinburgh and fell in love. Three months ago she came to me with palpitations and breathlessness, symptoms that surfaced during their separation for school vacation. Oh to be young and in love! They have become "serious," plan to be married, and intend for her to join him in Norway where he has been accepted at University. She is here today because they are pregnant. These stories touch me deeply; I enjoy the privileged place I am allowed in their lives and the pleasure they bring to my office, which I borrow back, treasuring it for its intoxicating effect. What can I give them in return? I ride as their "shotgun" on this careening stage, up and over the blind and treacherous passage. I am their witness and guide for the journey. How important it is for me to be here, for the companionship and the view and the sheer thrill that it brings.

The weather has gotten the natives grumbling, up to ninety degrees all week, and unmitigated by the offshore breeze. They are talking air conditioners. I remind the office staff that we're not living in Florida or on the Mississippi Delta, where Hurricane Andrew has been kicking up his heels. On this morning, like the several before it, Belfast has been shrouded in a wonderfully soupy, smothering fog.

Yesterday morning, I met a patient of mine in the emergency department. She had been discharged from the hospital two days ago after passing kidney stones. Her diagnosis then had been "kidney infection" with associated left-sided numbness; the latter had been all but ignored. Now both symptoms were back. After a thorough evaluation, I could find no focal neurologic deficits to suggest a stroke. She had a fine tremor of her eyes when she looked in each direction (nystagmus) and an absent ankle jerk on the left, but no muscle weakness, sensory loss, abnormal reflex, loss of balance, or visual disturbance to accompany her vague sensation of "numbness" on the entire left side of her body. I spoke with the nearest neurologist by telephone, someone whose judgment I deeply respect. After describing the patient, her symptoms, and my examination, he reassured me that, whatever the problem, it was not urgent. I could send her home, and he would be happy to evaluate her tomorrow. This I offered to the patient. We broached the possibility of stress contributing in some way to her illness. Things have been mighty rough these last three years, she admitted, since her husband died and she must make ends meet on a fixed income and do for herself what her husband had always done for her. I talked to the son on the telephone. He would catch a ride to his mother's and be there waiting when the ambulance brought her home.

But the sister and son were stewing behind the curtains. After my dictation, I approached the bay and could feel their teeth sink in. The patient *would* be taken by ambulance to a medical center where they could see a kidney specialist and be admitted until we could be more definite about what was wrong. We had missed the boat on the first admission. We had no firm answers now. They wouldn't just sit back and watch Sis go on and suffer, or go home to die. I patiently explained that a proper diagnosis can take time to sort out, that I had consulted a neurologist by telephone, that he had agreed to see the patient in the morning. I could foresee nothing catastrophic happening until then, and, besides, I had no authority to admit a patient to another hospital. It is the doctor's onus to hospitalize a patient based on the apparent clinical need.

"But doctor," the sister insisted, "she's got the medical card and can afford it; *you* (she shook a knobby finger at my nose) have no right to put medical costs above a person's health. She needs a kidney specialist and you're going to call an ambulance to get her one."

I was livid. The *suggestion* that the medical card was preventing this woman from receiving appropriate care! Hadn't I spent forty-five minutes in examination, fifteen minutes in consultation, ten minutes haggling with relatives? And what about you? Why don't *you* drive her down to Pen Bay yourself, sit in the ER for two hours, argue with another doctor's indefinite opinions, ferry your sister even farther from home, and miss the one appointment that will benefit her the most. Your choice.

I was beyond reason, beyond discretion. Yet I instinctively grasped at the one straw that united us—the patient. "In order to help her," I began, "we must work together. I'll call the neurologist to see if he might be able to see her today, under the circumstances. And, if you feel insecure about driving, I'll call the ambulance to see if they could deliver your sister to the doctor's door and wait to see if she's admitted." The patient, sitting for the longest time mute and frozen on the cart, finally spoke in support of the plan.

Unbelievably, both the neurologist and the ambulance agreed. Later that afternoon, I saw a message on my desk, a request to call the patient at home. When I finally reached her, she told me that the neurologist had thought her numbness might be related to an overly restrictive diet for weight loss. No, he didn't talk stroke or suggest anything serious. Yes, she would be able to come to the office for a follow-up appointment. As we wound up the conversation, I waited for her apology, at least on behalf of her family, but it didn't come.

Yesterday morning Lindsay and I performed a pregnancy test that I had smuggled home from the office. She knew already, though I waited in agony for the second blue bar to appear that would signify a positive result. What mixed emotion; in Lindsay's words, "four more years." We agreed to tell no one, partly so that we could adjust to the news, partly to wait for time to prove the pregnancy viable. Would we choose amniocentesis, and if it revealed Down's syndrome, would we abort? Would we go to an obstetrician, or deliver at the local hospital, or move forward with remodeling plans, or wait to break the pregnancy news and make do with the space we had? There is much to think about, but the embryo growing inside Lindsay's womb will not give us long to ruminate.

I saw John Moulton in the office yesterday. He is the mentally retarded son of Elena and Harry and has the annoying habit of laughing when he is upset. Dad hauled him in for fecal soiling; he is now dirtying his underwear four or five times a day, something he hasn't done for years. Harry thought it sheer laziness. I suggested that stress at home might be a factor. It can cause both encopresis and the bad habit of stool retention, both of which are responsive to bowel retraining and positive reinforcement. Harry confessed that punishment hadn't worked; at this, John looked up at me sheepishly and laughed. In a week, Elena's brother will arrive from New York and we will attempt a family meeting. How, I do not know. The computer is working again, so Elena might try to communicate through that.

Over the weekend Anne, John, and their two children stopped on their way to Swan's Island. We adults have known each other for more than a decade. Lindsay and Anne go back to college days at Beloit, a history nearly twice as long. Anne and John are likable people: our age, our era, our dilemmas, our disaffection from family, our diffidence toward career. In them we see our own foibles more clearly (though fancy theirs to be far worse). We did not tell them that Lindsay is pregnant. Or, is she really yet? And will it last? She has no nausea or telltale cravings or a bulge to betray the baby's presence. Only symptoms of breast tenderness and fatigue.

I ran twice over the weekend. The long run on Saturday was brutal under a sweltering sun.

Last night I suffered another "choking spell." After falling asleep on Clare's bed as I read the bedtime stories, I awoke with a start. There, in my throat, was a plastic object too small to choke me but too large to cough out. If I tried to extract it, I would only succeed in wedging it down farther. I began somnambulating down the stairs and calling to Lindsay. She was in the kitchen chatting with our guests and probably felt embarrassed by my behavior, or relieved that others could witness what she had long suffered alone. At any rate, I received no sympathy, no show of concern, only the startled, curious, teasing comments of my wife and friends. As I began to awaken, I felt the keen embarrassment, offered my apologies, and retreated to the safety of my bed.

Lindsay believes that the spells are a result of psychological trauma suffered in youth. I wonder if it's not a "high hernia." The facts are these: the spells occur shortly after falling asleep, only while lying down (that's how I sleep), usually after a period of exceptional anxiety, and often after a large and late meal. Lindsay wants me to get hypnotized or seek serious counseling; I would prefer a trial of Maalox.

Yesterday I led a "family meeting" for the Wilsons. Roberta has multiple myeloma and less than a year to live. She is a picture of New England self-sacrifice, stoicism, and parsimony of speech. Walter is a ball of nerves, and talks (and weeps) easily about his wife's cancer. He has one of his own, in the prostate gland, but it is little cause for concern now. They have raised nine children, seven of whom gathered yesterday in the function room of the Hospice Unit for the meeting.

SEPTEMBER

People expect too much from speaking, too little from silence.

⁂

HENRI NOUWEN

The Genesee Diary

I had hoped to rest during the first week of September; or perhaps, at most to review the writing I have already done. I need to revise an essay on New England connected farms, and tape parts of the journal for a blind writer, Alfred Goodale, who expressed an interest in sampling it. But life stampedes ahead, and I need to make mention of my mother, who has settled into my thoughts these past several days.

About 3:00 yesterday afternoon, Cathy, the nurse-administrator at the Pocahontas Residential Care Center, called to express her concerns about my mother's impending departure. The break was planned for this weekend; my brother and his wife would be in charge. But Cathy feels that Mom is not ready: her memory is worse than when she arrived three months ago; she totters on toothpick legs; and, though her appetite is reasonably hearty, she has lost thirty-five pounds since her brain surgery, tilting the doctor's scales at a mere eighty-nine. Her sodium level has fallen despite fluid restriction and salt supplements. Although I haven't seen the test results, I believe Mom has the Syndrome of Inappropriate

Antidiuretic Hormone (SIADH), which often accompanies head injury or pulmonary disease (or both, as in my mother's case). The brain produces too much of a water-retentive hormone. This hormone (or a facsimile thereof) is also produced by certain tumors, and I worry about this latter possibility in light of Mom's unexpected and rapid weight loss.

After my talk with Cathy, I called one of Mom's doctors, John Rhodes. He confirmed reports of weight loss, electrolyte imbalance, and his suspicions about SIADH. He also expressed strong reservations about Mom going home but felt that her regular doctor (his son, John) should convey the bad news. Over the years, my mom (a head nurse at the community hospital) has kept her doctors at bay with her headstrong opinions. She has cajoled them into removing a bit of bad bowel that could not cope with her daily intake of animal fat, delivering cocktails to her hospital room, and prescribing more and more blood pressure pills to compensate for cigarettes and highballs. She has made this bed for herself, and must sleep in it.

After my conversation with Dr. Rhodes, I spoke with my brother, Jeff, and his wife. They are driving to Pocahontas this Labor Day weekend for "the move." Mom had called them two weeks ago and insisted upon it as an antidote to her depression and loneliness and withering self-image. We talked about strategies, how to say "no." The best way, and the one I argued for, would be to call it a matter of timing: The electrolytes must be treated first, and the cause of the weakness and weight loss must be found. A visit home this weekend, yes, and perhaps a more permanent move when I arrive in a few weeks. But the best strategy should include everyone working together, and the possibility that the option of moving home is not available. As I have seen in so many family crises, the doctor's role (and, I believe, his responsibility) is to present the hard facts, promote discussion, and argue for whatever he or she feels to be the patient's voice *and* best interest. I encouraged Jeff and Jane to enlist the doctor's help at any cost.

My last telephone call of the evening was to Mom. She expressed some reservations about going home and wanted to maintain a bridge back to the Care Center. But she insisted upon going home! How will you manage the stairs, or remember your pills, or get to the doctor's; how much worse will you be in a week or two with a broken hip? I urged her to wait, perhaps for my visit in a month, before settling on her plans to move back; I urged her to listen to the nurses and doctors, and to trust her kids. But Mom could not negotiate the facts, having forgotten in five minutes what we had thoroughly discussed. It will have to be a firm, nonnegotiable "no," spoken in a way that convinces her we are motivated by love, not self-interest.

I was depressed yesterday. Perhaps it was simply fatigue, as I stifled yawns all day and finally collapsed at 8:00 P.M. Or perhaps I am coming down with something, as I felt chilly and noticed a large knot in my stomach upon rising this morning. That is the way depression hits me, like soggy cardboard that I must cart from room to room. The day is reduced to a portage of body and mind, slogging through the bare minimum of my duties, fulfilling the obligation to listen and prescribe to the very last. I ended the day feeling dissatisfied and insecure. I could not talk to Lindsay; had no energy for Clare; and obsessed about my mother, her failing health, and the uncertainties and responsibilities that accompany it.

There is a temptation at the end of a busy weekend to tally all the feats of skill and endurance that I have accomplished in good humor. This is not simply the pride of a well-trained physician. It comes, too, from the need to serve, the need to be needed, the hope of reward in the patient's gratitude.

There is a discipline to medicine that every student rebels against, but that we all grow to respect and depend upon. It is the keel that keeps you righted, that holds you to your priorities, and responds to the undercurrent of time's passage. It reminds you of the value of a second opinion and the danger of a snap judgment or a cursory examination. It restrains your anger, turns a deaf ear to distraction, and checks the rising sense of dismay as you preview the afternoon roster. Tradition and training keep the ancient ideals in focus. They remind me of who I am trying to become.

I am breaking my fast, my long rest from the journal, with a note on Peggy's death. She died last evening on her eighth hospital day, shortly after I went to bed. Her family had been keeping vigil. I nodded to the granddaughter and her friends—who were still camping in the Hospice family room—when I passed by at 8:00 A.M. In Peg's room, I stood (for there was nowhere to sit) and chatted with her daughter, Shelly, and her constant companion, Clarice. Others, too, kept the night fires burning: Steven, a grandson; Bob, Shelly's husband; a niece from Portland whom I failed to recognize. We spoke of Peg, the plans for her memorial service, and the many memorable nights already spent waiting and listening to the shallow gasps and the occasional sighs and . . . the rarer pause . . . before she tugged for more air and bought another few moments of time. Only late that morning, when I bent over Peg for my habitual greeting, did she open her eyes and stare up with a glazed expression. It was a confirmation of her presence among us—patient and knowing and thankful—in these last unwasted days.

Peggy feared that emphysema would be the death of her. Every breath required a taxing, audible effort. Over the past several years it had become a conscious struggle that sapped her of strength, tethered her to an oxygen tank, occupied each waking thought and lent terror to the contemplation of her end. At home, we maximized her breathing medications, tried her on steroids, adjusted the flow of oxygen, kept fans running constantly, and prescribed Ativan to relieve the anxiety associated with her air hunger. How ironic that in the past week she breathed peacefully, with only a slow drip of morphine and a stream of nasal oxygen. No nebulizer treatments, no theophylline, no food or water or IV hydration. Our attention now—our gaze and conversation in the hospital room, *our anxiety*—was focused on that slow, irregular, shallow heave of the chest, the purse of her lips, as we kept watch for the final sigh.

As the first guest in our new Hospice Inpatient Wing three weeks ago, Peggy had been greeted by the hospital administrator, whose mother recently died in an out-of-state hospice unit. On the morning of her discharge, she was perky and hopeful. She ate a hearty breakfast, and we planned an excursion to Chelsea's, a new restaurant down by the water. But the ovarian cancer would not loosen its abdominal knot and, after six days of caring for her at home, Shelly could no longer cope. Plans for a home death broke down, and it was back to the Hospice Wing. Emphysema, that old and tiresome companion inherited from her grandfather, shared with an aunt and sister, and certain to come to her after years of inhaling cigarette smoke and poultry plant dust, had finally bowed to the cancer. Emphysema had distracted us by its nagging demands—the nebulizer treatments, oxygen tubing, and midsentence gasps—while the ovarian cancer took its less visible course. In the end, it robbed her of what little energy remained for shifting in her chair, moving her bowels, gulping her pills, or sipping ice water from a glass. Only a flickering spark remained, until at last the light went out.

Lindsay has been a faithful hospice volunteer during the six months since Peg's case opened, ever reminded of her mother's death from ovarian cancer. So Peg's journey has been for her, in some strange way, a reexploration of that death and mourning. She visited Peg twice a week, made pilgrimages with her to the shore where she grew up, brought her bouquets from the garden, plotted other outings, including the luncheon at Chelsea's, and sat beside her at the family meeting, and in many subsequent smaller combinations of family. Last night, after we were telephoned the news of Peg's death, Lindsay went over to the hospital to sit with Shelly and to acknowledge this momentous passing.

I have not had the same sort of deep attachment to Peggy, though I loved her as a patient, especially her transparent humanity. My detachment was made easier because she asked so little of me, and gave me so much. Her family, too, were always there, though not without their own pain, fatigue, guilt, and ambivalence. Perhaps, too, I recognized and accepted this as Peg's struggle, knowing that my day, with my family, will come soon enough. I did what I could, what the family had asked and needed of me: controlled Peg's pain, attended to her symptoms of dyspnea and nausea and constipation, visited the home regularly, supported her decision to quit chemotherapy, and shouldered that great burden of sorrow and regret that was stored in the family archives. My partner, too, did what he could.

He was there in my absence, emotionally as well as physically. I had made my goodbyes, expressed my love, held Peg's hand those several times before she finally turned her spirit homeward.

I will miss Peggy, and I will carry the memories of her signature gift (lollipops), of the two stuffed animals she handcrafted for the office, of the barren apartment she had packed and emptied in anticipation of her death, of her unblinking facing of death, of her desperate desire to open (so as to heal) old wounds, expose her pain, admit her mistakes, and offer her children all the love and regret her poor heart contained. It is hard to believe that she is not still dying, that we are not still in that slow procession to her grave, honoring and celebrating her life. She asks little of those who survive; only a brief memorial service and a few appropriate graveside remarks by her grandchildren. I risk remembering her now, and cherishing my memories of her hard and simple life.

I remember our first meeting six years ago when, over the weekend while covering for a colleague, I found her, ashen and struggling for breath, on an emergency room gurney. Her hospitalization was a brief one; we liked each other, and she transferred to my care. Over the years we combatted many bouts of asthma, a heart arrhythmia, chronic high blood pressure, and a detached retina. On August 29th of last year, she complained of a constant queasiness, and worried about colon cancer. She had recently lost five pounds (fifteen in the past year), and my hand on her belly acknowledged a firm mass. A barium X-ray suggested a tumor that had encircled the transverse colon. Later, the surgeons would find and debulk this pulpy mass, a papillary adenocarcinoma, but had to leave behind scattered seeds along the omentum and sigmoid colon and the uterine cul-de-sac. Though the ovaries appeared normal, they were implicated as the primary (cancer) and were the target of five rounds of chemotherapy. During that time, and on her occasional visits to my office, I did not broach the possibility that the treatments might fail. But in April, the oncologists assured me that they had. And Peggy no longer had the strength to deny it. She returned to me for her terminal care.

She was an enigma to me, one of the first to challenge an old prejudice (and an embarrassing one) about the kind of people who end up on Medicaid. Peggy was proud, tough, savvy, considerate, grateful; she grew up on the shore, knew her ground and defended it; she had earned my respect and gave respect freely to others. How was it, I wondered, that such a woman could be denied a decent life? I didn't know the circumstances. I didn't know the legacy of her children and grandchildren. Nor did I know then about the deep reservoir of love and courage that would sustain her in the final campaign against emphysema and cancer. She taught us all how to go bravely into the night. She accepted life for what it had offered and for what she had made of it; she tried to settle arrears with her children, knowing too well how unsettling it all would remain. She prepared to meet her Maker with a skeleton faith, without the trimmings of religious doctrine. What little she had in the way of material wealth she parceled out before she died, saving her family the bother, and giving generously in death as she had all her life. The more she wasted away, the more her presence was enlarged by a fierceness, a tenderness, a single-minded determination, and by love. Her gifts will not soon fade from memory.

After several days of a gravy fog, a full moon rose last night in the chilly, wispy air.

We called Kay and Kevin Drew to express our profound sadness at the loss of their son, Patrick, stillborn the day before. A cord accident at forty-one weeks gestation ended their hopes, expectations, plans of the last nine months. I could hardly allow the news to penetrate, given our own fears and ambivalences about the new pregnancy. Lindsay broke down in great heaving sobs after our telephone call; I could only hold her and lie next to her until the paroxysms passed. It was, however, touching, enriching to feel included in the sadness of these friends who had embraced us during our sabbatical year in San Francisco. We received separate phone calls from Charlie Moore and Ise Zopf to report the news. It was reassuring to hear their voices, Kevin's and Kay's, and in the background, the high-pitched chatter of their daughter, Emma. Life goes on, Emma teaches them in her four-year-old ways, with boundless energy, living for the moment, puzzling over her parents' mercurial emotions, shrugging off her own disappointment at losing her baby brother. Her solution: why can't mommy and daddy just plant a new seed tonight? She is their hope.

Today is Peg's memorial service at 11:00 A.M. It has been a week of hardship, with the loss of Peggy and Patrick, and another hospice patient, Hank, who died last night from head and neck cancer. I transferred an eleven-month-old boy to Bangor two nights ago, after sitting on the decision all day, worrying about his rapid, labored breathing from bronchiolitis. Two deliveries were crowded into my hospital mornings, one of which involved a hemorrhage before and after the baby. And as county coroner, I was called to a trailer north of town to examine the body of a twenty-six-year-old man. He lay on the forest floor, twenty yards from his home, illuminated by the ascending harvest moon. His face was split open from the blast of a twelve-gauge shotgun; a double-aught shell had exploded under his bearded chin and blown a crater between his eyes, causing the left orbit to bulge and stare eerily without blinking. I was stunned by the apparition, by my proximity to such a raw, violent, disposal of human life.

Suicide in this rural county is rarely the result of too many pills or a whiff of carbon monoxide. It is usually the explosive mixture of alcohol, speed, and guns. And one persistent impulse to end the torment that is strangling their lives. That evening, as I sat around the dining room table with his mother and half of the six older sisters, I absorbed the details of a sad life, of a boy who was thought "strange" by his family but never examined by a doctor or psychologist. One morning in ninth grade, he gave up school because of how painful it felt to leave home, and because no friendships drew him to school. He never attempted it again. He spoke few words, avoided direct eye contact, hid in his room when a girl would come around, and occasionally punched his fist through the trailer wall to dispel his temper. A couple of years ago he told a sister in New York State that he was hearing voices; this past summer, he ceased leaving home. His room was a jumble of pornographic and motorbike magazines, empty beer cans and dirty laundry, a bench press that occupied the center of the floor, an unmade bed beside it, and an arsenal of rifles in a corner cabinet. After inspecting the row of weapons and boxes of ammunition, I felt thankful that his was the only life taken.

Paranoid schizophrenia probably undid him. How much mental illness, I wonder, is allowed to fester behind trailer walls, under the cover of the Maine woods, far from the reach of the law, or from doctors, or from any test of social reality? The family and I talked that night as I tried to ease their sense of guilt. I explained that Bobby's behavior was a sign of illness and that emergence of similar behavior in other family members should signal a need to get help. I talked to one sister at length about her disturbed nine-year-old son, and I tried to help Bobby's best friend cope with the unfortunate circumstance of having been the last to see him alive, "the last hope he had on earth."

I am thankful when a religious service offsets the powerful, wrenching images of suicidal death. As a doctor, I rejoice in the delivery of new life, which balances the sorrow and pain and struggle of life's departure. Inspiration and expiration. It is no wonder that spiritual meditations focus on the natural rhythm of breathing, and that family doctors are drawn to these polar events—birth and death—for as long into our careers as we can continue.

Running yesterday broke new ground. It took me across the Passagassawakeag, around the tidewaters to the north, past the East Belfast homes that greeted first travelers over the Upper Bridge in 1801, and near a neighborhood cemetery at City Point. On Memorial Bridge, I could see the Lightship *Nantucket* berthing at City Pier and realized that it was she who had bellowed her foghorn twenty minutes earlier. When I drove the route later for an odometer check (7.7 miles, just 0.2 miles longer than the "long" run), I stopped at the cemetery, which was set back from the road by a small, freshly mown field. The setting was pastoral, demarcated by a log fence, shaded by an ample canopy of trees, and adorned with floral arrangements severally placed. The ground was uneven and lumpy from the settling of graves. The family plots kept a familiar configuration: parental tombstones in the center, flanked by the lesser markers of the surviving children, and a frontal phalanx of infant graves that bore only initials. As I left the grave-yard, an elderly woman slowed her Mercedes to ask me for directions to Belfast. It seemed a peculiar request; hadn't she just passed through town to arrive at this remote stretch of gravel? I asked her to follow me because I was returning to town anyway, and watched her through the rearview mirror as she turned into an art gallery, safely inside the city limits.

An unusual thing happened at Mass yesterday: I was moved by a sermon, for the second time in a year. Catholics go to church, under the best of conditions, to participate in Liturgy, to pray the parts of the Mass, to join together in Communion. The sermon is always icing on the cake, and there is usually little enough of that, ten or fifteen minutes' reflection on the Gospel reading. I often take that time to meditate, to focus on a hospital problem or a perplexing passage from Scripture, to take in the human element of the Mass, or to consider all the Church dogma and prejudice that I have accepted on faith.

A year ago, Father Ray Lauzon substituted for our vacationing priest. He drove up from the Franciscan Monastery in Kennebunkport to be with us. Though I don't remember the content of his sermon, his *style* was unforget-table, for he was a natural storyteller, a passionate preacher, a man of deepest sorrow and magnified joy. He returned yesterday. I report his story now so it will not be forgotten. The gospel reading from Mark was peculiar, and so unsuit-able for commentary. Somehow, Father Ray got off on "commitment," and then slipped into a story about his father, as if the story would be told no matter what Scripture had in mind, as if he needed, on this occasion, a whole church full of confessors.

Ray Lauzon returned from boot camp at age eighteen, a strapping, cocky, self-assured youth. It was during the Second World War, and he had only a week to visit his family before shipping out. Every night he went dancing, "good, clean fun," says Ray, paying little heed to his family's needs. On the last night, his mother begged him to stay home with the family, but Ray would have none of it. "I know what I want. I know what I'm doing, and I'm going out dancing." Ray's father overheard the conversation, or at least the tone of it, and brought his son to the bedroom. "Don't you ever speak to the woman I love that way again," he said. Then he began to cry out of hurt and shame for his wife. Ray was too proud, too strong, too self-assured to apologize. He went dancing that night and left on the morning train for the Pacific Theater. Before long he was captured by the Japanese. After his liberation from a prisoner-of-war camp, he suffered a deep depression. It was on waking from a shock treatment that he first remembers hearing of his father's death.

In a voice that could boom off the back wall of the church or whisper in tears,

Ray promised that the first thing, the *very* first thing he would do in heaven, would be to apologize to his father. That man was *committed* to his wife, his sweetheart, his friend.

The penitential sorrow that Catholics can carry in their hearts is a joy and a mystery to behold.

It rained most of yesterday, and the air was heavy and windy and warm. But a great weight seemed to roll off my chest. I would have denied its presence, could not supply its name, until the sudden departure sent my spirits soaring. There is no obvious explanation for the shift. I did receive some good news yesterday, but in trivial amounts: A patient's test for acute intermittent porphyria had come back positive, confirming my suspicions. It represents a tiny bit of egg on the face of the general surgeons, who opened her twice for abdominal pain but found no obvious explanation. I admit taking pleasure in their mistake for all the times they have relished mine.

I arranged the trip to Iowa to visit my mother and settle her affairs. Most important among these is her apartment in Rolfe, which must be closed down and emptied. I am anxious, too, to see how far and fast she is slipping. On either side of that visit, and as part of my Midwestern tour, I hope to visit Gary Ceriani in Denver and rent a car to visit his hometown of Kremmling. This sidetrack is to research a paper I hope to write on a Gene Smith photo essay that appeared in *Life* magazine ("Country Doctor," Sept 20, 1948) about Gary's father, Ernest Ceriani. I also hope to visit my favorite college professor and his wife in Omaha, Bruce and Diane Malina. Yesterday morning I finished my essay on connected farm buildings of New England, which offers a metaphor for family practice. In order to send it to Gayle Stephens for his editing (and his blessing), I called him at his Dillon, Colorado, home to be sure he was still summering there. He was, and we had a brief but engaging conversation about writing. He also said that he was hoping to visit Maine in December, perhaps on the tail of a Christmas visit to his son in Connecticut. Whether that visit materializes or not, I am honored by the intent.

A flurry of patients yesterday afternoon: A Hospice admission; an elderly patient with cellulitis who is accustomed to visiting me every several years; a woman with some sort of inflammatory rheumatism. I am less perplexed by the diagnosis than by the odd stance she takes toward her health. She is smart, pretty, runs a high blood pressure that she would rather ignore, and, for the past six weeks, has suffered silently from her swollen joints and muscles. She harbors the common delusion that eating and exercising and living properly guarantee good health. I will send her to a rheumatologist and not to the chiropractor that she requested.

Lastly, I saw a new patient whose profile is every doctor's worst nightmare: middle-aged, overweight, disabled by low back pain, and seeking refills of his pain relievers and muscle relaxants. I agreed to take him on because I believe his pain is real and his cause deserving. My assumption may be wrong, but I don't mind being duped if it means giving patients the benefit of the doubt. I expect, in return, their honesty and personal involvement in their care. We arranged a referral to the pain clinic, a return appointment here for a complete H&P, a signature to release his old records, and a transfer of his care to an orthopedic surgeon if the condition worsens. So I refilled his Percocet and Soma and hoped for the best. Last night I got the worst—a telephone call at 11:00 P.M. stating that the back pain had gotten worse, the pills were of no use, and would I call the emergency room to arrange for a shot of morphine? He claimed that his doctors in Florida left a standing order. "Sorry," I said. "You're on your own."

One last patient to remember. I saw her out of the corner of my eye at the emergency room window. She was registering at the desk while I pored over X-rays and laboratory results and examination notes at the nurses' station in an effort to justify my decision to send an elderly woman home. The minister at the window was a painful reminder of a correspondence I had shared four months earlier. She had come to me with a lump in her breast, and I evaluated it for the possibility of malignancy. It was not large, but firm, and had a history of growth in recent months and a slight irregularity to its margins. I recommended a biopsy; alternatively, we could watch it closely for the next three months. Either way was fine, I told her, but I leaned toward the biopsy.

On that same morning four months ago, a patient of ours had died of breast cancer. She had presented with an innocent bump, one that my partner had evaluated six months earlier and agreed to watch. Then, as now with the new patient, the lump felt benign, but it created too much lingering doubt to ignore. The biopsy came back malignant, and within three years, despite deep surgical excavations and chemotherapy, it got the upper hand. My partner felt terrible throughout all of this; had confessed, in the month before she died, his burden of guilt and grief. All of this I had remembered as I measured and palpated and scrutinized the reverend's lump. Because she was a pastor, an educated woman, a person aware of the psychological aspects of human decisions but nonetheless capable of making rational decisions, I told her of my patient that morning. I cautioned her that one adverse experience influences the rest and that this was a factor in my recommendation to excise the lump rather than watch it. Another doctor might properly decide otherwise. The patient shared my caution and agreed to return in a week for excisional biopsy.

She did not. Instead, she made an appointment with a local surgeon who would remove what the pathologist confirmed to be a perfectly benign fibroadenoma. Two weeks later I received her angry chastisements. She recounted our appointment in the office—accurately, in all fairness—and related the tremendous fear and anxiety she felt after leaving my office that day. What followed in her letter I wrestled with, discussed with my partner and a visiting psychiatrist, plumbed to the depths of my soul over the next few weeks:

> I believe your conduct in telling me of a possible prognosis before you had made a sure diagnosis was improper, irresponsible, unprofessional, and uncalled for. That is why my husband scheduled my appointment with the surgeon. You had no right to tell me all the things you told me related to someone else's diagnosis, prognosis, and death. I felt like you did everything but hand me a business card of a funeral director! What you did would be the equivalent of me, as a Pastor, telling someone who came to me in distress over their sins, that they had no hope of salvation and they were going straight to hell. I have been in distress and anxiety for two weeks because of your poor judgement. Only my strong faith in my Redeemer and prayers of my church family have seen me through. We only hope that you do not follow the same procedure with others.
>
> Because of this incident, I can no longer trust you to care for my health or that of my family. I know you have many more patients and one family not coming to you anymore may not seem that important to you . . . but it reflects on you as a doctor and speaks volumes to others.

My first response was shock, disbelief, self-reproach, outrage. Had I done this, and if not, if not *exactly,* why such an attack on my character? Gradually, after obsessing on the encounter, reviewing my office notes, rereading her letter, and talking to Lindsay, I boxed up what I would consider to be "the facts in the case," then composed this letter and mailed it, after first reading it to Tim and Mary Beth at our Thursday morning group:

> I received your letter two days ago, and read it with the concern and humility that it deserves. The greatest privilege of my work is the chance to help patients through their suffering. I was troubled to learn that I had magnified yours. For that I am deeply sorry.
>
> You could have simply transferred your records without any explanation, but instead had the kindness to express your feelings. Please allow me the chance to do the same. I remember the conversation we had that day, aided by my office notes, and trust that it proceeded along the lines you describe. Whenever I cannot make a certain diagnosis, or propose a procedure for which pain or other complications are possible, I routinely discuss

the range of diagnoses and treatment options. Even when cancer is among the possibilities.

I could have ended there, recommended surgery, and ushered you out the door. Instead, I told you about a patient of mine who died that day of breast cancer. The comment was made, to the best of my memory, in our discussion of treatment options: We could observe your lump or remove it. I recommended surgery to be absolutely sure that cancer was neither present nor could develop there. I wanted you to know that doctors make their decisions partly on the basis of science, partly on the basis of experience. We factor it in because we are human, because we find ourselves caring deeply for those who place their trust in us.

Perhaps I shouldn't have burdened you with that discussion. With perfect hindsight, it was wrong to have done so. Our experience will serve to guide me in future encounters. But I do feel obliged to say that your reaction seems exaggerated to me. I tried to separate your lump, which I assured you felt benign, from that of my cancer patient, whose memory would influence my recommendation for treatment.

There is a dangerous temptation to share a little of our burden with our patients, especially those in the ministry. I do know of many patients who have benefited from such a discussion, who wanted to know what "the doctor would do under these circumstances." Did I exercise poor judgment, or simply express myself badly? Did you over-react to the possibility of cancer? Are you judging me too severely, without allowing the doctor to make a mistake? I don't have an answer, only the belief that I did not act unethically: I did not breach anyone's confidence. And I did not knowingly, maliciously, try to frighten you, but offered every reassurance that your condition seemed benign.

All cannot be said in a letter. Just as my comments that day "reflect on me as a doctor," your reaction also reflects upon you as a patient. Perhaps we could get together to discuss it, not in an effort to "win you back," but rather so that I could apologize in person. Perhaps, in the process, we might grow from this complex relationship between a doctor and his patient, which has its parallel in the relationship between a minister and his parishioner.

Before the doctor lowers his guard, he must know the patient and be willing to accept the risk. Patients do not come to us to be burdened by someone else's problems, especially their doctor's. My comments in the office that day were partly in honor of our deceased patient, for the loss of a wonderful person and our missed opportunity to save her. But I also wanted to express the complexity of a medical decision, which is influenced as much by recent experience and our threshold of worry as it is by the medical texts.

Occasionally I *do* try to scare a patient who is destroying his lungs with cigarette smoke, or drowning himself in alcohol, or walking dangerously close to the brink of suicide. But it needs to come in the context of a trusting relationship, when the patient knows that the motivation is out of love, not ego. Yesterday a gentleman came to see me for a physical. He puffed through a tracheostomy tube, which a surgeon fitted two years ago during an operation for throat cancer. His wife had died of emphysema a year or so before, on every available drug, and strapped day and night to an oxygen tube. Still the man smoked two or three packs per day. We discussed methods of quitting, and I prescribed the nicotine patch. It only made him nauseous, as it will do if you continue to smoke while you wear it.

His addiction reminded me of a cartoon I saw a number of years ago in the *New Yorker*: An arm stretched out of a meat grinder, still attached to the crank handle. Upon observing this curious sight, one detective remarked to another, "It's the most determined case of suicide I've ever seen." I recall that absurd image every time I encounter a patient whose behavior seems suicidal. But this was only our second meeting. As my patient sat on the examination table—a provocative stream of air from the tracheostomy tube striking my face—I assured him that we could try again, try to quit smoking again, but in the meantime we might consider medication to relieve his air hunger. The first step is hospitality, to let the patient feel welcome, respected, understood.

I periodically reviewed our transfer notebook to see where the reverend would take her family for medical care. No transfer request was ever made. I timidly sorted the mail for another personal letter, both doubting and dreading her reply. It never came. Then three weekends ago, I spoke to her husband on the telephone for advice on tetanus prophylaxis. I mentioned our exchange of letters, his wife's and mine; he thought she would want to discuss matters more openly when time permitted.

The minister was no longer at the window, having seated herself until a room was ready. She had identified herself as a patient of ours. The prevailing custom and courtesy would allow me the option of seeing her. But I hesitated, turned the question around, decided that we should let the patient decide. "I would be happy to," I murmured to the receptionist, "but perhaps she would prefer to see the emergency room doctor."

"Doctor," she said, after returning momentarily, "it doesn't matter to her."

Then so be it. I took the chart, grabbed a deep breath, and strode in to examine her. We exchanged nervous greetings, then got down to the business of her visit: a sprained thumb. Old injury, not healing well, worried that something more serious might be the matter. An X-ray confirmed that it was only a sprain, and we agreed to splint it for a week. Then my gaze rested in hers, and we both saw that there was no avoiding the great mess that lay between us. "Your husband told me that you had received my letter, and I wanted to thank you for yours. He said you might want to talk about it sometime."

"Been awfully busy, but, yah, sometime would be good."

"Whenever. Give me a call in a week about your thumb, OK?"

We danced over it ever so lightly, in far less time than it had taken to tell of my patient's death. Would that be the last of it? Was there too much water over the dam, too much injured pride in our relationship, too nettled a path for any further progress along it? Would our lesson apply only to the next patient or the new doctor? That is all we get mostly, one chance, if we're wrong—one misjudgment, one burst of temper, one mental lapse, one uttered sorrow or sign of self-pity—and too often the only closure is our unacknowledged apology.

Sunday, and Tim returns. He has been gone ten days on a sentimental journey through the Midwest and to Chicago for a conference on the doctor-patient relationship. He will stop over in Cleveland (his home) on the return leg. The postmark on yesterday's letter confirmed that he was in Chicago, sightseeing at a few of our recommended spots: the Art Institute ("glass of wine and a plate of *hors d'oeuvres* at the museum cafe, after I asked for 'snacks'"); the Walnut Room at Marshall Fields ("Frango Mint Pie in a diminutive wedge that trembled before my manly appetite"); Jimmy's in Hyde Park (with a list of selected menu items). Tim included a final, cryptic note about the young Tolstoy and the relationship between knowledge and religion. Tim, with his solitary, unencumbered, and hermit-like ways, seems to live for trips like these; perhaps it is our mutual appreciation of time alone that we share most deeply. He guards and defends these opportunities with vigilance. I will see him tomorrow at our Monday morning meeting, and hope to find him invigorated, chipper, and happy to be back.

It has been harder on me, but I do not complain. Taking over the watch at Searsport Family Practice is part of our bargain. I enjoy the challenge, cope with the decisions, revel in the narrowed field of possibilities. No discussion, just decision. It is the doctor's gold mine, and his deathtrap. This week, our trusted head nurse of two years resigned. She did not tell me, only our office manager, Cathy, by way of a two-week notice. We all wondered why, blamed ourselves, and bemoaned the inevitable changes. Scott, in character, felt she quit because of his grumpy disposition this past week; I fretted over how little we paid her; Cathy, the maternal Cathy, probably worries the most about another child fleeing our dysfunctional home. It may be simply the need for more money, or for greater flexibility. We will probe at the exit interview in two weeks. Meanwhile, we have hired two new part-time nurses, who will appear on Monday with scrubbed faces, eager for orientation.

This weekend I have heard from two difficult patients, Isabelle and Janet. Isabelle has chronic liver disease, severe diabetes that led to the amputation of her left arm, festering sores on her legs, and a sandpaper voice that strikes terror into the hearts of her doctors. She has been calling our office daily about little complaints for which—she finally agrees—nothing can be done. Isabelle has driven away one home health nurse by her incessant demands. She needs human contact and knows of no other means to achieve it. She has sabotaged all attempts to heal her bleeding legs, so I tell her now, "There is no hope. You must live with these legs for as long as you keep them." Janet has had migraine headaches for two years now, resistant to every treatment except high-dose amitriptylene. But the amitriptylene caused twitching of the right eye, and worry that it would lead to tardive dyskinesia. She has been a regular customer of the psychiatrists, neurologists, the Lahey Clinic, and area emergency departments; yesterday I joined the list. I would have declined the opportunity, but she is a patient of Scott's. We spent an hour in the emergency room together, as I elicited her history, checked old records, reviewed tardive dyskinesia in the textbooks, examined the patient, and tried her on Compazine intramuscularly before giving her what she *really* wanted: Demerol. You might as fairly say *needed*, because thereafter the headache abated. What about the future? How many more trips to the ER: how many more pacing, moaning scenes in our waiting room and desperate phone calls late at night? We need to talk about these patients together, Scott and Tim and I. We need to have a "session for St. Jude." where we can discuss our growing hoard of hopeless causes.

This cannot be one man's burden, but becomes all of ours, as the weekend proved. What can be done to help her, or failing that, to protect ourselves? Why did the headaches begin two years ago? Why have so many doctors been involved? Why did the antidepressant work so well: because the headaches were migrainous, or because they were a somatic manifestation of depression? How will we approach this patient's needs, correct her habits and expectations, hold to a unified plan? Sessions for St. Jude. It's an idea, but one that takes time and energy and the correction of our own isolating habits.

Yesterday we harvested our enormous pumpkin, along with the miniatures, the eggplants, and unripened tomatoes. That is the last from our vegetable garden, the end of a productive summer. Swamp maples are already burning their leafy edges, and frost hangs in the evening air. We have been running the furnace every night now and have replaced screen windows with storms and transplanted the rosemary to a warmer perch inside. Had we still a wood stove, there would be that to bother with, too: the buying, splitting, and stacking of wood. We turn in, gather up, ready ourselves for winter.

Not a bad weekend, by all measures. I missed Mass because of other, more pressing obligations: a full morning on hospital rounds after a send-off breakfast for Cathy Rispoli. She announced her intent of returning to Maine within a year or two, if a job turns up, if conditions are right. Our dear friend is still smoking, and looking as gaunt and anxious and unsettled as ever. A friend of Cathy's has moved into the oceanfront house and will be working in Bangor. *Another* reason for Cathy to get back more often.

I tested my body with a long run on both Saturday and Sunday, after no weekday runs. On Sunday, my legs lost power on the last hill, where I broke into a purging sweat. Somehow I kept going, recovered, and ended strong. The yard got mowed, a baby was born, the emergency room quieted, and pestering calls from the answering service all were eventually laid to rest. We had a wonderful telephone call from the Drews in San Francisco, talking as in the old times when we shared a corner on Golden Gate Park. They are doing well. There is still a strong need to talk about Patrick's death: explanations, what-ifs, what-nows. The autopsy is not back yet; it will likely confirm the absence of major congenital anomalies or chromosomal defects. And then the doctors will say "it was a cord accident," as if they knew, as if they could picture the sequence of events, as if that crumb of inflated certainty would save anybody from their sorrows. I told Kevin and Kay of the feelings I had experienced on Saturday as I rode by the First Church on my bicycle. A wedding was letting out, and young, smiling, smartly dressed people thronged the boardwalk. How long it has been since I attended a wedding! How necessary are these concelebratory events to balance the laying low of funerals, the divorce proceedings, the disturbed family reunions. What one really needs is friendship, and the affirmation that life is full and good. Moments, fleeting moments, when love has penetrated us bone-deep.

I have been much too preoccupied with "things" of late—like the essay on connected farms, and a letter to the editor of *Family Medicine,* the official journal of the Society of Teachers of Family Medicine. Two recent articles have set me thinking: one entitled "Toward a Good Death," the other "Saying Good-bye: Termination of the Doctor-Patient Relationship." They are inextricably related, at least in the way I think of preparing for death. Other "things": a busy ten days of hospital work in the middle of the month during Tim's absence, which left me spent and demoralized; arranging the Iowa trip to visit my mom and dispose of her apartment; finalizing the remodeling plans for our house and borrowing the necessary funds. They came from my mom's estate, with an interest rate comparable to a five-year CD. I nevertheless feel like a vulture. This has been a bad month for depression, reaching a particular low this past week. I have no reserve, no defense against the insults and failings and demands of my practice.

Today I despaired over our pitiful cash-flow problem (Medicaid, which under-writes a third of our practice, is three months behind on its payments); today's St. Jude Conference was scheduled but never materialized. On this, one of my afternoons off, I fled home and collapsed on the sofa for over an hour, listening to a Palestrina Mass under the shroud of a woolen blanket. Now I must prepare for a family meeting with a woman dying of a brain tumor. She lies mute and motionless in the care of her daughters. We'll see what that does to my mood ring. I am not hopeful.

Autumn

※

A GOOD DEATH
IS HARD TO FIND

The telephone rang as I brushed my teeth, slipped into an overcoat, and sprang down the stairs for choir practice. It was the hospital. "Sorry," I snapped, "not on call."

"But doctor, I thought you'd like to know that Mrs. Johnson in Room 203 just expired." Alice Johnson was a hospice patient, her death sudden but not unexpected, and I politely thanked the nurse for her call. But before I could hang up, she continued. "Mrs. Pauling in Room 201 also passed away. Both exactly at 6:55 P.M.; we were with them both when they died!"

I was startled, too, by the coincidence: two of my patients, occupying the whole of the newly inaugurated Hospice Wing, ended their lives simultaneously. I flipped a familiar mental switch, one that cancels plans and shifts expectations, and acquiesced to the more urgent need. "Tell the families that I'll be over," I said, and headed for the hospital, ruminating on the Divine Hand that leads us into the heart of medicine.

Alice lay twisted in bed precisely where her husband and the nurse had hoisted her. As Hugh would tell it, she had felt gaseous and sick and motioned for the commode. Once seated, she turned ashen, clutched her throat, and gasped a final breath. No time for nitroglycerin; Hugh hollered for more nurses, more doctors, *anybody,* as his wife fell unconscious to the bed. I found him crouched beside her, stunned, and extended my hand and a few fumbled condolences. The sisters had gathered, too, and I hugged them and offered my sympathies. It was a blessing, we agreed, for her to have passed so quickly from this earthly pain. Hugh accepted my handshake but immediately launched into his familiar tirade.

"Doc, I'm not mad at you, it's just what this country has come to, when you can't do anything for a person's pain or even find out what's causing it. I spent three hundred bucks on a specialist in Saylorville—paid out of Medicare's pocket—to learn I would have to live with my dizziness, when he knew all along that there was nothing he could do, because all the other people from town who went to him were told the same thing. We're right here in the middle of the hospital, and you can't get a doctor to help when you need him, not that it would have done any good, but if we would have been at home at least I could have called the doctor to come, not that it would have done any good . . ."

Hugh's voice trailed off in an effort to swallow his anger, to avoid offending me further, and to cloak the bitter, lonely core of the man he had become or perhaps always was. His only bridge to the world had been Alice, and now that bridge blazed like a funeral pyre. Her death would further strand him in his bitterness.

We had tried to reach Hugh through two agonizing family meetings, countless hospice visits at home, and tedious discussions at the doctor's office. His shield was anger: the world had let him down. Alice had somehow made her peace. She locked herself away, kept her opinions and feelings and longings inside. The accelerating, inexplicable pain of these final weeks isolated her even more, and it distracted us, inviting ever-escalating doses of morphine.

In the adjoining room, the three children had kept vigil all day. Their mother trembled with fever spikes and focal seizures. They noticed, within Vanessa Pauling's cherubic face flushed from steroids, how her eyes darted, pupils widened, and arms frantically struggled to lift herself before that last bolus of meperidine. Vanessa relaxed, then gave up her ghost with a heavy, peaceful sigh. The children brought up the covers snugly, as they had done so many times before, even during the final feverish hours.

Katie, the eldest daughter, had been right in what she said about her mom in the hallway just this morning: "It's good for her to be here, to die here. She deserves it, this fancy room, all the added attention."

I thanked her for the compliments about our Hospice Wing and expressed my own gratitude for the hospital's gift to the community. But as I listened, she was thanking *me* for something, something she also found in the nursing care: our simple expressions of love. I hugged them all (save Gene, the barrel-chested, beer-bellied son) and felt an overwhelming surge of affection and admiration for this ordinary hard-working back-county family. They had struggled for months with their mother's brain tumor, shuttled her off to doctors' appointments and radiation treatments, juggled in the kids' summer activities and the start of school, somehow maintained an antique business, and dealt bravely with their own complex feelings about a "providing" mother who had difficulty baring her emotions or expressing love openly in a caress or hug.

Through it all, Vanessa was kept in the middle of the domestic flow of traffic, snoring in her Lazy-Boy next to the wood stove in the parlor. She was always the first to be hailed or hollered a "goodbye" as her family passed through the turnstile of a front door. Katie had requested the Hospice Wing only for these last eight days, as her mother's life began to flicker.

It was against this backdrop—the disturbing impact of contrasting deaths—that I came upon a curious title in the family practice literature: "Toward a Good Death: An Interpretive Investigation of Family Practice Residents' Practices with Dying Patients."* The authors had undertaken a study of residents' emotional responses to the impending death of their patients. It both delighted and disturbed me, fanning forgotten memories of my residency training, rekindling my profound sense of inadequacy to cope with the spectre of an impending death. During one week, while I was the senior resident on the inpatient service, three of my patients died. I felt abandoned by my attending physician, incompetent to care for the seriously ill, and suddenly embarrassed by the collapse of my self-confidence. The study accurately reflects, I believe, the terrible anxiety residents feel as their patients cross the forbidding divide between life and death.

On another occasion, I was chastised for not going to a patient's home to pronounce him dead. *That,* it was explained to me, is what family doctors do. Sometimes I go now, not compelled by law or even by a sense of obligation, but for the sacramental opportunities that abound there. No one had pointed these out to me; no one had remarked on the chasuble and stole that the doctor often wears to the deathbed.

The residents interviewed in Santa Rosa could recount only two examples of "good death" from among their experiences with thirty-one dying patients. The odds were stacked against them. In residency, and often there for the first time, physicians come to know death intimately, tragically, responsibly. The ones who die are vaguely familiar—is it our father, another patient, ourselves?—but the trappings are not—the strange diseases, the rigid expectations, the sense of time marching inexorably on. I was not surprised by what one resident said about a patient: "No one could deal with the situation, and [everyone] avoided his room." Or about the families: "It can be so painful that it can drive you to the point of feeling you must forget them, like you can't ever see them again, like you can't talk to them again." Or about themselves: "Death is a sign of my incompetence, the ultimate failure. I've been trained to go ahead and prevent death." But

---

* R. Dozor, R. Addison, *Journal of Family Medicine* 24 (1992): 538–43.

I was shocked to learn that "no one in the hospital talked about the nonbiomedical aspects of dealing with dying patients." Where *were* the attending physicians if not at the patient's bedside, or comforting the family, or supporting the residents during their tribulation?

Toward a good death. The phrase stuck in my throat as I tried to make sense of that evocative evening on the Hospice Wing, a double curtain call for those oddly contrasted lives. I am not sure what constitutes a good death. The authors did not define it. And I lack the convictions of my fundamentalist friends, who would cast the Grim Reaper in a cameo role and swing the spotlight toward an eternal reward. Growing up in Iowa, I learned that people died of natural causes, and natural was unquestionably good, even when my father died of a heart attack at the age of forty-nine. Coronaries ran in the family, like his cigarette smoking and his midriff bulge and his sedentary ways.

Once I entered the university hospitals, I saw life's unraveling with the cold, unblinking, cynical eyes of a physician. People died of complications, and complications were, well, complicated. My appreciation changed not so much because "the times" did, nor because I moved from the loping pace of the Midwest to a faster, more sophisticated East, nor because nostalgia sweetened my childhood memories. My *community* changed, from a rural farming population to a towering, technological, medical bureaucracy.

My community has changed once more, back to a small working-class New England village. Once again, many of my patients are dying naturally. Some have died at home, surrounded by their families, suffering no undue pain or worry, accepting their inevitable fate and bringing closure to their lives. But other recent deaths have left haunting, irreconcilable memories for their survivors: the stillborn son of our close friends, the shotgun suicide of a disturbed young man, the schoolmarm who withered away in her melancholia, and the victim of facial cancer who died in the saddle, so to speak, still leading the cavalry charge of chemotherapy. God bless Hank—one of our favorite patients—who would not give up until that last teary embrace, when his wife squeezed her blessings, and he turned his back on the pain and ignominy of his disfiguring disease.

And what can we say of Alice Johnson? What goodness can be found in her implacable suffering, in her undignified death on the commode, or in the rantings of her husband, consumed by anger? She reminded me of the old woman in Sherwood Anderson's "Death in the Woods," who froze to death in the deserted clearing, half clad and far from home, surrounded only by the primitive, mournful wailing of her dogs. Or Vanessa Pauling, who died in peace except for that one haunting moment when her eyes flashed the words of Kurtz, Joseph Conrad's antagonist in *Heart of Darkness:* "the horror, the horror." How would

I explain that unmistakable look to the family? Would I lie, and say with utter certainty that it was only the last physiological rush of adrenalin before the machinery seized?

I have no assurance that any of my patients died "a good death." The notion itself probably reveals more about our own needs and mental categories than those of our patients. Is it the longing for an easy death in an Age of Convenience? I try, instead, to withhold judgment and content myself in meeting my patients' needs. It is a role that feels clumsy and unheroic, like Tolstoy's Gerasim in the service of Ivan Ilych who sat with his dying master despite the unsightliness of his decay, and comforted him by resting withered legs upon his own broad shoulders. I know that I cannot create a good death where there has been "no real pleasure in life," as Grandmother learned in Flannery O'Connor's short story about the Misfit. He slew her family one by one despite Grandmother's appeal to his "goodness at heart." The goodness of death is always a matter for the patient to decide.

The least I can do for my dying patients becomes the most: choose not to abandon them, acknowledge their suffering, guide them at the journey's end. Ours is a supportive role. We are Sherpa guides whose strong backs and ready knowledge of alpine conditions help prepare the climber for his final ascent. This method, this mercy, must be learned and taught by example. We discover it in our painful attendance at the deathbed; in the awkward goodbyes we exchange when relationships rupture; in the mutual support we provide each other—doctors and caregivers and families alike—in the hope of surviving our losses, dying within community, and creating communities, like hospice, in which to die.

Good deaths are often tangled in complications, and bad deaths come as naturally (that is, as inevitably) as the change of seasons. Why not abandon our categories altogether, suspend judgment, break off our detached and empathic gaze? We would do well to check our stethoscopes at the doors of the dying and prepare to stay with them awhile, listening. We might be surprised by what we hear *inside us*. Is it our own anxiety, or sorrow, or perhaps a thin yet invigorated call to service, the voice that was calling us from the start?

Few patients will die "like they're being rocked to sleep in their mother's arms," contrary to the claims of a Santa Rosa physician.* And for these patients, our presence makes little difference. The challenge, the reward, the *mystery* lies more with people like Hank and Alice, who will cling to us, test us, and leave us with their frayed ends and unfulfilled desires. Perhaps it was for them, too, that Dylan Thomas penned these lines:

* R. Dozer, R. Addison, "Toward a Good Death: An Interpretive Investigation of Family Practice Residents' Practices with Dying Patients," *Journal of Family Medicine* 24 (1992): 539.

And you, my father, there on the sad height,
Curse, bless, me now with your fierce tears, I pray.
Do not go gentle into that good night.
Rage, rage against the dying of the light.*

* "Do Not Go Gentle into That Good Night," in *Collected Poems* (New York: New Directions, 1971).

OCTOBER

On the way to the family meeting yesterday, Jean Goldfine, the hospice social worker, turned to me and asked, "What's another name for nothing left to lose?" The answer (etched in my brain during the sixties) comes from the lyrics to Janice Joplin's "Me and Bobby McGee." Freedom. It was also the name of the village we had just entered, and our final destination. Jean and I had shared a perfectly serene twenty-five-minute drive together amid the rolling hills, gunbarrel-gray skies, placid lakes, and burning maples along the road to Freedom. It evoked a melancholy mood, a sense of isolation and abandonment, that I remember from childhood.

After the harvest, the skies over western Iowa can droop for months on end. Those who inhabit the land are pinned to it, to the fields and meadows picked clean to the bone. During the march of seasons—spring to fall—my classmates worked the land almost every evening and weekend. After my father's death, Mom went back to nursing. She became supervisor of the three-to-eleven shift at Pocahontas Community Hospital. My sister, two years older than I, soon left for college, and my younger brother became more my responsibility than my companion. So it was for me a time of brooding, a time to be gotten through, before the liberating day when I would leave for college. After my father's death, I noticed the look of abandonment and melancholia persist in my mother's eyes, that look of bleak midwinter, which slowly spread over the future of our family.

It was thirty-four degrees outside when I returned from the short run this morning. The frost would have been on the pumpkin had we not picked it last week. On the way to the office, the sky melted from periwinkle blue to salmon pink to pepper gray behind tissues of cloud that marched on the distant horizon. Again the mood returned, so forlorn and familiar. I mentioned it at Thursday morning group with Tim and Mary Beth.

Autumn's splash of color, washed in the crisp, dazzling sunshine of autumn, heralds the approach of winter. Today the sense of loss overwhelms me. I am frozen by fall's festinating gait*, which reinforces my own unwillingness, unreadiness, to move beyond the moment. These are the doldrums, from the first of October to mid November, when the countryside is cast in an Andrew Wyeth palette of charcoal gray and rusted brown, before the Currier & Ives snows of December. It brings me back to the deprivation and loneliness and loss I felt as a child on the Iowa plains.

Yesterday morning at 10:00 A.M., Lindsay called me at the office to say she had noticed dark blood when she wiped. I had all but forgotten about our discussion two weeks ago, when she had felt a trickle run down her legs. It was probably urine, I had wanted to believe. Now, her obstetrician was gone from the office but not yet home. He could not be reached at the hospital, where his wife had asked Lindsay to try; nor did his answering service provide any useful leads. I made the decision to schedule a fetal ultrasound examination tomorrow at the hospital, and met Lindsay there at noon.

The ultrasonographer was very kind. After we saw the large (ten-week-size) empty uterus, and the incongruously small echogenic flecks of a gestational sac, she suggested the transvaginal probe. It magnified the bad news: the sac was empty, the embryo dead. As Lindsay and I hugged in the parking lot and spoke at home last night before her meeting, we both realized more clearly what mixed and muted emotion the loss had created. It was not only the pregnancy but our expectations for it that had never gotten off the ground. We made plans, but hedged them in the possibility of Down's syndrome or birth defects, spoke only of inconvenience and adjustments to our lifestyle. We had not committed to the pregnancy; we were holding back. Did it fail because of this, I wondered; or because, coincidentally, Lindsay had run out of prenatal vitamins a few days before? "Next time get me a bottle of a hundred," she insisted.

---

* A gait characteristic of Parkinson's disease, where patients, once moving, accelerate their speed in small, shuffling steps and cannot easily stop.

So, then, she is willing to try again.

We had lost only ten weeks of time, and a nonviable pregnancy. Already I have forgotten about the empty sac inside her, awaiting its eviction. I expect that Lindsay will have a heavy flow in a day or so, but some miscarriages are more complicated than that: they can bleed heavily, get infected. Perhaps this impending ordeal will force our emotional hand and allow us to grieve the positive two-thirds of our ambivalence. Lindsay is looking forward to a large glass of wine and a cup of coffee tonight. I am looking down the road. The postponement will allow me to finish the journal and attend the Society of Teachers of Family Medicine Conference in San Diego this spring. We will be spending the afternoon together, comparing Victorian porches in order to model our own addition, and looking for a stained glass window to install in the new downstairs bathroom. I hope, if nothing else, that the miscarriage draws us closer, that our next pregnancy grows from a healthier bed.

News about town. Yesterday, as I went to get lunch for Lindsay and myself at Dexter's Dogs ("Over 17,000 Sold," boasts their sign), I noticed in the parking lot five large trucks belonging to the Atlantic Location Equipment Company. This would be an unusual sighting in Belfast, except that there have been rumblings, rumors, and local newspaper confirmation that Glenn Close is in town to shoot a Hallmark Classic sequel to *Sarah, Plain and Tall*. Two weeks ago, the Belfast Motor Inn called our office to see if we would back up the film crew as their "family doctor." How could we decline, especially since nothing will come of it, and hasn't so far.

Last evening we went over to the hospital to visit Marc and Cheryl and their new son. This is the third in an all-male cast, a healthy eight-and-a-half-pound squealer. Clare wanted to hold the baby desperately, which we permitted despite the warning label on the bassinet. They offered their condolences for our pregnancy loss, which still feels tiny and distant and unreal. Belfast has given the Stewarts precious little stability, or acceptance in the community, or professional gratification. But it *has* given them a family that will grow strong and healthy into maturity. I have less optimism for the congregation they leave behind. Marc still has not received a solid job offer, but there is yet time.

Yesterday, after devouring a sweet Italian sausage and a hot dog with spicy mustard and hot pepper relish at Dexter's, Lindsay and I went on a home-remodeling spree. Our mission was to find the stained glass windows for the new porch and bathroom, and to finalize our remodeling plans. We settled on an "airy" design, with slender, molded columns, no railing, wide steps: the classic New England porch fronting a kitchen-ell. Our carpenter accepted the decision contingent upon his finding turned wooden columns.

How marvelous it is to invest money in durable goods—"retail therapy," as a student of mine once called it—rather than the intangible changes that education or psychotherapy or consultation have to offer. Our lives need an uplifting, a "cordial for the drooping spirit," to borrow a favorite expression of Gayle Stephens. We need to work on the foundation of our marriage, our lives, before adding a sibling for Clare. Lindsay's pregnancy came too quickly for us (after one try); now we have the chance to retreat, regroup, recommit ourselves to the proposition.

Gayle's letter arrived yesterday in response to the essay I sent him about connected farms. It was wonderfully personal, yet erudite and intellectual, wide-ranging and constructively critical. Our exchange of letters has been the greatest influence on my pursuit of writing. We have chosen different modes of expression—he is an essayist and I more the storyteller—though the mediums overlap and conflate. He talked of the ethos of reform and the current fervor in farming. Toward the end of his letter he commented, "My summer here [in Dillon, Colorado] has been mostly desultory, although I have worked at writing almost every day. I enjoy the mountains, but I feel disengaged from real life. I have no duties, and I miss my connections to patients."

It is sad to reach retirement in good health but lacking a continued sense of productivity or fulfillment. Gayle is still busy with writing workshops, orations to family practice colloquia, writing and editing for the *Journal of the American Board of Family Practice,* and teaching students of optometry. But for most of my elderly colleagues, retirement is a painful adjustment; they tarry too long at their professional duties, puttering to the point where their skills appear to be inconsistent, outmoded, and sloppy. I know little of these things, but am privy to the whispers, frowns, and behind-the-back remarks of my self-satisfied colleagues, those of us who are in-the-know and thoroughly up-to-date. We are too fiercely independent in our work to ask another for help, or to offer it unsolicited. But in time our ears too will burn. And our privileges will be politely cropped. Though Gayle is nowhere near the edge, he—like the rest of us—must watch his step. It is easy to end up on the wrong side of an accusing finger, but better this than to be among those who project it from their own locus of insecurity and forget that "there but for the grace of God go I."

Weekend in review. The last three days have been free of work and filled with activity. It was a family weekend, with projects like gardening, the Church Street Fair, and leaf gathering excursions under clear, blustery autumn skies. I went on the long run Saturday, the short run on Sunday. After Mass yesterday I chatted with Mary Schmidt, a frequent "reader" at the 10:45 Mass, who infuses gospel readings with *passion*. She will be hosting a small faith-sharing group called RENEW. The program, she tells me, offers a structured, lay-directed, multi-pronged approach for parish renewal. I don't know what to make of it, but signed up anyway.

I have not *remained* Catholic because I was born to it. Nor have I stayed for the logic or beauty or purity of its teachings. I have remained Catholic because of my Catholic friends, those who have kept the fires of morality and sacramentality burning in their lives. I need my Catholic neighbors, need their support, need accounts of their struggles to remain faithful in spite of all the obstacles and excuses we strew in our paths. Perhaps RENEW will do that for me. The first meeting is in eight days.

Yesterday Lindsay completed the miscarriage. By evening, the pain had vanished and the bleeding slowed. It is done. I think we both secretly, hesitantly, welcomed this false start; it brought us square around to the risks of pregnancy, the change it portends for our lives, the commitment it will exact, the sacrifice it will require. It is not like the new addition on the kitchen-ell. We each had done too little preparation; we relied upon the first signs of pregnancy to pick up the slack. But before we petition God for a second chance, we will put our marital house in order.

I drove to Lincolnville on Friday to visit a hospice couple. Twenty-two years ago they built their home here, on a hill overlooking their land, with everything planned for a low-maintenance retirement: shingled siding, stained wood instead of painted; oil heat instead of firewood, a reliable septic, a deep well. This was my first visit to their home; likely, it will be my last. They leave for Vermont within the week to make a winter home under the protective wing of their daughter. Dot has metastatic lung cancer. And she is failing, despite her tolerance for pain, her trust in miracles, and the personal stamina of a woman half her seventy-eight years. With each office visit I document more weight loss, more erosion in the voice, more coughing and panting.

Dot had her children late in life. When they were still young, Edwin suffered a back injury for which he was awarded full disability. Dot supported the family as a bookkeeper, but that did not slow her productivity on the domestic front. Her handicraft fills every room of the house: curtains, rugs, blankets, chair coverings. Edwin's domain lies outside the four walls. Here he has planted, cultivated, pruned, and harvested to his heart's content: fruit trees, flowering shrubs, a large vegetable garden.

These parental attributes—Dot's strong will and abundant energy, Edwin's cultivated taste for gardening—were passed directly to their daughter, Connie. She is a hard-working optometrist who runs, along with her husband, a large greenhouse in Vermont. She has been indefatigable and dogged in her pursuit of treatments that might slow the spread of her mother's cancer. Clamped to the doctors' cuff, she cannot be shaken free once she is convinced that a treatment option might benefit her mother. At the time, I wondered if Dot approved of the lung surgery, the postoperative radiation, the herbal remedies, the Lourdes water. Or did she simply relent? But now, high on this Lincolnville hilltop, I can see that Connie is her mother's daughter, acting on her behalf. It will be a hard transition to pass from The War Against Cancer to the tenderness she deserves in the last moment's of life. The garden is dying before the coming frost. Edwin sees it, and Connie has inherited his sensitivities. She will be a strong ally and friend for us all during these final months.

It is easy for doctors to forget that the frail, stooped, hobbling patients in a hospital hallway once had important careers, raised robust families, supported the arts, enriched their congregations and communities, and grappled vigorously and successfully with the great problems of their day. In family meetings and home visits, or on a leisurely stroll through the past medical history, I catch a glimpse of this hidden past. I warm to the dignity of their lives, now mocked by age and disease and our unflattering hospital regimens. Dot and Edwin, still at home and surrounded by all that they created and loved, exude that dignity and deserve my respect and affection.

I will not forget that last gentle hug, and Dorothy's repetitive phrase, "It's good, it's good, it's good." Her life, yes, and our friendship, and even this opportunity to wrap it up in a manner that blesses all who have been lucky enough to cross their threshold.

Two days ago, as Lindsay and I caught a fast lunch at Dexter's Dogs, Channel Five News focused me in their Live Eye. Jeffrey Hope, the newsman who interviewed me, had long been a fan of Dexter's, ate here every chance he could. Now he was producing a "color piece" on the mother of all dogs. He relished the image of a doctor in bow tie and stethoscope chomping down on this little finger of animal fat. But I am not good at impromptu one-liners. My only credible reply came in response to Jeff's question about "where do you put the hot dog among your favorite meals?" Since my mouth was full, I merely gestured toward my stomach. But I could have spoken of the hot dog as "part of this complete meal," like the TV commercials that push sugar-coated cereals. I could have played with the Latin meaning of *dexter* by suggesting some slogans: "Dexter's, the *right* dog for you," or "Never any *left*-overs at Dexter's," or "They do you *right* at Dexter's." This is good publicity for Dexter, and it will keep me glued to the Channel Five News over the next several weeks until my seven-second spot is aired (if it is aired at all).

It has been a week in turmoil. Normally the chaos is capped by our evenings together, but this week Lindsay had a hospice board meeting on Monday, a hospice volunteer training on Wednesday, a bereavement support group on Thursday, and I will moonlight tonight at the emergency room to pay our property taxes. Last night the tension erupted in an argument over discipline. Before supper, Clare was swinging my jumbo brewing spoon perilously close to my head; I warned her that if it hit me she would lose it. It did; she did. There was silence for the next ten seconds; Clare stood beside me at the table, stunned and teary-eyed. Lindsay finally spoke up, "Aren't you going to say anything?" I balked. Clare had tested me, knew the rules, and now faced the consequence. But I knew Lindsay was right, too. No need to shame her, to reject her with my silence. I should reach out, try to understand, offer her now what she *really* wanted then.

I cannot say why, in that split second, I came down on the side of authority instead of mercy. I was dead tired; or needed just a half hour more of adult conversation and companionship; or perhaps felt compelled to curb Clare's misbehavior over the last four weeks by a decisive action now. Why can't parenting wait until you are fully prepared? Like our peers, Lindsay and I want nothing more out of the role than to avoid our parents' mistakes. Last night we could not talk to one another, let alone decide together what approach might be best for Clare. Tim and Cris, my partner and his wife, have a parenting pact to clean up individually whatever mess he or she steps into. It is the classic model of doctoring. The captain of the ship must pull *himself* from the drink.

We don't run the tightest ship in the shipping industry. Sticking together has been the most formidable, least expected obstacle in our parental path. We work better alone, but parenting in the modern age demands teamwork.

At the Thursday Meeting yesterday, Tim came in with his head a-hanging. He has been depressed since he returned from vacation and assumed the hospital helm. He has not enjoyed the work, not looked forward to his patients, not offered them more than a prescription and a warm body to share the exam room. No energy. No satisfaction. Tim has been here before, though rarely this deep. We acknowledge that there are differences between our styles and our commitment to doctoring. He is more restless than I, more poised near the exit of his career, it seems to me. But today I realize how much exhaustion and job stress contribute to the mood, to that common feeling of being used and violated, for little gain and no glory.

Mary Beth asked me if Tim's lament threatened me. It does not, or not nearly as much as it might have five years ago. I am ready to release Tim from the partnership, this practice, our utopian vision, if I knew that it would save our friendship and improve his chances for survival. These careers too shall pass: this sturdy building, our devoted patients, the able crew here assembled, and our fine conception of family practice. That it sprang into being, that it was once, is more the miracle for me than its perpetuation. It is a fine conception, but only an envelope to hold the friendships we have forged.

I am sympathetic to Tim's depression and have looked at it more honestly in myself since I began writing. At the office I have no time to brood, no right to expose my weariness, my exasperation, my anger, my emptiness. Patients expect the whole nine yards from their doctor, and the doctor, in turn, wants to give them their money's worth. So I bear the tension headache, the strapped feeling in my chest, the stifled yawns. I haul them all home at the end of the working day. I steep in them as I slump at the supper table or offer blank stares to the television.

But I can also bring my feelings here, to this journal, conjure them up on the black screen and mull them over and make them into something they are not: fixed and substantive. They are only mood and feeling, free-falling in my unconscious like Northern Lights. They are my interior, as real as the introspection you find in a Vermeer painting, as genuine a part of my "true self" as the exterior I project. They are a private and untouchable self, the hermitage to which I hastily retreat.

Though I started out in reasonably good humor yesterday, my work was especially trying. In the morning I saw three patients who returned with back pain. Only one had improved. The hardest part is waiting for improvement and being willing to accept even the faintest signs of progress, and resisting the temptation to blame every delay on secondary gain.

Pain is a wholly subjective matter, but muscle spasm is not. I took the limbs through their range of motion, palpated for trigger points, tracked blood pressure and pulse, studied gait and body movement. I steered to the objective. But it is not so tidy. How has this pain changed the patient's life; how is unemployment pinching his monthly budget? How is he regarded by his fellow employees, his spouse, the nurses and doctors and therapists who treat him? How has he come to regard himself? Workman's compensation is big business in the State of Maine, as it is everywhere. I'd just as soon wash my hands of it, the Darvocets and claim forms and mistrust exchanged between adversaries in this often contentious relationship. But for every malingerer and addict, there is a person in legitimate need and real pain. Many have been our patients all along. So I offer them the benefit of the doubt, and adhere as rigorously as I can to rules and limits and therapeutic endpoints.

There was also a string of long faces yesterday, those who have been herded into psychotherapy, others who are still being nudged. Their stories are legion, of incest and battering and abandonment. Their diseases carry convenient labels, like reactive depression, obsessive-compulsive disorder, agoraphobia, inadequate personality, major depression. Nobody is fooled. We will save a life or two, ratchet down the level of their anxiety, prop up a few rickety lives. But the suffering is so embedded in the broken homes, destitution, self-defeat, and pervasive gloom of their lives that the usual yardsticks for success are wholly inadequate. Doctors and therapists who work with these people must reach their own conclusions about the purpose and value of their labors. I have learned to settle for whatever crumbs of improvement I find along the way. Often I simply stand by the patient and hope that he or she will agree to stand by me. Standing in the face of misery requires a supportive community, and the pivotal part of that for me is Mary Beth. Her being here reminds me that we all must share the burden, pass around the pain and neediness of our patients and the doubts and frustrations that gather in our own hearts.

A word about this Mary Beth. She is a solid lady, and by this I mean neither stocky nor dainty, but someone who begs a reaction, engages your mind, allows you to depend upon her dependability. She can be loud and volcanic, arms erupting off the flat of her lap, her hair curled in a Sicilian rendition of Little Orphan Annie. Or she can steep in her thoughts, and project a sense of calm and reticence and satisfaction with the moment. That is a side of her that appeals to me most, connected as it is to her maternal side, and to her giving.

Mary Beth also hails from the Midwest, from the suburban Detroit and Catholic enclave that is her extended family. And she is devout, which is something easy to love about her. She is passionate about the faith she inherited from her father. His approach to religion was childlike and uncomplicated. Every night after supper he would disappear for fifteen minutes to pray the rosary. Someone would ask, "Where's Papa?" But they all knew where to look, and left him alone. Though her father spent long days at his grocery store, she was always absolutely convinced that "he loved me no matter what, just like the love of God." After a decade of knowing Mary Beth, I am beginning to understand her "thing about edges." People, she contends, need edges and definitions to navigate safely in the world. The Catholic Church fills this need for her. It covers the whole canvas; it portrays a world filled with good and evil, heroism and the dark side, salvation and grace and forgiveness. It simply makes sense to her, and has been affirmed through prayer. She loves the Church, and she loves her friends, and loyalty binds her to both.

For Mary Beth, Catholicism provided the logical path to social work. Any good Catholic girl of her generation was expected to become a teacher (which is what her two older sisters became), a nurse (the chosen profession of my own mother and sister), or a social worker.

She inherited an attraction to "fixer-upper" men from her mother. And her husband, James MacKenzie Thomas, squarely falls into this category. She says of him, "He was very unlike all the other charming guys I dated. My father was incompetent around mechanical things. But along comes Mac, the wonder man. He can fix anything, understand anything that is electrical or mechanical or computer-oriented. I mean, it was like 'this guy's smart.' That was appealing to me. My mother would have loved Mac. She married my dad, who is this sweet, ineffectual nincompoop, and her whole life was 'Oh my God, if only he could be like Uncle Henry and fix a lawn mower.'"

I appreciate something else that Mary Beth got from her mother. She says, "I think my mother made life a problem, and that was a legacy she left me. Well, I'm not going to make life a problem. Clear and simple." And she hasn't. She approaches her clients the way she engages life, with edges and the generosity of her full attention. A friend once commented about her work, "Oh, you help give birth to people's psyches." She replied, "Maybe your therapist does that, but I certainly don't. I think the greatest thing I bring to people is who I am. I try to be honest and real and present. I don't think there's any magic to it. But that's the gift my mother gave me. She had this thing about being direct. It was driven into us. People will either like you or not like you. That gets me into trouble sometimes as a therapist, but I think it's a good thing, and it works. To be a good therapist you need edges, and can't be afraid." This is the kind of commentary you might expect from the physician-poet William Carlos Williams.

Mary Beth, like Lindsay and Tim, is a humble person, which is something you can learn from helping people. "A lot of people wouldn't see me that way," she remarks. "They might call me arrogant, or allow themselves to be intimidated. But with people sharing their stories, you can't help but be humbled or you'd be a fool if you listened at all."

The air this Sunday morning is balmy, thick, and super-saturated. It is already fifty-four degrees at 6:00 A.M., and I am late to the computer. I have rushed through the cat and coffee chores and now position myself at my desk, as William Bird's *Mass for Five Voices* rises through the Kyrie and a cat scampers after loose beads down the hallway's wooden floor.

Yesterday afternoon I collapsed into a deep and disorienting sleep. I had sacrificed my night before in the ER, moonlighting. I needed the money; they needed a warm body. The night saw a steady drizzle of the worried well. Some of their problems were urgent and interesting: a fresh myocardial infarction, a Baker's cyst, a Bell's palsy, a syncopal episode. Most were not, and the whole experience bolstered my resolve to remain a family doctor, not a mercenary. In the ER, the money is good and hours snap off clean. But you cannot connect with your patients. There is time only for addressing demands, containing risk (of malpractice), and tying together a few frayed ends with a diagnosis.

A nap today left me hazy-headed and vaguely unhappy, and I putzed about aimlessly until the telephone rang. It was my best buddy from college, Bill De-Mars; his voice was balm for the aching heart. He called in remembrance of what I had forgotten: the fourth anniversary of Clare's baptism at St. Francis Church.

Bill and his wife, Therese, are her Godparents; we delayed the baptism until they could visit us from South Bend.* In return, I sponsored their first child, Daniel.

We, in our Godparent exchange, have honored a long friendship and a parallel journey. It was I who clung to the Church during college, drawing Bill in through the back door of music ministry (we played in the same folk group at Mass). But he chose other expressions for his faith. Bill joined the Catholic Worker House after graduation, studied theology at Loras College in Dubuque, taught religion at his old high school in Bismarck, North Dakota, contemplated a religious vocation but married with all the Catholic trimmings, and undertook graduate study at the most celebrated American Catholic university, Notre Dame.

I have always been a one-foot-in-the-door Catholic. My only parochial school experience was at a Jesuit university, Creighton. At twenty-three I married inside the church, but it lasted barely five years. After college I began skipping Mass without pangs of conscience (even on Holy Days of Obligation). I would mumble my way through the problematic parts of the Nicene Creed and avoid parish picnics and K. of C. (Knights of Columbus) recruitment suppers like the plague. Then I married Lindsay outside the Church.

Last night, for our Saturday home evening, we watched "The Song of Bernadette" on video, the story of Bernadette Soubirous and her apparitions of the Blessed Virgin at Lourdes. We let Clare play with the souvenir bottles—plastic Holy Water–filled vials in the shape of Mary—that we had fetched from there four years ago for a dying friend. Perhaps a seed was planted, because after her bath the next morning she accompanied me to Mass. Whatever her reasons, nothing could have made her father more proud as she walked up the aisle, her little hand in mine, dressed in autumn hues and poised with piety and charm. Clare has come before, with Lindsay at Christmas time, but lasted all of twenty minutes before curiosity, restlessness, and sheer boredom got the best of her. Now she is older and has volunteered to come, and consents to the terms: no talking out loud; no escaping the pew. For her part, Clare warned that she'd not be singing any "songs about God." I fully expected to haul her home fifteen minutes into the service, but she went the distance, well beyond Communion to the final blessing.

I hadn't anticipated the importance of Clare's coming. I didn't realize my need for a faith to germinate in her young heart, and for me to be passing along my Catholic sentiments: a sense of ritual, of grace, of God's great mercy. While she *wishes* to come, while she is still impressionable and imitative, I want her to know about this Mass and allow her romp in its spiritual realms.

* Bill is now on the faculty of the American University in Cairo.

Clare had a wonderful weekend, as all of us did, with much less rancor, violent shouting, foot-stomping, and entrenchment. She enjoyed helping us in the garden, playing with the visiting children next door, entertaining our dessert guests last night, accepting the limits we are laying down. Something has settled in her psyche: the passing of a phase, or the easing of parental acrimony.

The next two weeks allow no slack for smoothing out family wrinkles. I am scheduled for a double shift of hospital duty, and during the second week Tim is away and I'm on call for all of family practice. Thank goodness that most of the plans for Lindsay's thirty-seventh birthday extravaganza (on the eve of Halloween) have been made.

It is the middle of the first week, and only two new hospital admissions. The first real crisis arose yesterday morning when I discovered that we were out of raw eggs for the cats' breakfast. At first Kitty and Dinky stared incredulously at their gleaming bowl, then they protested bitterly, whining loudly, stomping about, until a new carton of eggs came through the door.

Last night was the first RENEW meeting. It was pleasant and sociable and worth missing the vice-presidential debate for. In our discussion, I talked a little about my depression, and about a God who whispers from the floor boards. I feel that he speaks to me loudest when I am low, when depression drags me to my knees, pulls me firmly against the floor, places me within the tidal sound of my own breathing, far from my self-important plans and purposes.

I want to know, likewise, how my fellow Catholics face their God, how they pray and posture themselves, what personal devotions they maintain and what articles of faith they contest. Though faith is a personal matter, I want support in my efforts. If RENEW provides me with some adult faith-sharing and a sense of connection to my Catholic neighbors, I will be satisfied.

It is Saturday morning, after a busy week that kept me—almost every evening—apart from my wife and daughter. I have decided to attend Mrs. Johnson's funeral (10:00 A.M. in Belfast) and telephone my sympathies to Mrs. Spaulding's family (whose funeral is at 2:00 P.M., and twenty-five miles away). Top priority goes to Clare; Lindsay and I have already arranged for a babysitter to give us the evening out. I had also hoped for a long run with Sam Mitchell, whom I met on the Memorial Bridge last week, and who might help me expand a brochure on the "Old Houses of Belfast." But that is optional, depending upon how the day delivers.

Leona returned yesterday for a preoperative physical. After our conflicts during her last appointment, she saw the orthopedist and agreed to have a total knee replacement. She is scheduled for surgery in ten days. Leona and her daughter admit—sheepishly and with appreciation—that they would have let things slide without my prodding, the pain and the hobbling and the progressive immobility. But I rushed to interject, "You must decide for yourself. Though your surgeon is good, the new knee may not work or may give you complications. It's the chance you take, but the odds are in your favor, and I admire your spunk."

It is easier—after the anger, consternation, and jangled feelings fade—to put a clumsy interaction in context. Context does not exempt you from the pain, but it can give it meaning and thereby soften it. Leona may get her new knee and walk the better for it, but I must still live with the truth: my goading stemmed as much from my impatience and anger as it did from compassionate concern. If the operation goes well, the doctor is the hero, the patient is grateful, and the intervention will be judged appropriate. If it does not, we are stuck in the muck together.

Jesus warned that the poor will always be with us, and the same holds true for those who suffer. There is no future in peddling cures or fishing for gratitude. Some patients are bound to suffer; that is their lot. If, on top of their injury, we heap our annoyance, our bitterness, our condemnation, this becomes a penance for us as well. Pride can be found on both sides of the healer's coin. Good doctoring is not simply a matter of making the right diagnosis or pleasing the patient. We strive toward these; we try to aim our arrow true. But we know too well that both the patient and our own categories for understanding are moving targets. The drudgeries, exigencies, surprises of family practice allow our eyes to adjust, to focus in the dark and at a distance, where the broader questions lie: Have we helped our patients understand their suffering? Have we extended them our love, our respect, and an undivided moment of our time?

Telephone calls are the bane of family practice. We minister in a borderland between well-being and incapacity, where every illness begins with the familiar refrain, "Doc, it ain't nothing, but . . ." or "My wife nagged me to call" or "It's been going on for a month but I thought you'd like to know" or "My dad complained of the same thing before he stroked" or "There was just a spot of blood when I wiped." We never know quite how to take it, with what seriousness or urgency or perspective.

The ideal would be to see every patient personally. There is no substitute for absorbing the nonverbal cues, refreshing the bonds of intimacy and trust, and taking the first few steps beside the patient along the road to recovery. But today there is no time, nor tomorrow, nor the next day. My partner is on vacation for ten days; I must dispense the emergency slots with scrupulous discernment: There is only so much of me, so many hours in a day, and the rest must go to the ER, or wait.

Of course, even when you create time for your patients, they may politely decline. It is too expensive, they say; they can't catch a ride or leave work early; they don't want to bother the doctor; or (my personal favorite) they're too sick to come in. What do they *really* want: an appointment? an antibiotic? advice? or just a sympathetic ear?

We have a "trickle-down" policy in our office for routine telephone calls. They are taken by the receptionist, recorded, passed to the office nurse, and returned by her as soon as possible, chart in hand. If the nurse cannot satisfy the patient's concerns, or has more of her own, she gathers appropriate information and discusses the case with me. The protocol is not rigid, but it spares me most of the simple requests for medication refills, laboratory reports, or appointments.

Only six shopping days until Lindsay's birthday, or so I was reminded last night. The supper table has been little more than a feeding trough all week, with my late returns from the office and our early departures for RENEW, Pen Bay Singers, and Bereavement Support Group. The hardest part has been the relentlessness of the work. As if seeing patients were not enough, I must also sign all the charts of our physician assistant, return telephone messages for those who cannot be seen, take calls for our family practice group (six out of seven days this week, by some twisted turn of fate), and juggle Hospice and our hospital practice all the while. Fortunately, the latter has been slow. Save for a nursing home patient—a faceless, bedridden, incontinent soul, lying stroked in the ER—I would have attended all of last night's choir practice. Ah, well, the weekend approaches, and Tim is five days from home.

It was a good week for Lindsay. Two days ago, she had her ads approved by the owner of the kitchenware shop in Camden. Lindsay had been asked to come up with a few ideas, something to generate interest in a store now under new management. It's Lindsay's *forte,* her gift: arranging words like a floral bouquet, in an understated and refined and intriguing way. The surprise for Lindsay was being paid over twice what she had imagined. This week, too, she began "week two" of teaching French in the high school with a local surgeon, David Crofoot. The class is, to my reckoning, more of a French language interest club, but it pays $15.00 an hour and keeps Lindsay's hand in teaching and in French.

This week she nears the end of a bereavement support group she has been co-facilitating. It has been a disappointment for the facilitators, more of a social outing for the participants than good "grief work." But today more glamor: a Hospice workshop on the death of babies. She'll be carpooling with a friend of hers, the undertaker Marlo Bunker, who is young, lively, an accomplished flautist, and owner of two of the local funeral homes.

During Lindsay's meeting last night, I took Clare out for fine dining and entertainment. As has been our custom, we went to the hospital cafeteria, where the only appealing items on the menu were rice, beans, and a cookie. Then off to the physical therapy department where they keep the weight-lifting and conditioning equipment. Clare loves it. I slotted the steel pins into the lighter weights, and Clare was able to work most of the gismos. The evening ended at Jack's Corner Store, where she selected bubble gum, Tootsie Rolls, and Gummy Bears from the penny bins. Finally home to the ritual of teeth-brushing, pajama-wrestling, and bedtime stories. I wonder what memories the hospital will hold for her in ten years, or thirty? Will she remember the darkened rooms on the second floor where we tiptoe long after visiting hours have ended; or the ER, where she collects stickers while I speak in solemn tones to my patients behind the curtained bays; or the nursery, where wee ones squeal in their delicate and wrinkled skin; or the occupational therapy play room, which has become the reward for managing an "inside voice" and exercising patience while daddy is busy doctoring? Or will she remember what strikes me most dearly, the compliments and cries of "Gracious, how she's grown" that the nurses and patients lavish upon her, and that set off a blush and a face buried against my leg or a spontaneous gallop down the hall?

The long weekend is over, and tomorrow Tim returns from Costa Rica. I did not run once, or rest my eyes at the computer. All weekend the oppressive gray skies shed their tears, soaking the leaves so thoroughly that raking was impossible. The hospital and answering service rang just enough to keep me on the string, but in the aftermath, only one delivery, one hospital admission, and a handful of ER visits. Not an overly productive time. But the job is done, and I can return to my routines and my partnership and my patches of freedom. I recount the highlights: escorting my daughter to a local performance of C. S. Lewis's *The Lion, the Witch, and the Wardrobe,* working out a three-part arrangement to Bobby McFerrin's "23rd Psalm," and surviving a quarrel with my dear wife.

It began Friday night, when, as we walked out of a downtown restaurant, Lindsay suddenly complained that she had something in her left eye. Blinking and tearing did not help, nor splashing her eye with cold water, so I attempted an examination after we returned home. Flipping the upper lid with my daughter's paint brush handle, and crouching underneath a glaring bathroom light, I could see no dark foreign body; nor did I beneath the lower lid, which was easily retracted. "It just feels as if you have something in there," I reassured her, "but you probably scratched your cornea, and it'll clear by morning." This seemed the sensible approach, since a slit lamp examination in the ER would cost over a hundred bucks (applied to our deductible); my history and cursory exam provided a likely diagnosis, for which waiting would do no harm. I rummaged through our pill drawer until I found something for pain, squeezed antibiotic drops in her eye, and rolled off to sleep.

In the morning, the pain was no better. Since we were both up before Clare, I shooed Lindsay off to the ER for a proper evaluation. The doctor found only scuffing of the cornea—diffuse uptake of fluoroscein dye in the blue gaze of the slit lamp—and simply offered to coat the eye with antibiotic ointment. Lindsay was upset when she returned home. The pain, impairment, and the imposition completely frustrated her. She had desperately hoped to attend today's Annual Hospice Meeting; now she couldn't even watch Clare while I executed my hospital duties. I already had three patients waiting in the ER, a panel of inpatients to visit, and the uncertainty of weekend call stretching before us. I sensed Lindsay's collapse into utter helplessness and had no time for it, no emotional reserve of my own to compensate for it or to respond with an ounce of compassion. "You'll just have to accept it" was the advice I meted out. "Accept the pain and go to the meeting in spite of it, or suffer here with your medications." I knew—a second too late—that advice was altogether wrong.

Lindsay missed the first hour of her meeting, but I drove her to attend the remaining three: she was feeling a little better and couldn't bear missing the events. My day was still holding together respectfully, and I was in a position to watch Clare myself or let her play at a friend's house. Lindsay had a wonderful time at the convocation, and, by the next morning, the pain in her eye had all but disappeared. But not her heartache.

I reopened the wound by asking, much too matter-of-factly, "so what did you learn from your illness?" "What did *you* learn," she shot back. We talked. I told her that advice was what I thought she needed, but, more honestly, was all I had to give. Hadn't I expressed my concern, scrutinized her eye, encouraged her to have it examined, administered medication, cooked the meals, watched Clare as much as I possibly could?

"But you didn't offer one kind word; you fulfilled your duty, did only what was necessary, cold and clean and safe at a distance. I got more sympathy from my hospice friends, more, even, from the emergency room doctor. That's what I wanted, not your God damn advice." Clare raced into the kitchen from the living room where she had been watching cartoons. This tension, this argumentation, she disliked, and she glared at me: "Daddy, da-deee! Why can't you stop it now?"

"We need to talk, Clare; it will be OK," I tried to reassure her. "Mommy and daddy need to discuss some important things, but we'll be done soon. Please try to watch your cartoons." She pattered back to the living room, but kept one ear trained on the kitchen.

What was I reacting to? It was not just the plight of the cobbler, whose family is always the last to be shoed. It was not simply the overwhelming responsibilities of the weekend, to which another patient was added at home, along with a child to tend. Was it the long drought in our relationship that has seen so little mutual

support, so little affection, so little investment, and that cries for a monsoon? Lindsay complains, and rightly so, that I pour out my heart to Tim and Mary Beth in our Thursday morning group, or to the impersonal face of my computer before sunrise, but so little trickles down to her. I feel that absence, too.

Was it Lindsay's collapse, her sinking incapacity, that triggered old memories, that transformed her pain into another duty under my charge? Was it my sister's helplessness I was balking at, or the helplessness of all my patients who cannot, will not, get better? "Of course I care about your pain, and your feelings, Lindsay," I whispered as we held each other at the kitchen counter. "And I'm sorry for not saying it more clearly and more often. But I didn't, couldn't, under the circumstances."

Neither of us could wriggle outside of our own pain enough to connect with the other's. We expected the other to know, to touch, to heal us. It is easy to say that, under different circumstances, I might have said the right thing, might have found and better expressed my love. So I did it now. And afterward I shouted to Clare to join us for a family hug, which she did gladly, wrenching herself away from the TV. In my parental home, arguments never ended with resolution, only with bitterness and exhaustion. But arguments seem a necessity in a world full of disagreement and pain. I suppose the trick is to see, and to reach for, love waiting on the other side.

Three days until Lindsay's birthday. Yesterday Clare and I went to a garden store to pick out her birthday present for Momma. Lindsay has wished for a bird feeder that fastens to the window. But after thinking things over, Clare decided that Lindsay would rather have jewelry, and so would she, and why did all the presents have to be for Mommy, anyway? "Lindsay *loves* birds," I tried to explain, "and it's too far to drive to find fancy earrings that Mom would really like." Clare finally accepted my explanation, though she was decidedly unconvinced about the feeder. That evening, after a long pout that followed her late nap, she decided to "paste things." And she composed a lovely assemblage of rubber bands, stickers, tiny paper parasols, and polished pebbles, all taped to a piece of paper. This was Clare's gift, and surely it will make Lindsay the happiest.

Clare is a great keeper of secrets. So I had no hesitation explaining to her the plan for the weekend festivities: Friday afternoon I would pick her up from day care early so that she and I could bake the cake together; Friday evening, Tim and Cris and Rozy and Scott and Debbie would come for cake and ice cream; Sunday evening the grown-ups (Mary Beth and Mac and Mom and Dad) would go out for supper, and Clare could have Erin come over to babysit.

As I look at these plans, I am struck by how the autumnal season persuades me, nudges me back toward Lindsay by focusing me on the family: her birthday, Halloween, Thanksgiving, Christmas. Cosmic timing. I am also struck by the

staple friendships we seek for celebration: my office partners, Tim and Scott and Mary Beth. Have I narrowed my world too severely, or am I fortunate to have this kind of support through the struggle of my medical practice? Some of both, I suspect. And though I vow to open myself up to new friendships, to explore a wider field, there is already too little time to commit to it and still fertilize the friendships in my own back yard, or appreciate the joys of solitude.

The month is closing down. With the end of daylight savings time, it is now completely dark by 5:00 P.M., and the sun reemerges only during the waning moments of my morning chat with the computer. Yesterday a blustery, chilling north wind swept down the coast and stripped the trees of their last remaining spangles. The furnace races most hours of the day. Winter is pokin' 'round the corner, although we will likely have another month to prepare: Check the woodpile, put up the storms, add the antifreeze, pull out the boots and coats.

Tim is back. By all accounts, he had a wonderful time in Costa Rica. Three years ago, he left our practice to teach in an inaugural family practice residency program in San Jose. Thus began our cycle of sabbaticals. His first class had now invited him back for a visit, in gratitude for all that he had contributed to their education. Tim had become a father to them during these formative and challenging years. Fortunately, the residents grew to appreciate that, just as Tim became more self-assured in his teaching role. I'm glad that Tim has found some affirmation in medicine. We have both sought it through the back door, I in my writing and Tim as teacher in a foreign residency program. Neither of us has sought stature in our community or become a leader among our peers. Our patients show their gratitude, but we realize it is for the basic services, for which we have already received their payment in dollars.

It threatens me to hear of Tim's celebrated teaching status. Will he leave Searsport Family Practice permanently to pursue it? If he does, will our friendship survive? I worry like a Catholic who sees his parish priest on the lam. How can *we* survive when the pillars of faith crumble around us? How can we make it without the comforts of Catholic devotion, or the support of our Catholic friends? In our empty hearts, can we find the tiny mustard seed of faith that God planted there before our birth?

Much of my friendship with Tim is born of the work we share. I despair at losing it. I worry that our friendship will not survive the distances. But life is full of adjustments and compromise. And my endless worry threads through it.

Despair hung upon me heavily yesterday. I worried about Lindsay's upcoming party, the cake recipe and supper menu and social gatherings and final gift gathering that would make the birthday package complete. I was so distraught that I somehow became convinced today was her birthday instead of tomorrow. Now

everything was instantly upon me. After wading through the morning rash of patients, I trudged home and lay down upon the sofa, half-listening to Geminiani's *Concerto Grosso* before drifting into an uneasy sleep. The feverish infants, festering skin wounds, routine blood pressure checks, and endless flu vaccinations gave way to the heavy pressure of sleep. My dreams were interrupted an hour later by the ringing of the telephone. It was Lindsay, warning me that Clare would expect some Fruit Stripe Gum when I picked her up from day care today.

I lay back down for a moment, could not settle in, so rolled off the couch and struggled to regain my focus. Running, yes, running would do me good. So I wriggled into some running pants, a hefty T-shirt, and one of our own Searsport Family Practice sweatshirts, then loosely laced my shoes and set off on the short run. It was good to stretch my limbs, to head in a purposeful direction, to suck in the cool, clear, late-autumn air, to let my feet pat-a-pat a mantra against the leaf-cushioned asphalt. The winds and rain of the past week had decimated the remaining foliage, and now, with the Great Shedding nearly complete, I could grasp Waldo County with a piercing and wide-angled view.

After a run and shower, I knew that writing was out of the question. What to do besides languish alone, sulking in self-pity and wasting time? I decided to study cake recipes, weighed their merits against the anticipated bother of baking them, and settled on a hazelnut torte with butter cream frosting. I tackled other items on my list of projects, considered the depression that had momentarily capsized me, and arrived at no satisfying conclusions. Give it up, I thought aloud, give it to God who knows my pain and emptiness and will wash it all away.

Lindsay came home at 5:30 P.M.; Clare was already watching "Rug Rats" in the living room, with her afternoon snack and glass of milk, and perched on the sofa in her blanket. Within a few minutes she would be out for the night, completely and unexpectedly collapsed on the spot where she had toppled. As Lindsay and I prepared supper together, she asked me directly, "Why are you so depressed?"

I gave the answer I had been rehearsing: "I am worried about your birthday, and about comparing my life to Tim's, and about the gulf I feel in our relationship—the sense that we have stopped trying to understand it or bridge it." We talked. We meandered for over an hour, without a goal of finding solutions. Then I packed up my sheet music and trudged to choir practice.

We understand that our interests do not merge completely. I respect her gardening and her hospice; she respects my singing and my running. Where we overlap is significant: in our family, our daughter; in the physical structure of our home; in the social milieu of friends and activities and events; in the pursuit of exotic cuisines and foreign films and traveling together.

But I felt a keen absence, a void in the spiritual realm and a longing for physical intimacy. We cannot solve the problem tonight. The problem, we both know, lies in the frayed state of our relationship. We must work at mending it, over time and with vigilance, tend to it and care for it and redeem its value. Our commitment: to spend one evening a week together, alone and away from Clare. And, at my request, we will say grace at supper, not necessarily with a Catholic formula, but with words that acknowledge the sharing of a meal, the blessing of our union, and thanksgiving to God.

Last night Lindsay held me in a way she hasn't for months. It felt wonderful, as if we were trying again.

NOVEMBER

Living in community is the only asceticism you need.

꙳

KATHLEEN NORRIS

Dakota: A Spiritual Geography

The birthday weekend is over, after all the anticipation, preparation, and frenzied running about, leaving in its wake a lingering sense of satisfaction. Lindsay's two organized events—dessert on her birthday, supper at Nickerson Tavern—went off without a hitch. Even the birthday cake managed to rise for the occasion. It was my first-ever attempt from scratch. I didn't understand basic concepts, like the difference between a cake and a torte, or how butter cream frosting got its name. In the end, I chose a recipe for a hazelnut torte that called for eighteen egg yolks, a pound of butter, several splashes of rum, instant espresso, and a smidgen of flour. But it was tasty, and it provided just deserts for each of our three weekend nights. I think Lindsay was pleased.

Sandwiched in the middle of all that was Halloween. Clare was ready, all witched up in green face paint, broomstick and caldron, a black skirt, turtleneck, and cape. We toured the neighborhood by car, the heater blowing gale-force, but it wasn't enough to stave off the chilblains. Clare had resisted her afternoon nap, so she was on the verge of collapse an hour into the hunt. Her favorite house featured a walk-in dragon. His head and neck were fashioned from sheet plastic stretched around a metal frame. He sported electrified yellow eyes and a forked red tongue that draped the sidewalk as a kind of welcome mat.

I learned over the weekend that the enormous tree at the James P. White house is a copper beech, the largest in the state. Little wonder the name, with its large, waxy, and penny-colored leaves. I also ran the long run twice under crystal blue skies with temperatures just above freezing. It nearly spent me each day. But what clarity the run now affords! I can examine the entire opposite shore of the Passagassawakeag River as I run through the stripped-bare trees. I can study houses in relation to their land, peep at the rubble and rusted machinery that otherwise enjoy their summer privacy, appreciate the composition of stones and slopes and meandering streams. All of this acuity, oddly, without my glasses. Just a sense of openness and of another layer peeled back.

Tomorrow is the election. I am rooting for Mr. Clinton, no matter his hairstyle or the much publicized reports of his womanizing. He has tried to keep the focus of debate on the economy. The race has become too close for comfort, and I dare not think that George Bush can pull it out. I will be glued to the returns tomorrow evening, which almost certainly means no journal entry the following morn. And after Tuesday I must make serious preparations for my trip to Iowa and Colorado.

At 11:00 P.M., the Governor of Arkansas went over the top in electoral votes, so Lindsay and I retreated to bed. Ross Perot may have carried Waldo County and 30 percent of Maine's popular vote, but the nation went for Clinton. At long last, the Reagan-Bush juggernaut has broken down. I couldn't stay awake to celebrate the final tally, or enjoy the speeches of concession and acceptance, or follow the outcome of races in the Senate and House. I had been fighting a cold for two or three days and was dead-tired, thick-headed, raspy-voiced, and aching for sleep. It rained all day yesterday, including the half hour I waited in line to vote, partially exposed to the elements. But the experience was worth it.

The Ward One polling station was in the basement of Peirce School, an old-fashioned, three-story Romanesque brick schoolhouse around the corner from where we lived. Polling stalls had been fashioned at one end of a brick room that had been painted sunburst yellow and decorated with tiny American flags and citizenship posters. Galvanized steam pipes, the originals from 1915, fanned from the boiler room. One attached to a clanking radiator overhead. The large room was now stuffy with bodies, moist and dripping in their overcoats and umbrellas, and pressed close in a line next to the boiler room door and away from the soggy entrance.

The room was dotted with familiar faces—neighbors, friends, and patients who served me their nods of recognition, commentary on the weather, and updated health reports as if conversation were the hors d'oeuvres at our gala reception. But there was also reference to the candidates, to the situation we'd come to fix, traveling nervously up and down the line in brief electrical bursts.

There was a guardedness about declaring one's preference—an extension, perhaps, of the taboo against mixing religion or politics with public discourse. I remember my parents' evasiveness during the Kennedy-Nixon election. I was seven years old but still knew that Jack Kennedy was the Catholic choice and that no love was lost on Mr. Nixon. But to them the polling booth enjoyed the confidentiality of the confessional. Years later Mom admitted that she had gone with Kennedy, but "not because he was Catholic." "Never entered your mind," I winked.

Rocky died yesterday. Old Rock is the mutt retriever who wandered into my partner's life ten years ago. Over the summer, he was diagnosed with bone cancer in his left front leg; the limb was amputated, but no one expected the dog to survive. He rallied after the surgery on a burst of steroids and—I cannot help but believe—our introduction of a strict diet of Snausages. We began buying him these processed dog food snacks in a sausage shape to perk up his appetite. Truth is that Rocky would have eaten *anything* gleefully. But he especially favored the Snausages. First we bought him the original flavor, next the Cheese-Wrapped kind, and finally the Big Dog variety. Then we ordered him a serving container (shaped like a dog) that repeated, over and over in a monotone voice, "snausages, snausages, snausages . . ." until the lid flipped shut.

Rocky went with the Hughes everywhere. He could wait patiently in their car for hours while Tim made hospital rounds, visited friends, or sea-kayaked. At the office he would sprawl in the doctors' back room, perfuming much of the hallway and laboratory with his personal chemistry. During the brief decade he was among us, Rocky staked out a wide territory with the scent of his body and breath; it permeated both of the Hughes's cars and their entire house, and even our own home on that one occasion when Rocky (playing dumb, which he does naturally) got past us at the front door and terrorized our poor felines. The eldest literally scampered five vertical feet up an enamel refrigerator door to escape his gnashing incisors.

Over the last month Rocky has been dying. When he could no longer hobble up and down the stairs, Tim carried him; when he could not raise himself to defecate or escape his own emesis, Tim scrubbed him clean. With the end in sight, the elders plotted to lace his Snausage with potent barbiturates. Rocky refused. Did he smell a rat, or had he gracefully chosen to starve himself? Yesterday Tim drove Rocky to the veterinarian's office for a lethal injection, and buried him that afternoon in his lawn.

Tim and Rocky, Rocky and Tim. Plain, simple, smelly old dog with indiscriminate tastes and a reputation as a cat terrorist. I will not forget Tim's gentle praise, bestowed daily with a rub on the chin or a pat on the side, "Good boy, Rocky, good boy." They were a pair, those two. Now what will become of the survivor?

A woman waits in the labor suite for my decision: will I resume her oxytocin induction? Her second pregnancy, now at term, has been complicated by ruptured membranes and the need to initiate labor. Yesterday's induction produced reasonable progress: the head descended, the cervix thinned, and dilatation widened to three centimeters. Overnight I discontinued the oxytocin drip so that she could sleep, hoping that labor might resume spontaneously in the morning. In an hour (7:00 A.M.) I will seek a progress report. OB hangs. The problems, the worries, the due dates all float in your mind and shade every thought and action. Fortunately my patient is handling labor well; she is making progress. But we shall see what the day decides.

Yesterday I made satisfying incursions into my patients' lives: A minister whom I recently met returned yesterday for a complete physical examination. I reassured him that his heart attack, suffered nearly two years ago at the age of forty-three, had healed. He could tolerate exercise and now desperately needed it. I encouraged him to see a therapist in order to deal with his occupational stress, wondering all the while if I could accept the same advice. There was a parade of new babies, waddling mothers-to-be, sore ears and throats and shoulders. We celebrated the thirty-eighth birthday of Bonnie Allard, our head nurse, with a traditional cake and ice cream combo during our lunch break.

At the end of the day, an old drunkard returned to the office, intoxicated. He needed his blood pressure pills refilled. The pressures were up, though improved, and I began steering our conversation toward his cigarettes and booze. But his ears were plugged by booze and stubborn pride, and he would hear none of it. Should I throw the bum out, or place some conditions on his return (e.g., that he be sober)? Should I enlist the support of family, or neighbors, or anyone who still gives a damn? Am I wasting my breath? Should I move on to those for whom there is still hope?

There are too many drunks and pill-poppers and welfare mothers, the legion of depressed and lonely and incurable souls who will, regardless, wither and die in neglected trailers along forgotten country roads. Am I soft or stupid or crippled by some fatal flaw, or do they not deserve a second chance, the courtesy of my attention, and some connection to a world of kindness and possibility? In our practice, we have tried to respond affirmatively. Through mutual support we have kept the needle oscillating more to the side of hope than frustration, more to surplus energy than exhaustion, more to love than anger. All patients deserve kindness and caring, as much as we can provide. Our vocation to serve the sick relies upon this mercy to take us beyond the shortfalls of justice and reason.

At the IDT meeting today, I read a letter that I had just received from a family member of a hospice patient. I am proud of it; it is both gratifying and reassuring to hear from people who appreciate your efforts. I only regret not sending more of these myself.

Thank you for being involved in hospice. You truly have compassion, heart, warmth. It was a very tough time just talking about Mom's impending death. I was very hesitant to speak of it with her, or have anyone else speak of it in front of her. You made it not only possible, but almost enjoyable. Your support (sitting close beside her) and your comforting way was very special to see.

Our entire family was given support, making Mom's passing as acceptable as possible. With family, visiting nurses, and hospice, we are a richer people blessed with an almost unbelievable support. Even Mother's funeral was *special.* My uncle was part of the remembrance and the readings. The Reverend Wood was a warm and caring man.

Mom left us all with a lifetime of wonderful memories, even the last year of quiet strength, courage and faith. It was very nice to be able to honor her memory with a memorial fund given by her family, friends, and neighbors to Hospice totaling eight hundred dollars. I thank God for Dr. Loxterkamp, home health nursing, hospice, Waldo County General Hospital, and for the way they work to comfort those who need comforting. The way the program and the people work together to make the entire process a success! Thank you on behalf of Mother and the family.

On the back of the envelope she scribbled a verse: "I have given rest to the weary and joy to all the sorrowing" (Jeremiah 31:25). This is the ideal toward which we should strive each day in hospice.

I was testy at the meeting. We discussed a memorial book in which to gather artifacts, remembrances of the lives of hospice patients we have cared for. The question of confidentiality came up, as usual, so I suggested (tongue in cheek) that we obtain "informed consent" before we include a loved one in the book. I was also testy because certain hospice patients are still denied The Benefit. It seems that expensive services (home oxygen, palliative radiation, chemotherapy) automatically exclude certain patients from even being considered. I understand the economic realities, but let's call a spade a spade and admit who is the real beneficiary of the Medicare Hospice Benefit.

I am no expert on the history of hospice, and what little I provide here can be found elsewhere, in greater depth and with more clarity. It is important, first of all, to realize that the word "hospice" is derived from the Latin word for host, *hospes.* It shares that root with other words like hospital, hostel, hotel, and hospitality, which allow us to circumscribe its meaning. The Latin alone is sufficient:

hospice has to do with hospitality for the dying, a readiness to help and comfort them (and their families) in an age when society often ignores, displaces, or fears them. In this way it is a philosophy, an approach to the care of the dying.

Many in the hospice movement see its origins in the Knights Hospitaller, which were organizations formed during the Crusades to defend and aid the sick and wounded. The oldest and most famous order—the Order of the Knights Hospitaller of St. John in Jerusalem—began as the Hospital of St. John and was founded by Italian merchants in the mid-eleventh century to serve the growing numbers of pilgrims visiting the Holy Land. At one time it accommodated more than two thousand guests. After Jerusalem was liberated in 1099, St. John's became an order of knights, and its rector, Brother Gerard, its first master.

The movement of the Knights spread to Cyprus, Malta, and Rhodes, and their tradition of hospitality for the wayward and dying persisted for over six hundred years. They attended to both the physical and spiritual needs of their guests, and prepared the dying for a journey to the higher, infinitely more important plane that the medieval mind anticipated without question.

In modern times, Sister May Aikenhead of the Irish Sisters of Charity (and a co-worker of Florence Nightingale) opened a hospice in Dublin in the 1800s, modeling it after houses she had observed in France. In 1906, the English Sisters of Charity founded St. Joseph's Hospice in London, where, in the 1940s, a nurse named Cicely Saunders came to work. After training to become a physician, Dr. Saunders founded St. Christopher's Hospice in London in 1967, where she blended the ancient tradition of hospitality with modern palliative techniques. She visited Yale University, where her work and teachings inspired the establishment of America's first hospice in 1974. It was initially home-based, and funded in part by a grant from the National Cancer Institute. Connecticut Hospice (as it is known today) later opened a free-standing forty-four-bed hospice unit to support home-based services around the state. Hospice of Waldo County was created in 1984 as a volunteer organization whose members dedicated themselves to providing the dying with comfort, companionship, and family support. Hospice care is now an integral part of services offered by Waldo County Home Health Agency, though the volunteer group is still a separate entity governed by a separate board. In 1992, the hospital inaugurated the inpatient Hospice Wing—the first in the state—to supplement home-based hospice care.

So, as one can see, hospice is more than a *philosophy* applicable to everyone who faces death. It is also, in a more limited way, a *service* provided by a home health agency. Such a service may involve nurses, home health aides, hospice volunteers, social workers, ministers, or whoever is available to meet a particular need. And finally, less often but equally important, hospice is a *place,* the Hospice Wing at Waldo County General Hospital. Here the dying can go in their final hours, or when their family needs respite, or when doctors must tame intolerable pain. It is situated on the hospital's north side and contains two of the most elegant patient rooms in the house. In addition, it has a function room and bedroom to serve the families. The Hospice Wing proclaims in physical terms what those of us who enter it carry in our hearts: the dying deserve no less.

But hospice was not always this way. It arose as a movement. It mobilized volunteers who were drawn to aid the dying for their own varied and deeply personal reasons, including social commitment, personal loss or a spiritual calling. During its evolution, it was used by those who stood in opposition to the abuses of institutional care and defended the right of the dying to remain at home. It has been supported by health care financiers who saw it as a way to lower the costs of end-stage care, by academic institutions to study stages in death and dying, and by health care providers who sought to remedy the shameful lack of pain control and continuity of care that many dying patients have encountered.

Hospice is fundamentally about being a *hospes,* or host. It is, moreover, for those of us who labor by its philosophy, about becoming a privileged guest in relationship to the dying (as the Latin meaning also implies).* It is about our personal beliefs surrounding death, about our concern for the dying and our willingness to help them, to talk to them, to visit them and remain hospitable even when society tells us they are no longer valuable.

7:00 A.M. I discover we are out of milk and caffeinated coffee. I will subsist this morning on two slices of cinnamon toast and decaf coffee. Lindsay asked that I drop Clare off at nursery school today. She is weary from yesterday's name-hurling and obstinacy and arguments at every turn. I begrudgingly agree.

By 8:00 A.M. I have inserted prostaglandin gel in the OB patient I saw yesterday in the office. She is nearly due, but the head is so high, the cervix closed, and I anticipate a long induction with intravenous oxytocin if we cannot first ready her cervix. The external fetal monitor strip showed a few scattered contractions; the fetus is "reactive." Bishops Score was 0. Prostaglandin gel has the look and consistency of Elmer's glue, but I was able to squeeze it easily out of the syringe between the tongs of the speculum. Afterward, I dictated yesterday's hospice admission and returned to the emergency room, which had been paging me for two new arrivals. One has a badly sprained thumb and is awaiting X-rays; the other has blood in the urine, with back pain, and is waiting to be catheterized.

9:05 A.M. Clare, bedecked in her insulated blue coat, is pacing the driveway in search of tiny colored leaves. Both of us, Lindsay and I, must join the hunt if there is any hope of budging her. With coaxing, we head off to nursery school in "the golden car," Daddy's 1984 Toyota Tercel. She was happy to find her friends

---

* Lewis' *Elementary Latin Dictionary* lists several meanings, including host, entertainer, guest, stranger, and friend (especially one bound by the ties of hospitality).

Hillie and Lucy and quickly joined the other kids who were racing about the barn. Eventually they turned their attention to the giant, plastic three-wheelers. As Clare positioned herself for her suicide trip down the hill, I seized the opportunity to kiss her goodbye, give her a hug, and creep away.

9:30 A.M. The X-ray and catheterized urine results are back, and I examine the two patients who are waiting in the ER. Everything is normal and we all go our separate ways. My OB patient is having mild contractions every two minutes. It is amazing how quickly the prostaglandin softened the cervix and allowed the head to descend. Bishops Score is five. We could not give a second dose, but the patient was far from being in active labor. I sent her home with provisions to return in the morning for a nonstress test. I visited my hospice patient on the Wing. Her blood was too thin, so I slowed the heparin drip and listened to stories of when she was an LPN in the old Bangor City Hospital. Her favorite memories were of the nights when the interns worked, when they would spend hours swilling coffee and laughing in the nurses' lounge.

11:00 A.M. I drove to the nursing home to examine a patient whom I had seen several times recently for bronchial inflammation. She was doing fine except for prominent lung sounds that suggested bronchitis. I ordered an expectorant and nebulizer treatments. The director, Betty Barnaby, asked if she could speak to me in the capacity of medical director.

In her office, I learned that one of the attending physicians has continued to write progress notes and dictate H&Ps without examining his patients. He has been warned once. More disturbing were comments that he allegedly made to the patient's daughter-in-law, admitting that "we get along famously because I never see her." It was the daughter-in-law who sounded the alarm to the administrator. The patient has remained in perfect health throughout the period of so-called neglect. Malpractice is not at issue, but rather misrepresentation of the facts, breach of protocol, billing for services never provided, and an apparent disregard for the feelings of the patient and her family. I know the doctor, trust his judgment as a consultant, and sense his frustration and disinterest in caring for nursing home patients. But before he digs his own grave, I must talk to him and help him hand off his nursing home practice. I let the administrator know that punitive action on the hospital's part is another matter, one that is theirs to decide.

12:30 P.M. I arrived at the office early, and luckily so because a patient had been worked into the schedule. She is in her second trimester of pregnancy and is being treated for cervicitis, with complaints of bleeding and cramping. She says she feels better today except for the nausea and gastric distress caused by the antibiotic.

6:00 P.M. I got home at a reasonable hour, thankfully, because chills and fatigue have drained me utterly. The telephone rang and it was OB to report that another patient had arrived with ruptured membranes and early labor. We agreed to keep her. Lindsay, Clare, and I took off in the Jetta, beeper in tow, to buy groceries and get cash at Shop 'n Save and order a pizza-to-go. Then a relaxing, family-home-evening over pizza, Blossom Hill Chardonnay, and Dan Rather followed by the McNeil-Lehrer News Hour (with special Friday night guests Gergen and Shields).

9:00 P.M. After Clare was tucked in, I took off for the hospital and the OB ward. My patient's cervix was thin and two centimeters, and she had developed an active labor pattern. It would be a long night, I warned her (and the dozen or more family members who choked the hallway). Back at home, I kissed Clare good night and joined Lindsay in bed, and we read for fifteen minutes before unconsciousness overtook us.

11:30 P.M. OB called for a pain medication order. The patient was in hard labor and now wanted to rest in bed. I ordered intramuscular Vistaril and Demerol. Sleep returned, but it consisted of fretful dreams, intermittent coughs, trips to the bathroom, and forays to the refrigerator for juice and water.

3:00 A.M. OB called again: my patient was nine centimeters. I dressed and drove to the hospital, flew up the stairs to the maternity ward, and found madame pushing uncontrollably. On examination, the cervix was completely dilated, and so I let her push while I dressed and scrubbed. Justin Scott was born at 3:42 A.M. with Apgars of nine and ten. Almost immediately he emitted a beautiful lusty cry, with great skin color and alert eyes peering all around. The family was ecstatic, and so was I. After the placenta was evacuated and the perineal tear repaired "in the usual fashion," I finished the paperwork through puffy eyes.

4:15 A.M. The drive home took a minute along Northport Avenue, down that deserted, familiar, welcoming path. I felt ready to begin the new day, to mix the eggs, grind the coffee, chime the Powerbook, and listen to the Masses of William Byrd. First I slipped upstairs to turn off my alarm, which was set to go off in ten minutes.

And by 6:00 A.M., the sky outside had become tiger-striped in pale yellow and violet, with a faint belt of crimson crossing across its middle. A clear, cold day was dawning. I penciled a note to myself to visit my hospital patients, sign out for the weekend, and enjoy the rest of the day with a run, raking, and the preparations for tonight's dinner guests.

As I walked to the the compost pile yesterday morning, frozen blades of grass crunched under my feet, portending the advent of winter. The pile was heaped high with leaves, already lackluster and matted by the weekend rains, steaming their musty, earthy scents of decay.

In the evening, in the long luminescence of autumnal dusk, when the prickly rim of the western horizon was backlit by a yellow as deep as squash, I set out for a short run. The full moon, rising in the east, darted high into the starry night like a kite on a string. The bare branches of my neighbor's magnificent black locusts and maples and beeches offered no barrier; they could not snag it from my view. It kept perfect pace with me through the run, hugging my shoulder as we circled the town. I drenched my sweatshirts and stocking cap and Handy Andy gloves but needed their several layers in the crisp, cloudless evening air.

Leaves were piled everywhere. The moonlight revealed a few stragglers left on the trees. Beams of light from the approaching cars sliced over great piles in the gutters and on the parking, and the air was thickly laden with smoke from their distant smoldering fires. The resplendent, multicolored glory of three weeks ago had given way to this, the pyres of fall.

My weekend, now quickly fading from memory, was rich. I went for a long run at noon on Saturday, a wonderful jaunt along the Passagassawakeag River, eight miles around its banks. We had dinner guests Saturday night, three new acquaintances and potential friends, a stockbroker, a realtor, and an artist. It passed without sensation, except a few good laughs and some serious conversation with the artist, Jennie Baker.

On Sunday morning we attended a memorial service for Rocky Hughes. Over two dozen friends and neighbors attended, drawn by their connection to this great dog's life and, possibly too, the promise of pancakes and sausage. The format was familiar to me from my days as an altar boy when funeral and interment were followed by a big spread in the parish hall served by members of the Rosary Society. But Tim reversed the order. As we gathered on his back porch overlooking Penobscot Bay, he quoted the lines on Ernest Hemingway's grave, Debbie Bailly waxed eloquent about Rocky's unrequited love for their dog, Rigel, and Lindsay read the poetry of Isaac Watts.

Sunday afternoon I practiced with Scott Bailly and Jean Goldfine for the Advent Masses. We worked on marvelous harmonies, tight and dissonant, that Bobby McPherrin had set to the 23rd Psalm; old tunes from Taize that are essentially polyphonic chant; and responsorials to the Mass that acquire vitality in triplicate voice. We will gather for an hour this morning at Scott's home before the workday begins.

Last night Lindsay and I fought over grace before supper. Why do I insist that she join us in prayer? She wants no part of something that was forced down her throat in childhood. Lindsay would prefer silence, or dialogue, or some personal thanksgiving. I had hoped that the prayer might join us together as a family, but my hard line destroys any chance of that.

Yesterday gave us a full moon and one of my hardest days on record. One patient after another had problems with nerves, marriage, work, bills. But the most time-consuming and troublesome tale came from a lady whose husband was mentally ill. She cried throughout the forty-five minute visit. I knew that I was over my head, so placed calls afterward to Mary Beth and the local psychiatrist. Eventually I reached them both, discussed the desperate situation, and arranged for consultations with both of them later in the week. Since my patient had recently disconnected her telephone, Lindsay drove out to her home with the appointment times. Now the cogs were in place before my western trip, two days hence.

After the end of that long, unsettling day, we entertained fifty kids—in our waiting room for school physicals. It was the largest turnout in memory; it took three of us, working steadily, more than two hours to complete. How can you orchestrate a meaningful interaction with an adolescent in seven minutes? My narrow goal was to move the children through, perform the basic checkup, fill out the forms, and leave a door open: come back again if you need me.

I raced from the office to RENEW, stopping long enough at home to pick up a bible and acknowledge my family. We had a babysitter tonight because Lindsay wanted to attend a Hospice support meeting; I'd grown to like Mara very much even before we discovered our common birthday.

RENEW began in that awkward, stiff way that groups often do, with a formula prayer and the invitation for "any observations you would like to make." Our regular leader was away, so the meeting was run by a delightful lady (a patient of mine) whose insecurities drove her to incessant chatter. The discussion remained light and topical. We spoke about food kitchens and homeless shelters, genocide in the Sudan and the fascist right in Germany. The readings finally got us back on track, especially the story of the Good Samaritan. We were challenged to think about individualism and community, differences and similarities. It occurred to me that it was "difference" that made us "individual" and defined who we are. Perceptions of similarity allow us to form "community" and create the basis for relationship. As human beings, we must entertain both simultaneously, while living within our center. Here in Belfast, the issue of difference and similarity is often cast in terms of who is native and who is "from away."

Last night we talked of anti-Catholic smears during the Nixon-Kennedy campaign, when JFK was accused of plotting to import the Pope and create a Roman Catholic state. Is this fear so different from concerns about the Islam Nation in Sudan? And is the Church's good name hurt more by the slander of non-Catholics or the chilling tales we insiders tell of sadistic nuns and pedophilic priests?

We are being drawn together by our shared Catholicity to celebrate, enlarge, and challenge our religious beliefs. What will become of it? Will we expand the circle, discover unknown similarities, dissolve accepted differences? I have found that the easiest way to widen a circle is to listen. Listen to the stories of people's lives. Find in them some unexpected resonance and ground for mutual respect. Family practice situates itself on the margins of many circles, in the hazy area between truth and illusion, the familiar and the unknown, in a genuine effort to treat people in the context of their community. What a wonderful vantage from which to see the hand of God at play!

The first snow of the year fell yesterday, not much to speak of—one to three inches according the weatherman. It has been cold, and I'm getting accustomed to the deep guttural moan of the furnace from the cellar.

I am back from my journey to Colorado and Iowa. As always, I now have many loose strings to tie and thank-you letters to write for the hospitality extended to me while in Kremmling and Denver. There are new leads to explore, and the business of Mom's estate to handle. I still must ship a few of Mom's personal belongings to my sister, which I saved in her absence: a suitcase, quilts, family photos, and keepsake owls.

Lindsay has been much more affectionate, to my pleasant surprise. Despite the frantic pace since the return, we have found time for each other, and she has fussed over her appearance. Perhaps it is all my imagination, born of my missing her, too. But it feels wonderful.

Lindsay asked what I thought was the hardest part of the trip. No contest: losing Mom's rings. Before leaving her old apartment, Mom handed me her heirloom rings and asked me to divide them among the children. The request unsettled me, partly because my sister and Lindsay were both absent, partly because it was another onerous chore. So I placed them in a jewelry box on the top shelf in her bedroom closet and awaited for a more opportune time to return.

Meanwhile, friends and neighbors traipsed through the old apartment to help us pack and transport Mom's belongings to her new apartment. All of this, of course, without direct supervision. When I returned to the new apartment, Mom inquired about the rings. Her bedroom closet was bare, the key drawer contained nothing more, and the safety deposit box that the hospital held contained only yellowing certificates of stock, rubber-banded treasury bills, and the musty odor of cigarettes. "Don't worry Mom," I reassured her (though not myself), "they'll turn up."

Mom ruminated and stewed and worried about the rings, asking after them frequently, forgetting when she last inquired, making the rings a focal point for the larger scope of worry brought on by the weekend. Their importance was magnified with each turn of the screw. I combed the new apartment, but they were nowhere to be found. We scoured the old apartment again but doubted that anything could have been overlooked in my sister-in-law's careful cataloguing of its contents in preparation for the estate auction. Finally, in an effort to deflect Mom's preoccupation—to give her peace of mind—I resolved to tell her that the rings were safe. In the privacy of our ride to Rolfe that Saturday morning, I gave her "the good news."

"You mean you found them?" Mom pressed hopefully. "Oh God, David, you don't know how worried I've been, how relieved I am to know you have them." Tears streamed down her face, and she spoke in anxious little gulps.

"I talked to Lindsay, and the rings are safe," I repeated. And later that morning lied again at the dining room table with my brother and his wife. This was not *exactly* a lie, I tried to convince myself; I *had* spoken with Lindsay, and no doubt the rings were safely stored *somewhere,* in someone's hands, though I didn't know exactly where. Mom sensed the doubt, noted my hesitation, and set her sights on the jugulars.

"You have them in Maine? You wouldn't lie to me, David?" Oh, the danger of half-truths and best intentions. They require the perpetrator to hold an unwavering commitment to, even a self-absorption in, the lie; it must be defended to the last.

I took the plunge. "Mom, Lindsay has found rings in her jewelry box back in Belfast, and believes they are yours. I can't be sure until I return, but I'll let you know."

"I'm from Missouri, the show-me state, so promise me you'll send a picture when you get back. David, I sure hope you're not lying to me. You wouldn't do that, would you?"

By then the lie had acquired a monstrous life its own. It was leading me down the road to disaster, and I was on the loose gravel at the treacherous edge. Once my wheels had locked into it, I felt the headlong pull to the ditch. Even if I found the rings, the lie would persist. And I had been accused and convicted by my own mother, in her frailty and forgetfulness. The rings were trivial to my sister, my brother, and me, and to our wives who wear no jewelry. This whole bother had been blown out of proportion. But to Mom the rings were all that mattered, something she could pass, tangible and precious, from one generation to the next. They were infinitely precious to her, and so I felt devastated at the thought that I had lost them.

The next evening, after my return to Belfast, my brother called to say that they had found the rings in a jewelry box pushed to the rear of the closet shelf in Mom's new apartment. He would send a picture that could be forwarded to Mom that would complete my little deception. Thanks, but no need for that, Jeff. I'll just tell Mom the truth.

Yesterday began with the Wednesday morning meeting, where Cathy sobbed. She is the canary in the miner's cage, the bellwether that warns of an approaching storm. She was distraught over the way yesterday's staff meeting had proceeded. What went wrong? The conversation seemed stilted, splintered, newsy;

our two new employees were officially recognized but not personally welcomed. Our idea of mixing business and pleasure at a local restaurant had failed. Tim and I now agreed that we should take in the reins and run the meeting; it is our responsibility to set the tone of the meeting, to insure that "process" is part of the agenda. And we realize that Cathy is under enormous strain as she pushes us to become a rural health center, plans her daughter's wedding, and attends to the daily details of running a practice. We need to support and assist her more; and vowed to do so.

We ended the first round of RENEW Tuesday night. For some reason, non-Catholics have become a topic for conversation. That night, Witnesses took the stand. Why do they make us feel so insecure? Is it the force of their convictions, their inability to acknowledge another viewpoint, or the evangelical spirit we lack in ourselves? For a long time I felt intimidated by the proselytizers who darkened my door, yet invited them in anyway, and braced for a good argument.

Now I welcome the door-to-door evangelists as I would a pharmaceutical representative at the office: on the condition that we discuss anything but what they are peddling. I don't want a pitch. I'm not in the market. And if I were, I have my own sources, thank you. It has taken me too long to achieve some flowering of faith to allow strangers to manhandle it. My belief in God is shot through, like a wedge of Swiss cheese, with doubts and despair and my own mental dullness. But it's all that I have. And I would rather patch it with God's grace than a preacher's putty, with a greater love of neighbor, with humility, with the pangs of loneliness that lead me back to the good company of my patients. Mine is a fragile faith, something as insubstantial as tissue in water, dissolving with a wave of the hand. But it locates me in the universe. It's my gamble on eternity, and a source of hope for this lifetime.

Until yesterday, I thought the running season was over. But temperatures climbed into the mid-fifties, and the road beckoned to me once more. Sam Mitchell swung by at 11:30 A.M. to use our computer and talk hospice with Lindsay. The conversation turned to running, and we conspired to make a long run. Within an hour we had set off in leisurely strides through the balmy, almost steamy November air. We talked, on that Sunday jaunt beside the Passagassawakeag, about his current job (real estate) and what mine might have been. Would I have professed theology in some university department, or gone into advertising or editing with my love of words?

Idle speculation, because my entry into medicine was an arranged affair, a done deal. It was not simply that my father was a country doctor and I the eldest son; or that he died when I was thirteen and medicine became the means to know him, to honor him; or perhaps to earn his love by carrying forward his burden in some symbolic way. I recall the words of my younger brother, who was only five years old when our father died: Jeff proposed that I marry my mother in order to make everything right again. The theme recurred as I left for college. After a wrenching family argument the night before, we loaded the car and set off to Omaha and Freshman Orientation Week. "David," my mother confided, "if you should decide against becoming a doctor, I'll feel as if I let your father down."

Medicine, like many things you enter for all the wrong reasons, finally became something I had to take or leave. There were no staggering loans or "an accustomed lifestyle" to hold me. I had been given no more than a taste of medicine from my father; luck and circumstance played their considerable role. But in the end, it was up to me to commit to it. There would be no one else to blame.

And medicine has provided well. It has given me a job and job security. It offers a wide menu for the indecisive. And, from behind closed doors, the socially insecure can meet the public confidently, veiling their doubts or misgivings, fears of rejection, and private wounds that we somehow hope our patients will magically heal. Society has strong notions about its doctors. It purports to know who we are personally and what we value. Doctors, for our part, project a powerful social image. Like it or not, we are groomed for the role and share a common identity in the eyes of the public.

But who we *are* behind the starched smock and the stethoscope is something else again. I partly love medicine and the Catholic Church because they are both solidly institutional. They create automatic associations; they are connected to the seats of power; they permit access to the most intimate thoughts of strangers. And yet they allow me—the devoted G.P., the devout Catholic—the freedom to go about my business with a surprise or two up my sleeve.

Since last sitting, I have written letters and thank-you notes to my mother in Pocahontas, my brother in Iowa City, my sister in Wisconsin, Gary Ceriani in Denver, and Georgeanne Pineda in Kremmling (whom I had visited in Colorado). I have practiced music for the Advent Masses, helped ready the office for our Rural Health Center inspection on Tuesday, entered all of Mom's financial transactions onto the computer, and nearly finished reading *Virgin Time*. And yesterday I finished the brick sidewalk for Lindsay, leading from our new back porch to the asphalt drive.

I despise few patients, but one of them resurfaced over the weekend while I was covering for the family practice group. He appeared in the emergency room on Friday at 9:00 P.M., complaining of epigastric pain and requesting narcotics. He is a bad apple: a thoroughly irresponsible, intimidating troublemaker with juvenile-onset diabetes mellitus. He was my patient until he pushed me too far. It is true that he may have recurrent pancreatitis, which the record shows; after its course has become chronic, the objective signs largely disappear, and you fly by the seat of your pants, on the patient's word that he is in pain. Doctors are rightly reluctant to prescribe narcotics unless the need is clear and temporary, as with kidney stones or a postoperative wound. Beyond that, we require a trusting relationship with the patient before taking chances. Never would we prescribe them for a sociopath.

He slouched on the gurney half-clad in a hospital gown, kicking his feet with an obvious and advertised impatience. He had been waiting two hours by the time I arrived. During the interim, he had received the mandatory battery of tests, a half liter of intravenous fluid, and a shot of Toradol, the intramuscular equivalent of ibuprofen. It hadn't touched his pain, this veteran of the trenches, this frequent flyer on the narcotics trade. So I faced a man with an ironclad ticket for admission: nausea and vomiting for four days, uncontrolled epigastric pain, and a blood sugar of 870. But I smelled a rat. No one had witnessed his vomiting (though the patient had been in the ER for three hours). He exhibited none of the usual signs of pain. He had stopped taking insulin (a whopping eighty units a day), which would account for his remarkably high blood sugars. And even these fell to below 700 with a bolus of saline.

It wasn't so much the question of narcotics, or his menacing stare and vulgar tongue. I hated the manipulation, the relish he took in playing this game. His appearance in the ER late at night—when doctors are tired and the ER crew is skeletal—was calculated to bypass an outpatient trial of therapy. His own negligence in taking insulin had run the blood sugars to a critical level. His avoidance of routine medical care (he hadn't seen his family doctor in months) obviated any chance for a doctor to participate in his plan of care and give him a fighting chance to avert admission. This was health care on the patient's terms only, including narcotics on demand in doses that he dictated.

"I'll help you with your diabetes," I began in a voice as cool as I could muster, "but I won't give you narcotics. And don't expect them here, from me or the other doctors." I laid down the rule unilaterally, one that I knew was impossible to enforce. Perhaps it was heartless in the face of the possibility of recurrent pancreatitis. But did he really have it?

I knew that if I admitted him to the hospital he would badger the nurses until I prescribed narcotics. What fact could stay that order? There was a total lack of trust between us—it kept coming back to that. His repeated abuse, his lies, his calculations . . . perhaps anything more was beyond him, no matter who the practitioner. As for me, too much water had flowed over the dam to avoid a harsh and hardened judgment.

So I discharged him from the ER, ignored his threats of "Hey, pal, I hope I don't ever meet you in a dark alley" and the pangs of guilt that stemmed from sending home a sick diabetic with a high blood sugar. He was stable, I reassured myself, and nobody ever died of pain. He must meet the doctor halfway. And if he cannot, what then? Then I'll share the burden of his care with the other doctors but not suffer it alone.

We leave today for our Thanksgiving holiday: an overnight stop in Boston to visit friends and divide the traveling time to New York; then three days in Hastings-on-Hudson, where Lindsay's sister and her family live. Lindsay's father will be riding the rails from Washington, D.C., to join us on Turkey Day. The only stormcloud on the horizon is Clare's fever, most evident last night, coupled with a hoarseness over the past week and a stye that is receding from her lower eyelid. It is a watershed day on two other accounts: our office jumped the last hurdle on the way to becoming a rural health center, and I finished reading Patricia Hampl's spiritual travelogue, *Virgin Time,* last night.

Ms. Hampl is a wonderful writer. Her strengths are her lavish but controlled use of metaphor (not as rich as Annie Dillard's but more digestible), the historical detail in which she rests the life of St. Francis, and her portraiture of the pilgrims who join her en route to Assisi, Lourdes, and Rosethorn.

Her beautiful lines still cling to me like moss to stone, especially the descriptions of her convent school in St. Paul, where, "At intervals during the day, from the cloister side of the second-floor chapel, the choir nuns reeled out a taut line of Gregorian chant into the school corridors as they sang the Divine Office, troling by hour and season back and forth over the fathomless pools of the psalms." She writes of two lovers in a Lourdes restaurant, one of whom we learn—surprisingly—is quadriplegic; and of poverty in the time of Francis: "In the Middle Ages, begging was a job, or at least an occupation with social meaning. For in a society where charity is not merely kindness or tenderhearted guilt but an acknowledgment of the giver's even greater need—for salvation—the beggar performs an essential function. He provides a way for the rich man to get to heaven. Beyond that, the begger is a *memento mori,* and his ravaged face is the Face of God . . . Poverty is the big thing Christendom has traditionally held against Christianity."

My head is turned by the beauty of her prose. I squirm in my seat at her sumptuous table, so full of smells and pastels and convent bells. I am lost reminiscing in my own Catholic childhood, and race to read more about the mystic Francis. Why—I begin to wonder—did Hampl take us to *that* grotto or *this* shrine? Can I believe her claims about mysticism, monastic life, Franciscan spirituality? When will Ms. Hampl reveal some of the interior of her own life, with its doubts and aspirations, sorrows and misgivings, false starts and second guesses? Does marriage supplement her experience of God, or challenge it, or transform it? And if there hadn't been a book, would the journey have been worth it, all the pretense and piety and exquisite Catholic fare?

Patricia Hampl ends her journey high above the convent at Rosethorn, California. We climb to a moment before dawn, wait in the long grasses drenched in dew, observe a meadow that once inspired Thomas Merton to write, "For the birds, there is not a time that they tell, but the virgin point between darkness and light, between nonbeing and being . . . when creation in its innocence asks permission to be once again, as it did on the first morning that ever was."* It was here, at that virgin time, that Ms. Hampl uttered her first prayer. It seems almost an afterthought, not the fuel for such a long and beautifully crafted book. But it is a book worth giving and reading again.

Edwin called yesterday to report that his wife died three days ago in New Hampshire. Dot went peacefully, I am told. And without pain, only a week after giving up food and water. She chose to be buried on Mount Desert Island because of her love for the sea. Edwin will be back in Maine this Summer, and, yes, of course, he'll look me up.

I am happy as a clam this morning, sitting alone in Anne and John's darkened kitchen at 5:00 A.M. A mad kitten purrs at her unexpected company. A flowering narcissus bulb is potted on the kitchen table by which I, too, am planted; it awakens my nostrils with a sweet scent and presneeze tingle. And my glowing Powerbook is booted and running silently beneath my fingers. I do not intend for this to be a "productive" trip. But this morning I continue the familiar rhythm of solitude, nourishment, reflection. Perhaps this day I will be more attentive to Lindsay and Clare.

When the rains came two days ago, I had been caught with my car window down. They thoroughly soaked the driver's seat and filled the handgrip in the door panel with water. Though the seat quickly dried out, this tiny water well remained. Remarkably, every time I opened or closed the door yesterday, my fingers dipped into the cold water, triggering an instinctively Catholic urge to cross myself.

I read in the Bangor *Daily News* that Ross Perot finished second among the presidential candidates in the state of Maine, ahead of our "favorite son" George Bush. In every other state, he was dead last. We also had 73 percent of eligible voters exercising their franchise, the highest turnout in the nation, and the highest in Maine's history.

Thanksgiving Day. We arrived safely in Hastings-on-Hudson after a four-hour sprint from Boston. Clare survived the ride wonderfully. Today we will board an in-bound train for Macy's Thanksgiving Parade. This afternoon, after Lindsay's father arrives, we will slice turkey and avoid politics. Ray is a rabid Republican, inconsolable over the loss of The Great Communicator, Mr. Reagan, and deluded by the belief that Reagan's only failing was the placement of a few bad apples in his cabinet. End of discussion.

* Quoted in Patricia Hampl, *Virgin Time,* p. 206.

I set up the Powerbook in Barbara and Don's study, surrounded by neuroanatomy atlases, social work texts, and IBM-compatible computer parts. This is not home: no cat chores or icons or sweet strains of sacred choral music. I am off to a slow start and might do better to reclaim my warm depression in the futon where Lindsay and Clare lie slumbering.

But I am trapped! The outside door to the study clicked shut as I entered, and there is no inside handle. It is much too early to arouse the household with pleas for help. For a moment I content myself with the sound of drumming rain; it discourages my hopes for today's parade. Then I try jimmying the lock with a Citibank credit card and spare key I find on the bookshelf. It works; I am in the hallway next to Don and Barbara's bedroom, but swallowed in darkness. I grope for another door, another door handle, another elusive light switch. My eyes adjust to the glowing Powerbook and pitch of night; thin outlines appear, and I fumble for what declares itself to be a doorknob, then twist it and ease down the hall to our bedroom, slip under the warm wad of covers, drift back to sleep as the snores of my daughter envelop me.

Yesterday reminded us that there is no place like home. We donned our foul-weather gear, braved the misting rains, and marched to the Hastings-on-Hudson depot for a late train to the parade. The trains were running on an unlisted holiday schedule, so we impatiently reversed gears and headed for the City in our Jetta, down the Saw Mill and Henry Hudson Parkways and along West Side Highway.

All was going well: the threat of rain trimmed the crowds, and we quickly found a parking spot at 61st and Amsterdam. We schlepped the umbrellas, cameras, and kids to Columbus Circle. There we found not only the parade but the CBS Television booth and the smiling mug of weatherman Mark McEwen. The kids slipped under a police barricade to find a spot with a reasonably unobstructed view of the parade between downpours.

Our return to the car an hour later found the dashboard wires splayed like a medusa. The radio was an easy mark, smiling big-as-you-please in a car with out-of-state plates, and street-parked on parade day. The cruel irony is that we had purchased the radio just two weeks earlier with the savings anticipated from driving to New York (instead of flying). Fortunately, the police were already filing a theft report on a van up the street. As we angled back to Hastings I swallowed my anger and the I-told-you-sos. Yet I realize that the loss of a radio is a small price to pay for the reassurance it has given us about our decision to move to Maine.

We are back home in Hastings, but not *home*. Clare is becoming more easily perturbed by her cousin Emily, in whose company she has spent over thirty hours broken only by sleep. They have ceased to cooperate or share, or speak without name-calling, and tears flow like the afternoon rains. Finally, convinced that they cannot "work it out for themselves," we enforce a time out. Clare accepts stories from Mommy in the bedroom, but Daddy is told to "just go away." With an hour of quiet attention, Clare recovers and returns happily to the weekend festivities.

Grandpa Ray has arrived in time for Tom Turkey with all the trimmings, but the real focus has become the granddaughters in their party dresses and curling irons and necklaces. My misadventures in the study, the expropriation of our car radio, our daughter's collapse have all provided us with much to be thankful for: we have a home, close at hand and free of violence, one that graces us with solitude and keeps the world at bay.

Writing has not come easily today or yesterday, and I suspect the problem lies simply in the disruptions of travel. I require—more than I would like to believe—a familiar and secure cubicle in which to think. Or, as the doubts surface, is my body really craving more rest? Or have I simply run out of ideas and the facility to express them?

The first Sunday of Advent, season of longing and loneliness. It speaks to me with a deep and resonating call. It exposes old wounds and wraps them in the All who dwells among us. We are brought low to a primal place of dependence upon God and neighbor, but not with Easter's brazen pride, where Jesus occupies center stage and the crowds go wild for salvation. Advent is about the here and now, about the tangible loss of summer's light, autumn's harvest, the dying down of families, and the retreat to our interior lives. We will be singing at Mass today, Jean Goldfine and Scott Bailly and I. We have learned and practiced the music, but I am still nervous, and grateful for their support.

Before leaving Hastings, Lindsay issued an open invitation for Don and Barbara to join us in rural Maine. Plenty of work, nearly enough pay. And we have a handful of juvenile diabetics who could use a residential social worker. I recounted my story of the diabetic in the ER. Barbara replied that "I'm almost sure his behavior is organic, secondary to diabetes. He's partly a victim. When blood sugars are skyrocketing and the brain is starving, the mind becomes muddled and tempers flair. Common courtesy goes right out the window and you want to scream and make menacing demands and have your own way." Barbara speaks from experience. She developed insulin-dependent diabetes during her first pregnancy and lost Baby Katherine shortly after birth. She has since struggled with depression, a career change (from research neuroanatomist to social worker), and motherhood (Emily and Avery are now four and two years of age, respectively).

Of course, Barbara has a point. My diabetic suffers emotionally from his chronic disease. And, for all I know, he may have recurrent pancreatitis. He is alcoholic like his father, and a product of that dysfunctional environment. He requires medical care on a routine basis, not simply in times of crisis, but he cannot sustain a responsible partnership with his doctor. He has no capacity for a trusting relationship, hasn't a clue about social decency. He is a victim, yes, but also a sociopath who needs firm limits and clear penalties as the foundation for human interaction. And I have grown weary of providing them.

After our return yesterday, I set out on the long run. Then I helped Lindsay tidy the house, which sealed my sense of homecoming.

The latest edition of "Maine in Print" was waiting in the mail bin, and its lead story hailed May Sarton at eighty. She lives, so it is reported, in York, Maine, in a home called Wild Knoll. She granted the interview while reading her poetry at a three-day conference at Westbrook College in Portland, where gathered many of her most ardent scholars, critics, and fans. They attempted to bring focus to Sarton's long and prolific career (forty-seven books to date) and to give her "the recognition and acclaim she has so long deserved." I would add "and craved desperately." I am not convinced by the columnist's claim that "Sarton's faith in her talent sustained her." She seems to have needed, too, crumbs of critical acclaim and the praise of her enthusiastic readership. I have read two interviews with May Sarton, and both indulged her despair over a lack of literary acclaim. The reasons may be valid: that her sensibilities are too European, that she is the victim of misogyny, that the power brokers of literary taste have simply, inexplicably, perhaps unwittingly passed her over. But a tone of whining destroys all sympathy.

DECEMBER

Whenever I am reminded of death—
and it happens every day—I think of my own,
and this makes me try to work harder.

※

JOHN BERGER
A Fortunate Man

The first window on the Advent calendar opens today. It is also World AIDS Day. How curious that, after spending this morning thinking about May Sarton, I was asked to read her poetry this evening for the AIDS Memorial Service at the Searsport Methodist Church.

I visited the home of Elena Moulton yesterday morning. She sat smiling in her overstuffed chair, bound upright by crisscrossed straps of cloth. Her arms and legs, reduced to loose flesh and bone (except at the ankles, speckled red with edema), hung limply like a marionette's. Her breath showed in the shallow movement of her ribs, muscle withered here, too, leaving only a bony corrugation over the lungs. Her familiar pink nightgown had grown stained (though without odor) from drool.

I let myself in, stepping over Fluffy, their shaggy little dog who parks at the entrance like a doorstop. Elena bubbles with excitement as I approach her, motioning for me to pick up the alphabet board and sit down. I learn that her brother from Connecticut came to visit, at long last, for a few hours last Friday.

He'll be back, obligated to return a brother he borrowed from the Harbor Lights Apartments in Searsport. So there are three brothers, and one very close by! I have indicated to Elena that I would like to meet the Brothers Moulton when they return. Could she arrange it? There is much to discover about this family; I envision a bit of storytelling, with Elena present and, I hope, participating.

I pick letters off the message board, and Elena and I assemble them into skeleton sentences. "Aide hurt my neck. My balance is fine. Appetite OK." She reprimands me for guessing a word before she completes it. A matter of pride. I check her answers against Harry's, who firmly insists that her balance is off; she can no longer assist with transfers and frequently, more easily than before, slumps to the side of her chair. Elena had been eating well until two days ago, when her cough and choking spells began to frighten him. Weekends are worse because their son John is around, and because the aides are not. It is unbelievable that we are looking toward another Christmas, with Elena clinging to life by her cloth straps, supported by the love and attention of her husband, the visiting nurses, and the home health aides. From her kingdom on a stuffed chair, she has kept her fear and disappointments and losses at bay. She defends her high ground with an insistent, expressive grunt and a ready bouquet of smiles and laughter. Today the smiles bloom as I tease her about Harry's awkward tries at pivoting—crippled as he is with rheumatoid arthritis. "You can't get good help anymore, Elena."

The holy water remains in the door panel well, and as I dip into it with each tug on the door handle, I bless the pilgrim's path.

The poem I was asked to read at the World AIDS Day program touched me deeply. I was dubious at first, because of its author. Though May Sarton's recent interviews have soured me, her journals prove that we share much in common: something she calls the "sacramentality of the routine." I wonder at her choice of so Catholic an expression. But I understand it to mean the safety, the sustenance, the salvific powers of the simple tasks we perform each day that have become second nature to us, demand no attention, and, like an old parka, comfortably cloak us against the biting winds of change.

Celebrating the little things. Before "the cure" for AIDS is found or an effective vaccine becomes widely available, the little things—offered with love—are all we have. Like walking in tonight's candlelit procession in remembrance of those who have suffered and died from the plague; like becoming involved in AIDS education or befriending a person (or family) who suffers with AIDS; like lending our voice to the swelling chorus of those who challenge bigotry and fear and ignorance. Enough of *my* words, I tell the forty people gathered in this cozy church. You, too, are part of the chorus. The Searsport High School chorus sang, and one of the students delivered personal remarks about a favorite aunt and uncle who were dying of AIDS. Then I read a beautiful poem by May Sarton, who exhorts us to counter our fears of AIDS—of contagion, of homosexuality, of the suffering of the young—with love.*

A gentle, powdery snow is falling, the first lasting look of winter. It is predicted for all day—a fitting but slippery stage for the Christmas Concert today in Camden. Tomorrow we will be in Belfast, performing the sweet, melodic lines of Charpentier and Palestrina and Vittoria, Old World carols from Germany and Austria and Italy, and a modern (1911) piece to close, Harold Darke's setting of "In the Bleak Midwinter," and, as an encore, a chorus from Handel's *Messiah.* Sandwiched between is our date at St. Francis to sing the Mass of the Second Sunday of Advent. And tomorrow evening we relight the family Advent wreath, with prayers I will awkwardly propose.

My writing yesterday morning was deterred by earlier events. At 9:00 in the evening I was called to evaluate a drunk in the emergency room. He had a potentially lethal blood alcohol of 406 but, more importantly, was displaying bizarre posturing behavior that he claimed to be seizures. "Alright," I told the ER nurse, "I'm coming in for an OB patient anyway."

The disheveled gentleman in the first bay was my age, thirty-eight years old but insisting he was forty. Every detail he spewed was drunken bluster or bold-faced lie. The "seizures" were curious events: he would announce a bad taste in his mouth, stretch out on the gurney trancelike, momentarily rise with wild staring eyes and arms repetitively pointing to some imaginary vista, and, seconds later, collapse. All of this in the passing of ten seconds. He would perform only for the nurses and doctors, though, not for the police, who (thankfully) waited outside the door, or to an empty stall. When he wasn't seizing, he would boast about his income or his prowess, complain pitifully about his years in 'Nam—with their shrapnel and surgeries and, later, the post-traumatic stress, make fists and shake them at passing nurses or attendants, blame the drinking on his divorce (rather than the other way around), moan his regrets and wail his willingness to reform, and come full circle back to a lame challenge that began, "If you're so smart, doctor, then tell me why . . ." I left after a repeat performance of the seizures to visit my patient in labor and delivery, and would later admit him.

I got home at 1:00 A.M., and did not so much as budge at the alarm. I returned to the hospital at 8:00, finished rounds, and learned that my drunken friend had signed out AMA (against medical advice) overnight. As I was leaving the hospital by way of the ER, who should roll in by wheelchair but last night's bad actor, requesting an X-ray of his ankle. I stepped into the hallway to meet him and settle arrears.

* "May Sarton to Ronald McClinton with my love, Feb 29, 1992," in *AIDS.*

"You had one last night," I reassured him. "You don't belong here; please go elsewhere for treatment. I'd recommend AA or a drug rehab program."

Glancing at his sad mother, he moped, "It's clear they don't want to help me here."

"*Can't* help you," I corrected him. "Help *yourself*. Stay off the booze. Quit blaming Viet Nam or your divorce or your bum ankle. If you would meet people halfway, there are plenty of us who would go the rest of it for you."

At Thursday morning meeting with Tim and Mary Beth, we talked of Tim's cutting back. A few days ago he had expressed a definite intent to do so. He would abandon OB and take off another full day every other week. We had tried an asymmetrical arrangement like this in the past, but it failed because the burden of responsibility fell disproportionately on the more available physician. Mary Beth asked how I felt about it, Tim's trimming of the sails, his scaling back. Her question struck me strangely, for it seemed exclusively Tim's decision. My own feelings must be buried, bunkered against the worst-case scenario.

And I have seen the worst case already, when my natural parents left me at an orphanage. Again, when I was thirteen, my father died of a massive heart attack. And again, after four troubled years of marriage, my first wife walked out during the second year of residency training. Tim's departure is set unavoidably against this backdrop. I felt as if a close neighbor, the kind you could borrow a cup of sugar from or holler to over a picket fence, was suddenly moving out of town. What would hold us together or reconstitute our friendship? Will it change utterly as a result? Another fear, as Tim adjusts himself in his chair: does it mean he is ready to bolt, or that he is settling down for a long chat?

I have always preferred partners, enjoyed a close working collaboration more than solo or committee work. It began in college with my best friend, Bill De-Mars; continued in medical school with George and Pete; persisted in my attempts at marriage (the first a failure, the second still miraculously alive); and reached full stride in my practice with Tim. We have been two rebels against the armored divisions of the American health care industry, two rogues on the margins, two friends committed to the trenches for too little pay, against an enemy that is neither death nor disease but boredom, indifference, and the comfortable life. What will become of me if I lose this friend, or if our practice topples from lopsidedness, or if Tim steals away in the night?

Mary Beth spoke of her work with the wives of sex offenders: "When you work in the muck, it spatters everywhere." It is true of every job like ours, where doors open onto private lives, and scars are revealed, and you hear the time bombs ticking. We need companions to share the grief and the strain and the self-doubt, to help repair the damage to each other's self-confidence and vow of commitment. But when a friend leaves, we have no place to turn but inward, where we face the dark alone. Is our interior empty, or is it full of knickknacks and inspirational messages, or does it replicate the parental home of wood paneling and oil-on-velvet paintings and discounted plastic parts? My worst fear is that I would find I had no friendship there at all, that I had been deceived. These are irrational thoughts, I know, based on a broken life that hobbles along from on encounter with betrayal and loss to another. This is how I am feeling, Mary Beth. Where do we go from here?

It was a day of mixed blessings. Despite drifting snows that fell throughout the morning and early afternoon, we sang the concert in Camden. Sixty hearty souls joined us in the Chestnut Street Baptist Church, the quintessential New England house of worship, replete with white clapboard, black shutters, and a towering steeple. It is always gratifying when the size of the audience exceeds that of the choir. There were no blunders, but little energy. I sensed a physical letdown from an exhausting week, and the beginnings of a tickle in the back of my throat.

At the end of the day, around 7:00, Lindsay and I hired a babysitter and walked down the street to a neighbor's Christmas party. It was surprising to find so many familiar faces: Dennis and Megan (parents of Clare's friend Evan, artists and brewers), Mike and Cathy (a fellow tenor in the Pen Bay Singers), Dale (hospice president and editor of *Down East* magazine), Bob and Cathy (piano tuner and librarian), Lib and Herb (owner of that venerable institution, Perry's Nut House). Others knew *me,* often as not through the hot dog spot on Channel Five News or my well-publicized forays into brewing. It pepped me up, this small band of revelers, made me feel part of the neighborhood, connected me as I imagine my father and Ernest Ceriani must have felt connected in their day, to their communities. Lindsay and I anchored ourselves in the kitchen, ate too much, drank copious amounts of ginger ale, and laughed like silly school kids. The bone-chilling walk home reminded us that winter is more than the season's artistic backdrop, and sent Lindsay into a fit of asthma.

Yesterday's concert at St. Francis was an emotional mirror image of the preceding day. The morning had gotten off to a good start, for we (Jeanie and the Medicine Men) sang well at 10:45 Mass, and afterward I successfully reversed the door on our refrigerator, which for me is a mechancial miracle.

Lindsay and Clare left for the *Nutcracker Ballet* around 1:00 P.M., leaving me a few moments of solitude before the concert. I occupied myself by doing the dishes, presoaking a load of laundry, and organizing the household trash for tomorrow's pickup.

At the concert, held in the parish church of St. Francis of Assisi, I felt at home. From the shadows of the sanctuary, the stained glass windows shone brilliantly in the low light of late afternoon; two Christmas trees stood alongside the altar, heavily laden with ornamental gifts from the congregation; illuminated stars twinkled overhead; red votive candles were placed on every windowsill, cradled in holly leaves and dotted with porcelain angels and Santa teddies (all too cute); and a manger (bedecked with strings of colored bulbs) was spread on the snow-blanketed front lawn. The church filled comfortably by concert time. Our opening piece—"The Song of the Birth of Our Lord Jesus Christ" by Charpentier—sprang to life, spry and lyrical, accompanied by a string quartet. We closed the concert with a beautiful carol by Harold Darke, a lilting, resonant, meditative hymn that sounded like a cello, its opening lines, written by Christina Rossetti, equal in beauty:

> In the bleak midwinter,
> Frosty wind made moan,
> Earth stood hard as iron,
> Water like a stone,
> Snow had fallen,
> Snow on snow,
> In the bleak midwinter long ago.

Never mind the botched Palestrina "Hodie," where one section drew the rest of us off. We recovered at the soprano entrance and never looked back. The concert *really* did not end in bleak midwinter. We had rehearsed an encore that was guaranteed to raise the rafters: the Hallelujah Chorus from Handel's *Messiah*. Tradition has it that, during the debut performance, King George stood up to rest his aching backside at precisely this point in the concert, thus establishing a Christmas tradition as enduring as the *Messiah* itself. But one can hardly sit through the piece, tradition or no. There is too much driving force, enthusiasm, soprano register. We sang it with as much gusto and vitality as our thirty-two untrained voices could produce.

Another concert behind us. Usher in the Yuletide season, get on with the holiday festivities and plans for the office party. The best is behind us, until Christmas Day.

It was ten degrees when I awoke this morning. At 6:30 A.M., steel-blue sky met matching snow at some invisible line, broken only by the black, twisted spikes of the neighbor's black locust trees. Winter creeps, too, on little cat's feet.

To my surprise, I spent most of yesterday with Clare. After morning appointments and noontime tea with Marc Stewart, I came home to find Clare watching *Beauty and the Beast* on video. Lindsay was entertaining guests in the dining room. I had missed Clare the day before because of Mass, the *Nutcracker*, and her nap that began on the car ride home and lasted through the night. Today she demanded my attention, and I willingly gave it. "OK, to Camden, but I need your help picking out Mommy's Christmas present," I insisted. But Clare had difficulty with the notion; What's in it for me? Why wait 'til Christmas? After a firm representation of our goals (and a compromise: I would buy her a candy treat after shopping), we started off on our adventure.

She did marvelously, tagging along from store to store, hiding between the racks of clothes, playing with whatever toys were within arm's reach. Only when it came to choosing Lindsay's nightgown did we come to loggerheads: she wanted a quilted, synthetic, flowered gown; I, a traditional flannel granny in pastel tones.

"Do you hate roses?" she asked baitingly. "Well," she continued, with an edge of irritation, hands on hips and head cocked askew, "if you don't buy this for mommy, I'm not inviting you to my birthday party. *And* if you don't buy this, daddy . . ." She kept upping the ante over my objections. Shouldn't we go with the natural fiber, Clare, even if the rose print is more colorful? Shouldn't we buy Mommy what Mommy wants? Fatigue was now setting in, as her afternoon naptime approached, and so we made the best of our differences: I bought the flannel gown. Clare collapsed in *The Owl and Turtle* book store next to the new releases, with loud and labored snores.

In the evening, Lindsay prepared a sit-down supper, which I blessed with the traditional grace "We give you thanks . . ." and a lighting of the Advent wreath. Later, she hurried to her hospice meeting while Clare and I contented ourselves with "projects." She painted my face (and her own) and created a collage of crayon scribbles, glitter glue, pasted feathers, and taped-on paper clips. Afterward, I supervised a bath. We had a marvelous jamboree of squirt-gun fights, hair lathering, and face painting of Mr. Potato Head and Rubber Ducky. I coaxed Clare into brushing her teeth, and she allowed me to trim her nails while we watched the rest of *Beauty and the Beast*. Too much excitement and fear ("I keep remembering the scary parts") kept Clare from falling easily off to sleep. By 10:30, I broke down and allowed her to climb into the "big bed" with me until Lindsay returned from her hospice meeting.

Yesterday was the Solemnity of the Immaculate Conception, a Holy Day of Obligation. "Holy Days" are those few great Catholic feasts in the liturgical year where the Church requires attendance at Mass. The Code of Canon Law (1246–1248) so assigns the following: Christmas, Epiphany, Ascension (forty days after Easter), Assumption (August 15), Corpus Christi, Mary Mother of God (January 1), Immaculate Conception (December 8), St. Joseph, Sts. Peter and Paul, and All Saints Day (November 1). But the Code also allows some liberties: the United States Conference of Bishops, in its wisdom and by approval of the Holy See, trimmed St. Joseph and Sts. Peter and Paul as days of precept

and transferred the solemnities of the Epiphany and Corpus Christi to Sunday worship.

I have always had trouble grasping or affirming these two propositions: a Holy Day of Obligation; the Immaculate Conception. Only yesterday, upon *listening* at Mass and consulting the Catholic Encyclopedia afterward, did I learn that the feast recognizes not the virgin birth but Mary's freedom from sin; in other words, it is *her* immaculate conception we celebrate. A feast commemorating Mary's conception was first offered in Constantinople during the seventh century, and in Rome by the ninth. But the Council of Trent (sixteenth century) sealed the doctrine by a decree that absolved Mary of original sin. It saw "the privilege of Immaculate Conception as the anticipated fruit of Christ's saving passion, death, and resurrection . . . Mary would be the first to benefit from what he would win for the whole human race."

It is Mary-born-into-perfect-sinlessness whom Americans honor as patroness of the United States. By the hundreds of thousands every year, they visit the National Shrine of the Immaculate Conception in Washington, D.C., in devotion and pilgrimage, and perhaps, too, as another stop on the Capital tour.

In his book *Crises Facing the Church,* Raymond Brown speaks of the Mary doctrines as the most devotional among Church teachings; for Catholics, the very image and thought of Mary inspires prayer. Since she was the first to respond to God's call, we pray the Angelus and seek Mary's intercession in t Church's search for vocations. Apparitions of the Blessed Virgin still continu do pilgrimages to the Marian shrines around the world where the pilgrims e miracles, and where the greatest of these is their own faith.

Last night I attended evening Mass. Why, I cannot say, except as a re the growing need for devotion in my life, for focused prayer. Mary-ahistorical of biblical personalties—symbolizes that need and po need begins in the search for a right relationship with God; it is ex cally on bended knee; it is veiled in silence; and it always leads o unanswerable mysteries of faith.

The cry for "Mommy" just rang out from the upstairs be I race up the steps and, stumbling over books and stuff lying still in the darkness. I hoist her from the covers tions ("I want *Mommy"*) and wedge her between Lir Bed. Then I softly pad downstairs, pour myself the begin playing our recording of the *Messiah,* and re

Last night, after returning from Mass, we br tions. I untangled the light sets in search of wire that had spoiled the entire string, all empty sockets and delicate bulbs, and neg

bedroom or help with the Sesame Street Christmas puzzle or companionship while she sorted through the ornaments. All of this taxed my patience, despite the supplemental graces I received from Mass, despite a Geary's Pale Ale, despite my mental preparedness for the holiday strain. Christmas has been synonymous with stress, at least in my parental house, and especially during the final years.

Was it apathy or apprehension that I recall? Was it the homecoming, gift giving, going to Mass, or the electricity of our moods converging? I cannot be sure; memories of those times tatter and tease apart. I only know that some of my worst memories linger there, along with the best. I remember how tensions rose in earnest in the years following my father's death, after my twelfth birthday and in the throes of my adolescent rebellion. The bitter, intoxicated fights between my mother and sister. What did they mean? Were they distorted expressions of love, or marks of disease, or products of the times? Amazingly, the anger would always blow over by morning, slept away and forgotten in our unspoken domestic policy of "live and let live." Covered and sealed as if the tempest had never roared, never roused my brother to tears or tossed me in restless sleep on the waves of each verbal assault that crashed below. When I finally realized that Mom and my sister were co-conspirators, that the fights were only alcoholic rage, that they wanted no truck with "solutions" or healing, the damage had already been done.

And so it is that, ten years into our new traditions, the old instincts die hard. I vow to talk about them with Lindsay this morning. I'll ask for her help and her patience and her understanding. Once the tree is up I can stand back and relax. There is added pressure on me this week: I am off-hospital, and now's the time. But I must use it efficiently, and lovingly, on behalf of the family for whom I labor.

A total eclipse of the moon was the celestial surprise of the evening. Edged out of the limelight at 6:15 P.M., the moon was back with a vengeance, blazing torch-like at 9:00 when our choir let out. The shadows on the lawn were stark and long, the snow iridescent blue. As one meteorologist noted, it is far easier to predict accurately these cataclysmic phenomena, moving in precise eighteen-year cycles, than tomorrow's weather.

Our furnace is getting its first taste of winter, running at a steady (and no doubt thirsty) clip because of a recent cold snap. In turn, we have been blessed resplendent etchings of ice on the lower pane of our bathroom window: sweeping ferns, fleurs-de-lis, delicate crystalline trumpets. Oddly enough, crystals on the *upper* panel are a homogenous layer of frost.

Julie returned to the office yesterday at my insistence. I had examined her a in the ER for a persistent bellyache. Laxatives and antacids and anal-

gesics had been tried in turn, yet she remained edgy, sleepless, and miserable. I have known Mamie for five years, and recognize how anxiety can twist her bowels. Her living situation over the past few weeks has been, by report, an emotional nightmare, but now she is back in the county and in the keeping of her son. "OK Mamie," I offer reassuringly, my hand resting on hers, "I'll prescribe something to calm your colon, but because we know that you have an aneurysm, we'll take a peek at it before you leave, just to be sure." I left for the office while the secretary scheduled an abdominal CT scan.

It confirmed my gnawing suspicion: the aneurysm had ballooned from a diameter of eight centimeters across to seventeen and had begun to leak into the retroperitoneal space (an often fatal complication). Two years ago the patient and her family had decided not to pursue a surgical repair, and her heart and lungs and mind were that much older now. After conferring with the son on the telephone, I prepared the family for eventualities, prescribed liquid morphine for the pain, and postponed telling Mamie the sobering news.

My invitation to the office today was meant to rectify that omission. I also wanted to discuss pain control, the need for hospice, and my desire to say "goodbye" before a rift in the aneurysm robbed me of the chance. Mamie was a peculiar sight, hunched on my examining table in her bathrobe and snow boots, with makeup plastered thickly upon her demure, innocent, deeply contoured face. I hadn't intended to tell her, at least not so bluntly, and had reassured the family of these intentions. But I at least wanted Mamie to know that I knew the cause of her pain.

She looked me squarely in my eye. "Doctor, is it going to burst? I'm not scared, you know. We all have to go sometime. I just hope it happens quickly." From the corner of my eye, I could see the son and his wife flinch, then embrace each other, and I could hear their whispers and the wiping and sniffling of tears. Would they feel that I had betrayed them?

"It likely will, Mamie. But I don't know when. It could happen anytime, whenever the Good Lord wills. I'm just thankful that the morphine is controlling your pain, and that your mind is sharp, and that you are in a safe place, well cared for and loved. I remember telling you two years ago, when you were hospitalized for a heart attack, that you were lucky to be alive. It was not only luck, of course, but plain stubbornness and a lot of family support. You haven't lost any of that, and I know you'll make the best of whatever time you have." She nodded without wasting words.

We talked about hospice, about the possibility of a family meeting, about what the final moments might be like, about home visits from now on. I said that Mamie or her son could call anytime. And then the next patient captured my attention, and the day led on.

On this day, in 1941, Thomas Merton entered Gethsemani Abbey, and died twenty-seven years later in Bangkok by accidental electrocution. His memory I honor today.

I know the jig is up, and I am spending the last few, quiet, focused moments of the month at the computer. Today will be a frenzy of UPS packaging, Christmas card writing (to beat the UPS deliveries), and last-minute shopping before I return to hospital duty next week. Then Christmas. I should resign myself to an absence, but cannot; too much happens around the holidays to forego commentary. There is always a tension between enjoying life and examining it.

I have two brief, shining memories from the day with Scott Bailly. Yesterday at noon, the employees gathered in the library to eat our salads and Italian subs, which Trudy had so thoughtfully procured for us. Somehow I came around to referring to Scott as George Bailey, owing, of course, to the obvious similarity in their names. It prompted a discussion of the movie *A Wonderful Life*, which has always annoyed Scott. "Too much, too much," came his critical cry (this from a man who devours garlic by the clove and relishes the flamboyance of baroque music). I had the same reaction to *Terms of Endearment*, which to me seemed to paw at the audience's heartstrings. What is the difference between the two? Why does one appeal to our emotions while the other seems to manipulate them?

I met Scott in 1986. He was working at a rural health clinic in Brooks, Maine, several miles to the north of Belfast but in a world unto itself. Scott had begun there eight years earlier; Tim and I had just been hired a day a week to see patients and supervise the physician assistants. Then, a year later, we persuaded Scott to join our practice in Searsport. My memory of him then still holds true: sandaled feet, pants with an elasticized waist band, a broad and brightly colored tie in jungle motif, reading glasses from the local department store, bushy mustache, and a Peter Yarrow hairdo that acknowledges the march of time.

Even then, Scott was a curmudgeon-in-the-making, a man bound to habit and quirk. He would fuss and putz over piles of winter wood, a batch of beer, variations in a bird song, or titrations in his bottles of allergy extract. He has hardened in his habits that include a morning jog with his neighbor Jean Goldfine; his tardiness to work; his noontime sardines; his nature walks at Moose Point State Park, a quarter mile down the road; and nature shows on TV in the evening with his wife, Debbie. He is a man of fixed speed, fixed capacity, fixed swings in mood. It is no exaggeration to say that Scott has defined the personality of the practice, with his Buddhist nature, his playful conversation that engages you between patients, the office music he has personally arranged, his colorful quips about black ice or "hardware" that causes the death of cattle, or his propounding of a unified theory of endorphins that establishes their ebb and flow, release and inhibition, as the driving force of the universe. This is how things work, Scott assures us, from acupuncture to allergy desensitization to the calm that enshrouds even violent death.

Scott is another Midwesterner, Fargo-raised but not Fargo-proud, the second son of a successful businessman. After college he escaped a certain future in the Rotary and Jaycees, and the expectations of his father and the high school class that voted him "most likely to succeed." He joined Vista and worked for a year in West Virginia, where he met Debbie. Scott describes it as the most desperate time of his life. He recalls the morning he learned of Uncle John's death. "I was in Pittsburgh and heard how he had gotten up one morning and died of a massive heart attack. I was devastated. I was working on my C.O. at the time, angry at everything but especially at a country that educated its young and sent them off to die in a stupid, senseless war. John's death threw me into profound depression. I didn't know how to react; didn't communicate with the family; didn't resolve it at all. He was the one I had always wanted to be like. He was jolly and overweight, smoked and drank, did everything wrong. He died at a crucial time when I, too, felt sentenced to death. When everything was being sentenced to death before it got a chance to live. I just buried myself in Vista, dressed in black, played Dylan and Leonard Cohen. Eventually Debbie became a source of support. More recently, in my work as a P.A., there have been so many people who have touched me. Every year I open myself up more and more. I'm more receptive, less uptight about what patients think of me, and willing to spend the time simply chatting with these fascinating people."

Scott's conscientious objection to the Vietnam War has been a metaphor for his life. He chased butterflies to escape the noise and confusion of his childhood home. He fled North Dakota and his family's high hopes and gravitational field. He became a P.A. to skirt the prestige and responsibility of a medical career. And he still retreats to the woods around his Swanville home, to the trails of Baxter State Park, or to the broad beaches at Cobscook Bay, preferring nature to all the amenities of urban life. I am indebted to him, his poetry and stories, his humility and passion, and his sensitivity, which is transforming my life simply by its presence.

So this, then, is my constellation of saints, made visible each day: Lindsay, Tim, Mary Beth, and Scott. I see in their lives a reflection of my own failings and inadequacies; I see through their lives a likeness of what I desire to be. They have taught me humility, the value of stories, and the indispensable truth that out of their love and companionship I am not alone.

Yesterday I finished the compulsory exercises for the holidays: shipping packages for my Mom and siblings and nephew, and shopping for Lindsay. Some impulse-buying lies ahead, but the major purchases are over. Gifts are so very hard. Maybe a magical notion lingers from childhood: If I only can give the *right* gift, every wrinkle will smooth, every wound will heal, and my empty heart will overflow with others' gratitude.

I remember the Christmas I bought Mom an expensive watch. As she unwrapped it, her eyes filled with tears; the *perfect* gift to show my love, and show it off. Except that it overshadowed all other gifts, including a foot massager that my sister had bought for Mom's aching, calloused feet. All was ruined, all was undermined, in a single pass around the tannenbaum. Christmas came crashing down, as it seemed to every season until we abandoned the effort four years later. Now I stay away for the holidays; wait, instead, for Mom's expected offertory. The check, as they say, is in the mail.

Money, as a gift, has its advantages: no lines at the gift exchange, no quibbling about who got a nicer present, no bother, really, in an Age of Convenience. And it is always appreciated, even by those who claim they are cheapened by it. I now admit that, with a little mouth to feed and a perpetual cash-flow problem, it comes in handy.

My insecurity has not deserted me. I obsess over gifts: are they enough or too much? Are they too sappy or serious or silly? Do they say what I have failed to say out of sloth or preoccupation or embarrassment, or because the truth is too painful? This year I bought Lindsay clothes, which she needs desperately and buys rarely except for an occasional splurge at an underwear sale. So I tried my hand at sweaters (a good bet in earlier years), a black alpaca wool cardigan and a mail-order heavy cotton crew in a color as close to eggplant (Lindsay's new passion) as I could find. But wouldn't earrings have been more personal, a dress more daring, Deruta pottery for the kitchen more exciting? I must lay down this burden. I have slowly learned, with Lindsay's help, that she remains supremely satisfied with whatever I give her.

Last night's wine failed to douse my headache and only accentuated this morning's temporal throb. Tylenol with codeine will provide relief for today's undertaking: "doing" the tree.

I am still alive, the tree is up, and nobody is dead. Praise the Lord Protector. In my family of origin, the tree symbolized everything traumatic about Christmas. It was the battleground where we opened presents; it was a lightning rod for the family's friction; it provided opportunity for contention about who would assemble it, decorate it, and dispose of it each Christmas. In later years we had a screw-together tree, the kind that enjoyed a wave of popularity after metallic trees went out of vogue. So convenient; no needles in the carpet, no danger of fire, no assymmetry to the shape. And it fell to me—the eldest male and heir apparent—to put it up. So I carry some resentment, some injury and defensiveness, as Lindsay and I prepare to raise our evergreen.

While Lindsay stepped out erranding, Clare and I brought the tree into the living room, lopped off the top, and secured the trunk in its metal stand. So far so good. Lindsay returned, and Clare scrambled for the ornaments. I strung the lights, then lifted Clare to hang ornaments on the higher branches. An ornamental teddy bear shattered when I inadvertently brushed it from its piney perch. Clare rushed to my defense—"Daddy, that's OK; we can get another"—and lent me one of her cherished glass crystals as a consolation. I realized how badly she must feel when *she* breaks something, whether we scold her or not. Lindsay played a Raffe Holiday tape, then joined in the decorating without so much as a critical word, note of rancor, or strong opinion.

What is wrong with this picture? Except for Clare's racing around like any normal four-year-old, and my failure to find the one dead light bulb that spoiled the string, the other shoe never dropped. Whatever waves of annoyance, insecurity, or pressure I was feeling never breeched the seawall. Instead, they lapped inside me and were noticeable only as a bit of chest tightness that denied me a deep, satisfying sigh. From here I can coast to Christmas.

Yesterday was comfortably full. Scott and Jean and I sang at Mass, and Tim made a guest appearance with his rowing partner, David. After lunch, Lindsay and I escorted Clare and Tim's daughter, Rozy, to the closest showing of *Aladdin,* at the Bangor Mall. I look forward to these animated extravaganzas that burst upon the silver screen, especially when Robin Williams takes a leading role. But *Aladdin* seemed a remake of *The Little Mermaid,* with the voices (and even the facial expressions) of Eric and Ariel substituted for Aladdin and Jasmine.

Afterward, we went to the Bangor Mall, and outside the Porteous Department Store we found St. Nicholas high on his throne, an accomplice to a photography scam aimed at the children who sought out Santy's knee. We resisted, despite a nudge from Ol' Nick himself. Clare, burying her head in Lindsay's coat, could not think of a thing she wanted for Christmas, so Santa pledged to surprise her.

It is disturbing to see such a graphic display of Christmas profiteering. Give us back Jesus in a manger, who could at least decry the plight of the homeless right here in the Bangor Mall, or hand out bumper stickers that read "Jesus is the Reason for the Season."

When we arrived home that evening, Tim and Cris invited us in for beer and sangria and a long fireside chat. I loved how this day unfolded, relaxed and informal yet sandwiched between the bustle and regimentation of the workweek. There are many jobs that might be more informal and flexible than medicine. But they would not fill my need for a purpose, a *role,* and a clear set of expectations. Yet, within the code of ethics, there is still ample room to be your own man, a great doctor, or both.

I realize that I have become a cafeteria-style doctor as much as I am a cafeteria

Catholic, picking and choosing what suits me. Many of us "in recovery" from (and of) our Catholic faith have a stripped-down system of belief, a skeleton cosmology. In beating our retreat from Mother Church, we packed light. We abandoned the rosary beads and Lenten fasts, blessings before supper, and the last threads of guilt that bound us to our annual confession. We shed every outward sign of Catholicism without realizing that God, in His mystery, had hooked us at an early age. Patricia Hampl once remarked of her rediscovered faith, "I wasn't fallen away anymore; now, magically, the Church had fallen away. What remained of its colossal architecture was a frail structure of wonder, long forgotten." Only now, slowly and self-consciously, have I begun to liberate a sacred domain that I had long ago abandoned to secular cynicism.

Midstride in the month, and a week and a half until Christmas. Tim's indecisiveness is bugging the hell out of me. At our brief Monday morning meeting, where we hand off the hospital baton, Tim suggested that the office hold its Christmas party at Nickerson Tavern, present awards, then return to the office for dessert and carols. It bothers Tim—it is not his style—to stand center stage and entertain others. He would prefer audience participation, even during his reading of our traditional Yuletide poem. I presume there will be awards, but we have not yet discussed the specifics.

My first anxiety attack of the season jolted us from sleep last night. It happened early in sleep and shook us from the books and journals and pillows that we had piled around us. As always, I bolted out of bed and hunched on the edge, clutching my throat, absolutely convinced that I had something lodged there. Best not to move lest I jiggle it down beyond the tracheal bifurcation, where even the intercessions of St. Blaise, Bishop and Martyr, would be futile.

Lindsay is of no help in this crisis: she either ignores the obvious (that I am choking to death) or shouts for me to see a psychiatrist. She is convinced that these spells stem from childhood trauma—a bloody tonsillectomy or errant fishbone or forced feedings that I have repressed from memory. After what must have been only a minute, I crawled back into bed hoping that Lindsay would forget the whole thing, minimize my brush with destiny, harp no more on the embarrassing recidivism of my attacks.

After picking up hospital duty, the pressure escalated: six patients in the hospital; five emergency room visits during morning rounds. Also, a call from the Adult Protective Services, who want to hear the poop on Mamie. Her daughter had lodged a complaint against the son's neglectfulness. She claimed that I had recommended that Mamie be hospitalized, but he refused it. She claimed that he had ignored his mother's need for oxygen and smoked inside the house despite his mother's emphysema. I haven't seen evidence of this. Mamie will die soon of her leaking abdominal aneurysm, though the last time I saw her (four days ago) she was pain-free, in no need of oxygen, emotionally prepared to die, and asking to do it at home. I recommended that APS widen the investigation, talk to other sons and neighbors, and find wherein the truth does lie.

Robert returned to the office yesterday, after several weeks of tests in Bangor. He has had CT scans of the head, chest, and abdomen; he had CT-directed biopsies and bronchoscopic washings, bone scans, blood tests, and an MRI scheduled for Wednesday. His large lung tumor must be growing in the meantime, but imperceptibly so. The cough persists as the only niggling reminder. Robert has retained a surprising amount of energy, and voices no complaints of chest pain or windedness. After two months with the specialists, he tells me he feels the need to reconnect. He requests my advice. "They told me, 'you have cancer,' then raced on with their medical mumbo jumbo; 'you can do this and you can do that, and we really don't know what to tell you,' and lost me cold."

So today Robert and I go over everything. I know only what the pulmonologists and radiologists have reported in their cryptic jargon. But I pledge to go the distance with him over the coming months. My talk with the oncologist was fruitful; Robert will be discussed at Tumor Board in two days, and from there firm recommendations will be made. He is a healthy man, but tumor had already spread to his regional lymph nodes and across to the opposite lung. He wants a cure and will take his chances with the pain and aggravation and the disfiguring effects of therapy. "So would I," I tell him. "You're retired. Bonnie and you are in good health, and you have time and a little savings to enjoy together."

I am aware of my pangs of guilt for having letting Robert's cough go by; I notice it especially as he and his wife bring forward the Offertory gifts at Mass, walking in faith with their God, and, by extension, the family doctor. A misplaced trust, it sometimes seems. The cost of unquestioned beliefs? I told Robert that I was sorry for not finding his tumor sooner. And I had hoped this would release me from my doubts and self-recrimination. It never does completely. Meanwhile, much work remains to help Robert through the turbulent times ahead, and to sift more thoroughly for my mistakes, and to help the legions of others who are in medical need and come to me for care, flawed as my skills may be, weak as I am. But I will give what I have to offer. As Mark the *pidvizhnik* said in *The Way of a Pilgrim*, "To pray somehow is within our power, but to pray purely is the gift of grace. So pray to God what is within your power to offer."

Two Christmas letters dashed off this morning to Bill and Therese DeMars and Bruce and Diane Malina. Bill is my dear old friend from college; Bruce, a professor of the same vintage. Now I am writing family and beginning the Brownian movement through seasonal correspondence to friends both far and forgotten.

Our office party is three days off, and we—Doctor Hughes and I—have not settled on the details. Tim is less convinced than I about the need for the rituals of reading our traditional parody of "The Night Before Christmas" and lampooning the staff with special awards. He would prefer something more spontaneous; let the evening flow rather than stifle it with our agenda. But ritual, to this Catholic mind, also allows one to express gratitude and favor where it has long been omitted, to act in spite of our inhibitions, and to celebrate in high style. Tim and I have work to do, but at least we are talking about it together.

Despite a draining week, I feel refreshed today after a deep and uninterrupted night's sleep. Yesterday morning I slept through the journal. A baby whom I had delivered the previous evening after thirty-seven weeks gestation turned sour during the night. We had feared respiratory distress but saw no signs of it except a slight rise in the respiratory rate and a disinclination to feed. The chest X-ray was normal. Oxygen saturation of the blood was an encouraging 93 percent on room air; blood sugar was seventy. Then at midnight the baby began to tug at its breathing, grunt, and turn dusky. I scowled when the nurse first called. She is a favorite of mine, quiet as a titmouse but with uncanny instincts and the courage to use them. She has attended hundreds of laboring moms, suckling babes, and pompous doctors behind the closed doors of our sleepy maternity wing. It is the foolish doctor who ignores or discourages such apprehensions, especially Polly's.

I had gone home to dispel that heavy, sinking, gripping feeling that lodges itself between my heart and stomach, in the region of the hypochondrium where doctors worry sick over their charge and play out worst-case scenarios before an imaginary crowd of jeering patients and colleagues and their own inscrutable conscience. Polly now alerted me that the oxygen saturation was falling: 87 percent on room air. I might have chosen another tack, such as ordering oxygen, to buy some more sleep, but that would not deflect the underlying process, which seemed to be playing out its hand with a poker face. I rose and pulled on my clothes from the pile at the foot of the bed, then called the neonatologist at the medical center. We discussed the usual possibilities: hyaline membrane disease (immature, unexpandable lungs) and sepsis. The chest X-ray argued against a diagnosis of punctured lung or congenital heart disease or pneumonia or a large hiatal hernia. Yes, I admitted, I'd feel more comfortable if we transferred the baby. Thank God, the transport team deployed immediately.

I trudged to the hospital and found, in the plexiglass isolette, exactly what the nurse had described: a dusky, grunting baby, chest tugging like the gills of a fish out of water. I awakened mom, explained our concerns to her, outlined the course of action I had already set into motion. She nodded her consent with heavy eyes that hid her alarm. My task now was to execute the plan: increase the oxygen concentration in the isolette; order a capillary blood gas, blood count, and sugar; prepare a transfer summary and copy the pertinent medical records. The neonatologist had also asked if I would place an umbilical venous catheter. It has been years since I've inserted one, and, since the baby was looking better (or so I convinced myself), I would save the stump for a more experienced technician.

I go back, in times like these, to ponder what my father would do, or the likes of Ernest Ceriani. Would they bull ahead, screw up their courage, do what needed to be done? Or would they ship out these little puffers, free themselves of the sickening worry, concern themselves with problems more within their purview? It is out of my hands, I realize. A large portion of neonatalogy, or the provision of any hospital service, is dependent on the self-assurance and skill of the nursing staff. But shouldn't I be more brave, draw upon the courage I once felt as a resident, when we never blinked at the long needles we drove into the bladders and spines and downy scalps of neonates, never declined a procedure seen once, under different circumstances, in the heat of an emergency? Have I lost the will? Am I slipping toward that stodgy inertia in which crusty old physicians wait at the bedside, cupping their patients' hands, too enfeebled to attempt anything more? I worry about this, feel the erosion of my skills and prowess, sense a betrayal of my patients' confidence. What wisdom weighs in the balance?

A report yesterday morning from Bangor: Baby Brandon is doing well. Our preliminary diagnosis of hyaline membrane disease has stuck thus far.

The week draws to a close. Yesterday I cleared my patients out of the hospital; today I must dictate the discharge summaries. No doubt the emergency room, or a bevy of urgent pleas from the office, will distract me from preparing for tomorrow night's office party.

Three long and momentous days away from the journal. *Scriptus interruptus* on December 19th was occasioned by a medical examiner's call at 4:00 A.M. A young man had been driving on the Marsh Road when he lost control of his car, crossed the midline, and flipped into the icy embankment on the opposite shoulder. The driver was thrown thirty-five feet into a ravine, broke through the ice, and was found lying face down, soaking in two inches of muddy water. The only mysteries surrounding the event: Did he drown or die of head injuries? And where was he heading at so peculiar an hour? He had been to a party until 1:00 A.M., had drunk excessively, and was given a ride home by a conscientious friend. His parents heard him rummaging around downstairs but drifted back to sleep. Then, inexplicably, he took his mother's keys and raced toward town in her 1990 Chevrolet Corsica. The telephone rang at 3:00 A.M. Was it he returning from a joy ride, foolish kid? No, Belfast P.D. "Sorry to disturb you, ma'am, but we've got some awful news about your boy . . ."

Saturday night, and the office party went off with only a hitch or two. Service was slow at Nickerson Tavern; we left an hour behind schedule but primed for the roast to follow. I offered a few words of praise for our employees, and presents for their labors on our behalf.

The last gift of the evening was reserved for Scott. When he came to us five years ago, he had been on the verge of receiving a Ten-Year Service Award at another health center. We hired him with no clinical *need* in mind, only the sense that he would fit well into our office. Over the past year we have joked about the Ten-Year Award, the missed opportunity, and the absurdity of it all. How could we, on the threshold of Scott's fifth year at the Searsport Family Practice, not honor him with the "coveted" Five-Year Award? We had a plaque engraved with the Latin *Amicus Medicorum Fidelis* (the doctors' friend) and presented it with some appropriate remarks.

The awards were to say what Tim and I say far too little: we appreciate our employees, recognize who they are and what they bring to our practice through their individual strengths and weaknesses; and we include them in any calculation of our worth and purpose. At previous gatherings, I have announced this openly and caused a squirm. Humor seems the more palatable method of expressing praise.

The party was a mishmash of personal preferences and design flaws. Tim chose to lead a scavenger hunt, asking us to find charts that exceeded two pounds, samples of urine, unpaid bills, checks in the mail, and the like. Lindsay and Bonnie ran a game show, their version of Jeopardy based on answers to topical areas about Searsport Family Practice. The most clever category was "medicines," whose entries contained the names or nicknames of each employee. All of this was good clean fun, nothing too sappy or sentimental. We even received gifts from Cathy and the office; Scott, the office tinker, was given a cap that said "Mr. Fix-it." The only real disappointment was our losing the chance to sing; I had asked Jean to join Scott and me about 9:30 P.M., but by 11:00 we were still embroiled in group games, and she left in frustration. I could have insisted on singing first but preferred to let the party take its natural course. Later, I apologized to Jean, but the regret lingers.

When you put a dozen eggs in one basket, some will break. I felt that I connected with too few of our guests, said too little of substance, failed to seek out those who were, for most of the night, tucked away in the corner by the eggnog and Budweiser Light. Next year we will likely juggle things around, gather in one of our homes, try something new. The party succeeded because everyone came and everyone stayed, and because Tim and I shared in its planning and execution, its unpleasantries and "the duty." It was imperfect, like everything else, but symbolic of our intention to do the right thing.

Winter Solstice. The longest night of the year howled outside our window. By the time I crawled into bed, it was nearly 9:00 and the sun had been down for five hours. It would not rise again for another ten. On my lap lay Anatole Broyard's *Intoxicated by My Illness,* illuminated by a solitary beam from the overhead spot. I could hear Lindsay reading bedtime stories to Clare in the adjoining room; the soft click of her consonants, the rising and falling of intonation, soon lulled me to sleep.

All Things Considered commemorated the Solstice with a book review on the lives and outlooks of Americans (some seven million strong) who work the night shift. Several curious comments: Some report that working at night helps them anticipate their death. Others appreciate the expanded horizon: if our thoughts are only as big as the sky, in the day we are limited to the edges of the earth, but at night we can see the universe. The Trappists rise for prayer at 3:00 A.M., chanting their glory to God while the traffic is light; they challenge Satan at the height of his powers and meet him on his own turf. As a Catholic stamped with an indelible image of Heaven and Hell, I am thankful for these foot soldiers who pray on the front line.

These two movements, the astronomical pivot of the earth and the spiritual trajectory of Advent, transect each other at Winter Solstice. This season I am reminded of them too little. But I have noticed, nevertheless, my almost imperceptible turn toward God. I have discovered that needs cannot be borne in isolation, or met by friendship alone, or fulfilled in marriage, or perfected through man's rational apparatus. Nor can they be satisfied through artistic or athletic acheivement, even fleetingly, as when voices rise ecstatically in song or limber legs hit their stride in the long run.

I ponder this development through the lens of faith in a season that longs for acuity. These Advent prayers amount to what, really? An acknowledgment of God's fidelity; thanksgiving for His graces; a plea for the dampening of temptation and for mercy at every turn.

It is 6:25 A.M. and not a single ray of light bleaches the eastern sky. Night's thick blanket wraps 'round and blesses this hour before releasing me, dove-like, into a bright new day.

There are two billion Christmas cards to write, with more return addresses added to the list each day. Two million presents to wrap, reconsider, and rue their ill-considered cost. Two hundred thousand seconds until Christmas morning, when Clare will rise supercharged to embrace the day. She has not been sleeping well; she seems unable to relax, close her eyes, lie still, and allow sweet sleep to come. More often than not, we have brought her into bed with us after exhausting the usual options such as bedtime stories, tales of Christmas past, good night kisses, photograph albums, and endless repositioning of "the guys," the lucky recruits Clare has selected from her platoon of stuffed animals.

Much is happening in our practice as the holidays approach. The ills of our patients gather in intensity. This tends to worry the patients less for their own sake than as a potential bother for their caregivers and an uncertainty for their families, who will put travel plans on hold. There is movement among our employees. Scott departs today for Connecticut; I discovered his gifts in my car as I left work last night. Tim will stay around until Christmas morning, when he leaves to visit his parents in Vermont. Tomorrow at lunchtime, in the office around a crackling fire, we will exchange gifts, goodbyes, and well wishes for the Yuletide. All is well. I feel happy, and very lucky, to have this extended family gathered around me and working together with such kindness and support and love. Alas, there is no way to acknowledge this delicate flower properly without risk of crushing it. So I will simply enjoy the Christmas party and let come what may. Now, with only seventy-five minutes left to write my cards, I must leave these thoughts for a later reckoning.

The last box on the Advent calendar will be opened today by Clare's nimble fingers. Her eager anticipation has translated into insomnia and a nightly pass to the Big Bed. Tonight, of all nights, we must bank on it. An unexpected light dusting of snow yesterday brought Belfast a white Christmas. This was the first time in nine Maine winters that the outcome was in doubt. Thank the good God, who hears our supplications.

I spotted Ralph Wiley today, making his High Street circuit in a wheelchair flying great fluorescent flags stiffened by the frigid air. Only here, in our Belfast, does Ralph keep vigil over the community; not in Camden or Bar Harbor or Kennebunk. Nearly every day, regardless of the weather, he sets out from Bradbury Nursing Home for his far-flung posts: Doug and Ray's Service Station, the corners of High and Main, the gift shop at Waldo County General Hospital, or the gates of City Park where he often lingers on warm summer afternoons. Mum's the word as he perches motionless on his amputated stumps and watches for hours as the city flows by. The wayward resident can find no more reassuring sign on his return: there is Ralph; he must be home.

A telephone call from the medical examiner's office interrupted our supper. Could I attend a highway fatality? I graciously declined but offered them my partner's beeper number. How unsettling are these calls! Death is a ring away. Since I am here, talking on the telephone, it is not me this time around. But for *someone* in Waldo County, the jig is up, and the possibilities narrow to twenty-five thousand. It is not Lindsay or Clare, who are coloring dot-to-dot in the living room, nor a friend of ours we just spoke with and agreed to meet for pizza tonight. Everyone else is fair game, and I worry about who my partner will find, ghastly and broken alongside the icy blacktop, and whose disbelieving, wide-eyed family he will confront on the day before the day before Christmas.

Now I must write a Christmas card to George and compose a note for Lindsay before the day warms up to its nervous pace.

Christmas comes but once a year. Now we can step back, let embers die, silence the solemn chanting, extinguish the Christmas candle-bags, finish the last drop of eggnog (which will vanish soon from every store), pack away the gay baubles, disperse the carolers, and get on with the "bleak midwinter" as the frigid and blessed month of Janus approaches.

Christmas Day was good enough. Clare's reticular activating system woke her at 7:00, and she stumbled downstairs in groggy-eyed wonder. A bright yellow beanbag chair, a Barbie-like doll of Belle (from Disney's *Beauty and the Beast),* and a Troll Box all bore Santa's insignia. One of her favorite gifts was a jewelry box laden with my mother's costume jewelry. Clare's loudest peals of delight came with the unraveling of the Mousetrap game, until we discovered that it contained two of the assembly parts #12 and none of #1.

It took two hours of snipping, thrashing, sorting, sampling, savoring, and reflecting to plow through our mound of gifts. The pace included frequent breaks for coffee and a nibble on the Danish Pecan Kringle a friend had shipped to us from Larsen's Bakery in Racine, Wisconsin. And such *music!* We listened to selections from Christopher Hogwood's recording of the *Messiah* and a sampling of chants and carols from St. John's College Choir. Lindsay gave me four marvelous books, including May Sarton's *Plant Dreaming Deep,* a book on saints, Marina Warner's *Alone of All Her Sex,* and the Audubon Society's *Field Guide to North American Trees.* She also gave me a shaker-knit cotton sweater and a stocking full of Christmas favorites, including Flavigny Violet Pastilles, Cavendish and Harvey Licorice Comfits, Curiously Strong Peppermint Altoids, and Perugina chocolate-covered cherries. In return, I offered Lindsay clothes and books and verse I composed on a card with an angel sprouting butterfly wings:

> I will miss you in Paris, your eloquent French,
> Eating chocolate croissants on a Luxembourg bench,
> Admiring the colors of La Sainte Chapelle,
> Remembering *our* glass in the bath in the "ell."
>
> But tending the home fires your lover will stay,
> Busy with Clare while her mother's away.
> And here, just a token, to blow on a spree,
> Is the money I earned from a late 'xaminee.
>
> I will miss you in Paris, but thrill in your joy.
> And when you return, can we make us a boy?

Inside the card was the blood money for my services on a recent medical examiner's case, which, at the time, I dedicated to Lindsay's Paris trip. The money is negligible, but the income is "extra," as is the expense of her upcoming trip, and the sacrifice it deserves. At Christmas time, seven years ago, I first proposed that we should start a family, and after our European vacation the following summer (and several months of therapy) we did. Perhaps a sentimental nudge will work again.

In my family of origin, opening presents on Christmas Eve stood emotionally apart from every other holiday event. We would gather around the tannenbaum, each of us clutching our Kodak Instamatic and our garbage bag, each momentarily suspending whatever conflict preyed upon our soul, each certain that we were blessed, and blessed without bounds. It was never in doubt that Christmas would reward us, anoint us with a material privilege, fulfill our dreams, and leave us with only an aftertaste of guilt for having been given too much—more than I deserved, surely, and more than my equally deserving friends; more than the basic need of the average American, and far more than the poor of the community who join us at school and in church and around the neighborhood haunts.

It is probably this flickering flame of embarrassment that kindles my community spirit. I am learning, gradually, to separate good fortune from a sense of unworthiness. I feel the warmth of love, too, amid the guilt.

After an exhausting morning, we made the customary calls to family and settled down to prepare Christmas dinner for the Stewarts. Another tradition, four years old: leg of lamb and plum pudding with hard sauce. I fetched a long table from the office, one that could accommodate the eight of us. We had a frenzied, satisfying, chatty, and reflective time. The kids behaved angelically, which allowed the parents to gab about upcoming moves and the seasonal stresses.

Early that evening, after we waved goodbye to the Stewarts, loaded the dishwasher, snuffed the candles, and unplugged the Christmas lights, we set out for Searsport to call on Belle Martin, a nonagenarian whom I met in the early years of my practice. She had adopted us as family. "Auntie Belle" had no other plans that Christmas (how often we were reminded!), though her collection of greeting cards suggested that she was not forgotten. We talked at a Gatling gun clip for nearly an hour, covering all the reasons she *must* move to safer environs, such as a nursing or boarding home, as much for social reasons as for the plain fact of age. Something *will* happen, Belle; better to decide on the future while you are healthy and have the time and money and mental acuity to choose your options. I will arrange a visit for her at the Debra Lincoln Home (formerly called the Home for Aged Women), which in my view would satisfy her social bill.

So concluded our day. On the way to the car, yawning and stumbling, I glanced at the driving snow in the streetlights. It was quickly accumulating, slick beneath our feet and the treads of our tires. It made for a romantic and spectacularly beautiful, albeit treacherous, Christmas drive home.

The alarm sang its *hodie* at 4:30 A.M., but my brain was powerless to respond. I lay rigid in my warm bed under an electric blanket and imagined every virtuous excuse for my indolence. By 5:30 I was able to muscle myself down to the silver screen with a mug of Christmas coffee in hand and several squares of thought to quilt into today's report to the accompaniment of Geminiani stringing his angelic baroque.

Sam called me for a run yesterday: twelve degrees at midafternoon. I bundled in layers but still needed half the run before I warmed enough to remove my stocking cap and gloves. Sweat-soaked hair froze on the backs of our heads, and our lungs ached from the arctic air we gulped with abandon. Our shoes crunched quietly against the snow, austere hues streaked the low-lit sky, a heavy stillness hung on objects frozen in the passing dooryards, and ice floes formed, broke free, and reformed in the tidal basin of Belfast Bay. Sam and I dropped our pace to a crawl, but still the run drained me and contributed to a sluggishness that persisted all day, adding a pleasant but curious stiffness to my joints and a deep ache to my muscles. I haven't run for weeks and deserve the penance.

There are three more days until the new year and I am resolute to get Christmas cards out by then. Yesterday I procrastinated for an hour by cleaning my desk. Now I intend to launch several cards a day until the duty is done.

The Year 1992 went out like a lion. By the 30th I was utterly worn down by the events "ticking off" (as former president Bush was fond of saying) in rapid succession. Most were minor, but they had the cumulative effect of striking home hard. I inserted my second set of Norplant rods, a set of six tiny contraceptive rods you position under the skin, above the elbow, with a large-bore trocar. Only its size resembles the original instrument, which the French had named for its three-sided shape. The instrument was used to siphon off the excess fluid of dropsy. The patient asked me how many of these procedures I had performed. "We're only getting started," I replied, deflecting the point of her question. "But I have studied the technique, and it's a simple procedure, not unlike others I have performed a thousand times." Fortunately, the operation went flawlessly and afforded me a focused half hour in the midst of chaotic afternoon.

I spoke with a new patient about her first pregnancy. She was married, insured, intelligent, a woman with choices. And she chose us. This should not matter, of course. I bridle at my insecurity, at this worst sort of professional pride that measures success in terms of the caliber of one's clientele. The poor and destitute need my services far more than the well-heeled, literate, and employed. Most patients, I know, will not appreciate my skills or understand what sets me apart from the rest. They read in me what they like: the old-fashioned generalist, a pious Catholic, their successful son, a young maverick, a sympathetic ear, or just one of the boys. It is still nice to have a patient *choose* you when they can afford the more expensive alternatives.

I try to remember that doctors must coddle patients and attend to their needs. Both. Ultimately, the patient will judge your success. In the meantime you concern yourself with the quality of the relationship. It is a sacred relationship, founded on trust and on the humility of the doctor, who is wise always to listen to what the patient says is wrong before he takes off in pursuits of his own.

Last evening I was detained at the hospital by an old patient of ours, Buddy, who had arrived by ambulance with a heart rate of twenty-six and intermittent mental responsiveness. Atropine and epinephrine were tried without benefit, and the cardiologist could not be reached. When I walked into the ER, Buddy was in Bay 4 surrounded by ambulance attendants and nursing personnel busy with their chest leads, IV tubing, blood gas kits, and oxygen saturation meters. The physician assistant who first responded to the wife's call was also there; he had found Buddy on the bathroom floor, summoned the ambulance, and accompanied the entourage across the channel by ferry and up Route 1 by ambulance. All in an hour's time.

"Why the heart block?" I wondered aloud. Myocardial infarction? electrolyte disturbance? medication overdose? The first set of labs were inadvertently drawn upstream from the IV site, and were thus useless. I didn't trust the initial potassium of 6.6 or the normal cardiac enzymes. But the second and third serum samples, drawn from the femoral vein and internal jugular, reported even higher serum potassium levels of 9.4 and 9.3.

In the ICU, the cardiologist had arrived, and immediately began to thread an electrode into the right chamber of the heart. The temporary pacemaker began to capture beats, and the heart rate rose to eighty. I followed *The Washington Manual*'s recipe for treating hyperkalemia: ampules of sodium bicarbonate were pumped through the IV, ten units of regular insulin were administered by vein, and Kayexalate (a resin used to bind potassium) was administered through a nasogastric tube. Gradually the potassium fell, Buddy's indigenous atrial pacemaker took over, systolic blood pressures rose above a hundred, urine trickled from the Foley catheter, and the patient rose combatively into the scrambling arms of nurses and doctors. I kidded Charlene, the evening supervisor, that she should lead Buddy in guided imagery. She located a supply of limb restraints instead, and sedated the patient with Phenergan.

By 11:00 P.M., when dictation was done and the last order cross-checked, the OR called with an urgent message for me to assist at an appendectomy. The patient was twenty-four years old, the son of our nursing director, who was home on holiday leave from Case Western Reserve University. Fortunately, though the appendix was hot, it was not ruptured. An hour later, as I pulled on my street clothes in the dressing room, the circulating nurse slipped a message under the door. The ER had a probable admission: forty-five-year-old woman with unstable angina. Another hour of history taking, body probing, order writing. Finally, slaphappy with fatigue, I stepped into the frigid night air and drove home. All was silence save for the crunch of compacting snow, the creak of the car door, the squeaky, stiff rubbing of the steering wheel and vinyl seat, and the car wheels drubbing on the frozen asphalt. Not a headlight between the hospital and home, and I dozed off moments after stretching out beneath our flannel sheets.

By the morning, Buddy's potassium was a respectable 6.6, he was making puddles of urine, and he had recovered a tenuous grip on reality. The boy-appendix was serenading the nurses with his guitar and the bravado of that uninhibited age. The lady with unstable angina was free of pain but not of her addiction to cigarettes. We discussed it long and hard; I accepted her reassurances and prescribed a nicotine patch. By 11:00 A.M., the hospital ranks had swollen by two: an old woman from the boarding home with influenza and a newly identified lung mass; and Bernitha, who returned to the Hospice Wing to die of her lung cancer. Busy work, this, but at the same time consoling, rewarding, and reaffirming of the unheroic nature of our job.

I enjoyed teaming with the cardiologist and surgeon last night. It is fine with me that they should take the lead, the lifesaving role. I was just happy to be there, secure within my limits, versed in the rules, comfortable with the roles and the players involved. There is something to be said for crisis medicine, the flush of adrenalin, decisive action, and focused aims. But the thrill could not hold me for long.

I was happy to be out of the saddle by 5:00 P.M. Scott and Debbie came over to share a New Year's Eve meal with us (*pad thai* and hot shrimp soup combo), and we cashed in the chips by eleven. But an hour later the telephone rang again, and at 1:52 I delivered the third New Year's baby in the state, little Ginger, who crowned occiput-posterior and was delivered, as they say, sunny-side up.

This Advent has struck me as no other has. It has become for me a season of preparation, not one of waiting. In other years, I succumbed to the solitude and interiority of the season, dwelt its darkness, lay dormant, waited for the Savior who would deliver me from evil. But I see now that the challenge is to prepare for our given role, however unheroic or unproductive or undignified it might seem to be.

I was once invited to attend a local symposium and speak about the concerns of the dying. My assigned topics were living wills and organ donation, but I also wanted to set the record straight. Dying patients and their families often ask the doctor to predict the impossible: How much longer? when should the family come? and why me? "Why you" is the bargain for having been born. Because dying is the inextricable conclusion to life. This is harsh reality, but the shock of it is merely the result of our successful efforts to segregate, medicate, and ignore the fact of death.

But I thought to appease the audience with three questions a doctor *can* be expected to answer: Will you tell me the truth? will you be there when I need you? and will I suffer? There was a time when doctors could offer little more than a visit and a diagnosis. These were essential acts, and they remain the pledge of every good doctor. But the question of suffering remains the most troublesome of the three. In the bureaucratic age of hospice, it has been pruned to a focus on pain. Our instinctive response to pain is "spare no morphine." But what of the suffering that comes with saying goodbye forever, with losing control over one's livelihood, one's body, one's mind, with imagining the grief that will follow in the wake of our death?

I remember a patient of mine, Roy, who seemed ever on the verge of dying from a blood dyscrasia. He never squirmed at the thought of it, but rather, with the deep consolation of his Christian faith, often spoke of his need to be "punctual for the appointment." For Roy, the worst kind of death was the one that destroys a family. And that was precisely the fuse his family lit on a cold November night, with an argument between a visiting son and the resident daughter. Whatever substance lay in either claim, Roy could stomach none of it. Somehow he pulled himself from his hospital bed, clad only in flannel pajamas, and stole into the night. He found shelter in a concrete culvert some four hundred yards from his house. The family searched the country roads for nearly three hours before Roy finally wandered back. I asked him that night why he had decided to return. Being a practical as well as a deeply spiritual man, he complained that "it was just too damned cold out there." But he knew also that his family still needed him. Somehow he found the courage, made the time, to help them before he died.

Advent and death share strange sympathies. Both are seasons of longing: we wait for God to enter our kingdom, and for the moment when we will enter his. Both cast the world into deepest dark, when life begins to wither, whole families are tested, and we cry out from the pain of absence. But Advent and death bring us, ultimately, to a proper sense of relation where we can discover our dependence upon neighbors and our place in the universal scheme. For those of us with any foresight or inkling of the changing seasons, they roundly warn us to prepare for leaner times ahead.

The privilege of my work lies in how frequently I can encounter death and appreciate its demands. John Sassall, a Welsh physician whom I came to know in John Berger's *A Fortunate Man*, once said that "whenever I am reminded of death—and it happens every day—I think of my own, and this makes me try to work harder." Doctors work not only to postpone death, which they know to be a futile though profitable enterprise, but also to buy time for their patients who have not yet finished preparing.

There are workshops and professionals who can sell you insurance, plan your retirement, arrange the funeral, and execute a will; most states now require that you at least consider a living will and an organ donation. But the most important preparations are those to which Roy returned in his final hours: the readiness of one's heart, and release from one's familial entanglements.

Winter

☀

THE WATCH

I scurried past him in the hospital cafeteria, the solitary figure who nibbled his lunch and studied the cigarette smoldering in his ancient hand.

"That's Frank," someone whispered with a nudge. "He's been here longer than the hospital. Still drives to the office every day for a few colds, walk-ins, older folks mainly. Since the wife died, he has nothing left but his old habits."

On those blustery winter mornings, I would dodge him in the mail room, the Slow Moving Vehicle who had come to claim his fliers and announcements. The Credentials Committee had denied him every hospital privilege save his cubicle. He would hover near it, stalled in the flow of traffic, while he creased papers into the pockets of his flecked gray polyester suit, or threaded them through the "V" of a blazing canary-yellow sweater. After morning rounds, I would spy him again as I breezed through the front door, his shiny pate and bristly mustache poking over a newspaper in the hospital lobby. That was Doc Dennison, one of the old guard who passed nearly as unnoticed as the time of day.

Occasionally one of Doc's patients would come to me for a second opinion, dragged by a distressed relative who feared that "mother was slipping." So it was that I met Mabel Towey. I had delivered two of her grandchildren; praised them fairly with the coos and cunnin's (as in "ain't she cunnin'") that befit all newborns. Thus did I earn the trust of her son; he returned the favor by delivering his mother to me.

Mrs. Towey was a frail, toothless soul who plainly displayed, in her furrowed face and tattered rags, the erosions of a lifetime in poverty. I set about discarding her "kidney pills," which she squirreled away in yellowed boxes bearing the archaic names of Ser-ap-es and ethycrinic acid. In their stead I substituted the latest drugs and ordered sophisticated studies, not noticing the pinch of their expense. Fortunately, Mabel's kidneys held their ground over the ensuing months, and her blood pressure showed me the courtesy of a favorable response.

On New Year's, the "toothache" in Mabel's left shoulder unmasked itself as true angina. A heart arrythmia had tipped her into failure and sent her family mad-dashing to the ER.

They would keep a tireless vigil outside the ICU, through the initial heart attack, the waves of recurrent chest pain, and the succession of complications that included fluid on the lungs and failing kidneys. Mrs. Towey survived all this and seemed to progress without further incident through her physical rehabilitation. Two weeks later, in anticipation of her discharge, she underwent a modified treadmill test. The only worrisome finding was a dragging tongue from her profound fatigue.

That night, Mabel was visited by incomparable chest pain and a clutch in her throat. Her family reassembled outside the ICU, as inside we worked feverishly to establish venous access, push the rounds of cardiac medication, and maintain her breathing. It was no good. Though Mrs. Towey lingered, her face never regained its color or her hand its grip, and she slipped without struggle into a deep coma. Organs fell like dominos. Each received a full measure of concern and the ponderings of a specialist. But on the twenty-seventh hospital day, Mabel's heart gave out with a flurry of ventricular beats that widened before our eyes into slow terminal rhythm. The code was sounded but our efforts proved futile. Mrs. Towey was pronounced dead at 2:50 P.M.

We removed the artifacts of our care and prepared the deathbed for its last gathering. I ushered the family in, offered a few awkward words in the doctor's Latin, and let them be. My backward glance caught the angular faces, taut lips, and averted gazes. What a terrible silence they made, their hearts pierced and outpouring with love for the stricken matriarch.

Time passed and all memory of that day faded. I returned to my well-appointed schedule but took no notice that Frank Dennison had abandoned his. Suddenly one day, the receptionist interrupted me for his call. A quavering voice at the other end pleaded for help. Mabel's son was bullying Dr. Dennison on the hospital grounds, accusing him of the murder of his former patient, riddling his sleep with telephone calls, and threatening him with a lawsuit, or worse. Could I help him; did I know of a way?

"The son trusts you, admires you, I know he does. I don't know where else to turn and I . . . I can't go on like this. If you'll meet with the son, I'll drop off my office notes . . ."

I flinched at the thought of another imposition, another innocent demand on my free time, but what else could I say? "Please," I interrupted, "you needn't explain; I'm happy to help if I can."

The meeting was held, as arranged, four days later in the hospital library. I arrived early to review the office notes that had remained sealed in my briefcase these last several days. They were attenuated entries, scrawled in custom shorthand, more suitable for jogging the memory than aiding in any legal defense. With the care of an archivist, I leafed through pages that documented a bygone era in medicine. I ruminated on the outmoded drug list, the conspicuous inattention to health maintenance protocols, a seeming stance of nonaggression toward the encroachment of disease.

But the notes sketched ten years of a faithful, fruitful relationship, doctor with patient, the kind that all of us aspire to and claim as our heritage. The serum chemistries and blood pressure readings and prescriptions all flowed in a logical order. Had every fact been recorded, every circumstance fleshed out, would they support the general plan of care? No irrefutable tenet of science seemed to have been breeched, and so I sighed, heavily and long, for having been spared a conflict in the old doctor's defense.

I pushed back my chair and glanced at the sober, magisterial faces that hung on the walls around me. Doctor Emmuel Johnston was there, modestly recalled by the epithet "Suggester of This Hospital." Doctor Gerald Hobbes, a "Lecturer, Author and Pioneer in the Field of Radiology," held court with his fixed, wire-rimmed gaze. What did they know of these unpleasantries; what would they utter now, in judgment or sympathy or scorn? Were the times so different, their conduct so unblemished, that they could not cast sympathetic eyes upon our prickly scene?

The contemplative silence was broken by the son's nervous rapping at the door. I motioned him in, and he took a chair opposite to me at the table.

"Bobby," I stammered, once we had inquired after the children, "Doctor Dennison gave me your mom's records. I've looked through them and could find no obvious wrongdoing. He used medicines that might be considered old-fashioned, did not push your mom toward the tests that I later performed, but on the whole he gave her very good care."

"But Old Doc, he never really *did* care. He counted her pills and took her money and pushed her out the door. How many times did he pay a call when she took sick?"

True, I could not remember him ever visiting, but I understood that he had learned of her hospitalization only in those final, difficult days. "I can't answer for his sociability, Bobby, only his medical care, and that seemed appropriate."

"I know Doc killed her, he *killed* her. She had been slipping for a long time, and he just stood by. But he's going to answer for it in court, goddammit." The son lurched forward in his chair, fuming with anger, his fingers flying open from a clenched fist like a skittish gunslinger.

Against Doc Dennison's better advice, I fanned out his office notes on the table before us, the pages sticking to my trembling fingers.

"See for yourself. He knew she hadn't much money, accepted her stubborn ways, and cared for her anyway the best he could. There was a limit to what anyone could have done. She lived a hard life, didn't get many breaks, battled diabetes and blood pressure and cigarette smoke for too many years. I know that Doc Dennison really *did* care for your mother, even though it wasn't his manner to show it. And she must have liked him, too, for as many years as they hung together. Patients and doctors decide on each other, Bobby, and both take their chances."

He sat fixed in his chair, eyes darting, limbs coiled. Suddenly he bolted upright and began pacing in a narrow arc behind his chair like a dog on a tether, poised against any intimations of reason.

"I'm really sorry your mother's gone," I chanced again. "In the hospital, we did everything we could. Still, she slipped away. Her old and ailing body would carry her no farther. Now all of our collective anger cannot roll back her life. It is a hard and terrible thing when a parent dies, as my father did when I was a boy. It is hard at any age, under any circumstance. All our lives they were there for us; suddenly they are gone. You have a right to be angry, Bobby, but please be fair to an old doctor, who shared your mother's friendship and respect and did his level best to help her."

The pacing slowed, and in time Bobby spoke again. The words were softened with kindness, and replayed his mother's final days in the hospital, the last year when she took sick, her life of toil and tenderness in the trailer on Back Belmont Road, her work as a "throater"* on the assembly line at the poultry plant, her hanging laundry in wintertime and the Christmases she always made good for the kids. An hour raced by, and the conversation drifted toward home and family. Finally we rose in one motion to make our goodbyes.

"We can sit with these records again," I offered. "Or you can file a lawsuit, if that's your choice. I don't know how I will feel when my mother dies, Bobby, but it won't be far from your own sense of anger and emptiness and grief. Let's talk again; will you come see me at the office?" We walked out of the hospital together, squeaking on the snowpack outside the hospital's main entrance, and shook hands goodbye.

The following day I called Doc Dennison to apprise him of the meeting and to offer words of comfort. He thanked me effusively for the generosity of my time.

"Doctors these days are too godawful independent. We stick to ourselves

---

* The job is named for the action of ripping the trachea from a chicken's throat.

and let the devil take the hindermost. And if you're unlucky enough to *be* the hindermost, it's too damned bad. Someday I'll reward your kindness. No, *no*," he insisted over my protests, "I won't forget you and what you've done for me."

I simply performed my professional duty, I later reasoned, took the higher ground, the easier path, the doctor's more natural role as helper. I was *not* the one, as the gospel hymn goes, "standing in the need of prayer." For me, it was reward enough to watch one man pass from crippling anger to supplicative grief, and help another find peace in his dreams.

Several months later, five days before Christmas, a package wrapped in plain brown paper arrived in the mail. It was identified only by the initials "F.R.D." in place of a return address. Doc Dennison and I had spoken not a word in the interim, avoiding even a nod of recognition that might have betrayed his shame. I opened his gift at the appointed time, as we emptied stockings and whittled away at our private mounds of Christmas presents. Inside was a greeting card with the printed message "Happy Holidays," and a jewelry box that contained the finest watch I have ever owned. Over my wife's objections, I kept it. These several years later, I still wear the watch with pride and privilege, and strive to earn the right to be its keeper.

The watch has become a symbolic reminder, a memento of what is expected, what is possible, within the life of a professional community.

Throughout our careers, doctors publicly conceal a secret, darker side of our soul where, banished, lies our lingering guilt, an embarrassing mistake, the intrusive fantasy, flashbacks of a momentary weakness, or waves of despair that lap at our pride and self-confidence. Though we live in dread that our secrets will become public, we gape with the curious crowd every time a colleague is exposed. We lock our dark side away, in the back of our minds, then feel the creep of its shadow over the mess we've made of a professional interaction, the stories we confess to a friend, or the misdeeds of a colleague we have lately discovered. An awareness of this other world—where all of us are citizens but none master—compels us to take up the night watch.

Thomas Merton, a Trappist in the Abbey of Gethsemani, closes his journal, *The Sign of Jonas,* with a description of a fire watch—the obligatory nightly stroll undertaken by the monks to guard against the threat of fire:

It is when you hit the novitiate that the fire watch begins in earnest. Alone, silent, wandering on your appointed rounds through the corridors of a huge, sleeping monastery, you come around the corner and find yourself face to face with your monastic past and with the mystery of your vocation. The fire watch is an examination of conscience in which your task as watchman suddenly appears in its true light: a pretext devised by God to isolate you, and to search your soul with lamps and questions, in the heart of darkness.

One day we may find ourselves on the fire watch. Coaxed, we rise from a cozy bed and stumble into the frosty air, while around us the profession slumbers. We keep the vigil to a chorus of coughs and stirrings in the night, the sounds of our comrades guilty in their dreams. As ours eyes adjust, it seems clearer now that we have taken up these nocturnal rounds for the sake of becoming our brother's keeper. We are drawn to the fountainhead of our vocation, where notions of professional identity and mission take on a human form.

The faces are familiar. I recognize them through the veil of decorum, can recount every whispered rumor and identify the festering wounds: The surgeon I assisted when his handiwork broke down; a colleague whose "product of a normal delivery" died en route to the medical center; my dispirited partner, whose father tosses on stiff, mitred sheets in some distant postsurgical ward, "just another broken old man." What could I offer them, what words would they not refuse? The watch becomes my rosary, my meditation on the grace that holds a community together.

We keep the fire watch—those of us who know the danger in our hearts—so that volatile egos and the tinder of careers will not go up with an errant spark. We have seen how indifference and competitiveness and arrogance within the profession can fan our misfortunes into a furnace of self-reproach. We know the flashpoint of a house of cards. We keep the watch in hopes that we, in our woundedness, will likewise be watched.

JANUARY

How do we tell the truth in a small town? Is it possible
to write it? Certainly, great literature might come
out of the lives of ordinary people on the farms and ranches
and little towns of the Plains, but are the people who farm,
the people working in those towns, writing it?

KATHLEEN NORRIS

Dakota: A Spiritual Geography

At the end of the month, a good friend of ours will be moving to Florida. Sunday evening he invited us over to share perhaps our last meal together. I was on call for OB and hospice but didn't think twice about it since it seldom disrupts our plans. But no sooner had we arrived than the beeper went off like a cicada. The day had already been interrupted with Roberta's self-imposed withdrawal from morphine, Noble's weight gain and breathlessness, and Elena Moulton's choking on her own secretions. During the night, another hospice patient of ours would die on the Wing.

The beeper directed my call to the maternity unit at Waldo County General Hospital. Claudia Marshall, one of my favorite nurses, answered with the news that Tammy had returned by ambulance, this time "right wild" and in active labor. She was contracting every three minutes, but the cervix was only two centimeters dilated. Tammy was still seventeen days shy of her due date, yet delivery—if it were to come—would be considered safe. Claudia reported poor beat-to-beat variability on the fetal monitor strip, but there were no decelerations and the baby was active. I ordered a sedative of Demerol and Phenergan, requested an hour's observation on the monitor, and urged Claudia to "call me if there are problems." Tammy and I had been 'round robin's barn with her abdominal pain throughout the pregancy; I saw it as just another wrinkle in her personality. She would stay in OB until I could be reassured that it was safe to send her home.

At 8:00 P.M., the beeper again sounded for me to call OB; Claudia was growing worried over the lack of variability on the monitor strip. Along with the amniotic fluid, meconium was passing in clumps, and the cervix had dilated to eight centimeters. "I'll be right in," I reassured her, but first rounded up my wife and daughter and made the appropriate apologies and farewells to our disappointed host.

When I arrived on the OB ward, it was 8:25 P.M., and Tammy's cervix was fully dilated. But something was wrong. Through a gloved hand in the cramped quarters of the vagina, I could feel a boney prominence and something surprisingly spongy and wrinkled. I ordered a pelvic ultrasound and reviewed the patient's chart. Our most recent office notes had not yet arrived in the hospital chart, but Tim had suspected breech lie a month ago. Had he ordered an ultrasound? No matter, for I would need a new look now. Twenty-five minutes later, the portable ultrasound unit lumbered into the birthing room and obtained a clear view of the fetal cranium in the upper right quadrant of the abdomen. The baby was curled in a transverse lie! I made arrangements for an urgent C-section and patiently explained its necessity to Tammy. Up until now she had been handling her contractions wonderfully, but now she insisted on pushing with every pain. To her cries of "I've gotta push, I've gotta push," the nurses replied *"No, Tammy, you can't push!"* Fortunately, the obstetrician had abandoned her crusade to have surgically trained assistants at every section. She agreed that I should assist, that the pediatrician should attend the baby, and that we should get underway as soon as the slippery roads permitted.

Within an hour, the spinal anesthesia had been administered, the patient rolled on her back, and her abdomen became a gleaming dome beneath the bright lights of the surgery. I warned the pediatrician of the patient's ominous tracings, the passage of meconium, the baby's prematurity. Then I turned to watch the surgeon's knife slit open Tammy's lower abdomen like a crescent moon. Layers were parted, bleeders clamped, the bladder dome shielded by my retractor, and I readied the suction tip for the surgeon's final nick into the uterus. The blade slid horizontally in careful, even strokes until, with a gush, cloudy yellow amniotic fluid poured into the operative field. Retractors scattered and the obstetrician's sure hands probed the womb for a boney handle on the baby. I applied fundal pressure and stood poised with a nasogastric suction tube. All at once legs followed feet, then trunk, arms, and head. But only after I had suctioned large strings of mucous and meconium from the baby's nostrils did I notice an unusual mass gathered at the baby's abdomen: his entrails lay outside like links of gray-green sausage. Gastroschisis: the belly had developed inside out.

We quickly finished our business atop Tammy's belly and handed the baby off to the pediatrician. He, in turn, placed him under the radiant warmer and suctioned the vocal cords more thoroughly with a laryngoscope. He would later wrap the intestines in saline-soaked gauze, then cellophane, then aluminum foil, and insert an umbilical vein catheter through which to replenish evaporating body fluids. That night, Tammy's baby was whisked to Portland in anticipation of surgery before infection or entanglement or dehydration could take their toll.

Many thoughts crossed my mind with my first glance at the abnormal newborn. What other abnormalities were hidden from view; will the mother adjust to her child's birth defect; how did such an obvious anomaly go undetected? In retrospect, what had I felt on my cervical exam, if not bony spine and loops of bowel? Did the flat line of the fetal monitor strip indicate anoxic insult (cerebral palsy) at some indeterminate time, or future risks for CP or developmental delay? Tammy had pelvic ultrasounds at nine and twenty weeks' gestation; shouldn't we have detected the gastroschisis then? A blood screening test might have detected the problem at sixteen weeks, but Tammy had missed that appointment.

As I scribbled my labor notes in preparation for the transport team's arrival, Tammy's labor coach sat opposite me and revealed tidbits of her tangled life: nine documented pregnancies by age twenty, six ending in miscarriage and three in elective abortion. Tragically, her uncle had fathered three of the pregnancies. She had known nothing but foster homes, streetlights, confusion, and tears. It is no wonder that she felt safe in the hospital.

After returning home a little after 11:00 P.M., I could not dispel thoughts of Tammy and her future—now greatly complicated by this crippled child. How rarely do we see major birth defects in our tiny hospital. How odd it feels to relay bad news instead of good to the hopeful parents. Morning came and went without the computer. I chose the absolution of sleep over memories of Tammy. The journal will wait.

We beat a hasty retreat to the northern Massachusetts town of Newburyport, where we met our San Francisco friends, Kevin and Kay and Emma. Emma's friendship with Clare is legendary; no kid has replaced her since we returned to Belfast. Their mutual adoration began at age two-and-a-half and continues despite the erosions of time and distance. What do we, as parents, vicariously draw from that friendship? Are we numb to the intensity of their joy? Have we lost our freedom to express it?

The six of us camped out in a lovely B&B near the downtown. The area was littered with colonial clapboards, their squat center chimneys looking very much like the foot of a clam poking from a bivalve. Our large brick lodging, "The Windsor," was built in 1786 as a wedding present for the owner's bride. It had wide plank floors, thick brick walls, and deeply set windows with interior wooden shutters. Our hostess appeared only as we were leaving, having taken violently ill with a stomach flu. Her husband served ably in her stead, fixing high tea at 4:00 P.M. and a lovely breakfast the following morning, with cantaloupe, scrambled eggs, biscuits, and coffee. We had the whole place to ourselves during this after-Christmas lull.

Our spirits were not dampened by the unseasonably warm gusts of wind and torrential downpours that inconvenienced day two of our travels. In fact, the swollen mud puddles provided more entertainment for Emma and Clare than did all of the belated Christmas presents we had lugged along. Kevin could not keep the camera clicking fast enough as our street urchins abandoned their umbrellas, stomped boot-deep in the large parking lot lakes, and soaked their hair with rainwater spouting from the gutters. Later, we walked the deserted beach at Plum Island, collecting razor clams, sharks' egg cases, sand dollars, and the ubiquitous "sea glass."

It was good to see the Drews. Our visit will be remembered for our meditative meandering along the shores of the Merrimack; for the tiny wooden booth at Fowles Soda Fountain that we somehow squeezed into; for fighting off sleep in the lovely parlor of the B&B after the kids were tucked in and storied; and for the breakfast table where we sat oblivious to the antlike march of pillows and stuffed animals that our children assembled into a collossal nest. We talked, of course, about Patrick, now almost three months gone, whose stillbirth picked the pocket of their dreams. And about jobs, and moving East (our perennial dream), and fantasy trips to Paris, and racking up credit card balances beyond the point of return.

I inquired about Kevin's father, an eighty-year-old internist who still practices medicine, and exercises, on occasion, his hospital admitting privileges. "Do you see a danger there?" I pressed. Kevin could see only the positive value of wresting him from stagnation. It is hard to imagine that one's father might lose his mental edge, fall behind on continuing medical education, or seem antiquated in the eyes of his patients and younger peers. He is a partner to Kevin's brother, also a family practitioner, who has expressed no concern about the quality of their father's care. But would he, as a son; or could he, as a colleague?

Doctors are unschooled and awkward in the art of criticism. In our myriad of hospital meetings—all held in the name of "peer review"—we stumble like schoolboys at a ballroom dance. What do we learn? How to blame the bureaucracy, rationalize our mistakes, express our loyalty, or conceal our own fear and insecurity?

Never mind pride, or worry over the medico-legal climate; there is an urgent need for gentle, respectful dialogue about the quality of our work. It must come from peers, focus on the patient, and be undertaken with the goal of preserving our clinical prowess, professional dignity, and moral culpability. We need support as we toil near the limits of our clinical abilities, remaining open to the possibility of error, oversight, or plain ignorance.

H. J. Van Peenen has reflected upon the unpopular, uneasy choice that older doctors face as they reach the end of their careers, having gone as far as they can go.* The name of a colleague—"not just another name, but a long-standing friend"—appears in the *Bulletin* of the Medical Disciplinary Board in a neighboring state. He has been entered into a "retired status agreement, without findings and order." The reader can only imagine the sordid details. The author himself considers the possibility of substance abuse, or a sexual offense, or Medicare fraud before dismissing all but the last.

He speculates on his friend's change in *identity:* what becomes of a doctor who does not practice? Is he remade in that instant when the public releases him from its gaze? Is he like a defrocked parish priest who can no longer administer the sacraments, yet is forever fixed by his solemn vows? All of us, Van Peenen proposes, are "sanctioned ultimately by time, fading powers, obsolete knowledge, the inevitable drifting away of patients, the diminution in status that comes with simple old age . . . At what age in our careers do we cease to be doctors and become undeserving of the honorific 'M.D.' after our names?" For those of us in the healing profession, is it when we cease to heal, or forsake our vows?

Some doctors never cease being. Van Peenen tells of old Dr. Glass, the "only physician in a small neighboring town who, at the age of eighty-five, finally gave up his last, very loyal contingent of elderly patients. He was an honorable man who had always practiced within his limits and maintained the affection of his peers until the day he died. But by the time I knew him he had gone from being a busy, competent, useful physician to a trembling old man, far gone in dementia. He lived in a chair in the nursing home, his withered hands holding an *AMA News* he could no longer read or understand. Yet even in the home, he was not 'Jim' or 'Bill' like the other patients; he was Dr. Glass until the day he died in his sleep, and he is Dr. Glass still, for his tombstone proudly portrays 'M.D.' after his name."

I am not judging Kevin's father—the Dr. Glass of Gliddentown—but fear for his good name and his increasing isolation. He walks on thin ice, needs

---

* H. J. Van Peenen, "Are We Always? When Do We Stop?" *Annals* 118 (1993): 69–70.

more than mere instincts and common sense to assure his safe passage. His failing senses will not warn him of the changing conditions, and his solitary ways mitigate against any reasonable hope of rescue should he be plunged into the icy waters.

This month, the *JABFP* will publish a story I wrote about retirement-age physicians. "The Watch" is a true account. An elderly, semi-retired GP was being harassed by a patient of mine who blamed him for his mother's death. Frank Dennison had been the attending physician. By the time I had assumed the woman's care, she was failing from decades of chronic disease and the ravages of poverty, and appeared much older than her fifty-eight years. My interventions only delayed her pitiful decline. Within six months she succumbed to a heart attack that was complicated by pulmonary edema, then pneumonia, then kidney failure.

I wonder if Kevin's father, or the thousands of GPs in his generation, will read the story. If so, what will they think? Could it apply to their circumstance, or the one which I, too, may face?

Yesterday I spent home alone. It was one of my every-other-Fridays-off, which are too often consumed by competing claims and distractions.

My writing was interrupted by telephone calls from registrants to Lindsay's hospice conference. She has invited two gifted speakers—John Stephenson and Bill Hemmens—to enlighten us about grief, especially the grief of children. A week ago, Lindsay had twenty-two registrants for the day-long event, eighteen of whom were local hospice volunteers, entitled to free admittance. Now there are ninety, the vast majority paying customers, and a sizable profit looms. She is cautiously ecstatic. I was becoming perturbed by the interruptions when a saleswoman from Augusta called about insulated siding. No, I replied bluntly, but would *you* be interested in a workshop tomorrow at 9:00, starring a couple of big names in the area of grief, twenty bucks for a half day and thirty-five for the shootin' match, including continuing education credits, a certificate of completion, and happy-face name badges? "Sorry," she demurred, "I've got commitments."

There was an hour left in the day, after my errands to the post office and before Clare and Lindsay would arrive home. I nickle-and-dimed it away in the Belfast Free Library, researching the grange in Maine (which seems strangely on the wane), looking up an old Waldo *Independent* newspaper column on Ralph Wiley (the wheelchair man with no legs), and browsing through old *New York Times* book reviews. Quite unexpectedly, I came across a wonderful piece by Kathleen Norris about small-town writers. How hard it is, she suggests, to tell the truth; how much easier to write a local history that "makes things nice" and creates a "harmonious whole." A rural author often finds herself out on a limb, which maintains her perspective but also sanctions her for using it.

She had this to say: "It is a truism that outsiders, often professionals with no family ties, are never fully accepted into rural or small-town life. These communities are impenetrable for many reasons, not the least of which is the fact that the most important stories are never told." Families that have staked their claim on the Great Plains *and survived,* have weathered a harsh, barren, solitary lifestyle and have resisted the steady drift of their young to the cities, of the old to Arizona, and have held to the best of times if only in their memories.

She continues, "a 'good story' is one that isn't demanding, that proceeds from A to B, and above all doesn't remind us of the bad times, the cardboard patches we used to wear in our shoes, the failed farms, the way people you love just up and die. It tells us instead that hard work and perseverance can overcome all obstacles; it tells lie after lie, and the ending is the happiest lie of all." Surviving families, the old names of the county, "have an exceptionally difficult time dealing with conflict and change. To them, change means failure; it is a contaminant introduced by outside elements. Such families have brought the local history mentality to life, and in sufficient numbers they dictate the ethos of their small towns." I agree with her, see it at work in my own small community, can easily imagine its influence on the farm towns of the Midwest, where erosion has thinned the soil far less than it has the indigenous population and rural culture. I will watch for the book, *Dakota: A Spiritual Geography,* when it is released later this month.

Yesterday I received a hearty letter from Gayle Stephens. I learned that he is taking up the piano, reading Irenaeus's *Against the Heresies* (somehow he got on a list of Catholic book publishers), and going to the spring meeting of the Society of Teachers of Family Medicine. It is so good to hear from this broadly read, philosophically inclined, wise yet humble practitioner of the art. He is family doctor foremost, passionately and self-critically.

I am curious about Gayle's premature departure from the battleground of academic medicine. A few years ago he stepped down from the chair of the Department of Family Medicine at the University of Alabama, Birmingham, to putter on the edges of the discipline. He has since been content with writing, lecturing, teaching, and practicing medicine through an occasional *locum tenens* in his brother's office. I wonder about his plans, regrets, sudden uprootedness. This paragraph was wedged into a letter I had received from his retreat in Colorado: "My Summer here has been mostly desultory, although I have worked at writing almost everyday. I enjoy the mountains, but I feel disengaged from real life. I have no duties, and I miss my connection to patients."

Did he expect that his fans, his patients, the communities for whom he sacrificed so much would remember him once the tail of his white coat cleared the door? Short-term memory is the first to go. And those who best remember him—the founders of family practice—are themselves, many of them, stepping back from the limelight. I intend to send Gayle a copy of Dr. Van Peenen's essay concerning old physicians, a late revision of one of my essays, and Kathleen Norris's article on writing in the rural Midwest. Gayle tells me that he grew up in a "culturally impoverished village in northeast Missouri" where the best literature was found in church songbooks and the King James Bible.

When I was a senior medical student at the University of Iowa, I first wrote to Gayle with my naive, half-baked, untested notions about the purposes of medicine. He responded to my letter then, and to each letter since, and has become for me a trusted mentor. I miss him already, my aging friend. I curse the misfortune of having embarked on my career in family practice when the field was already in full bloom, long after the first seeds were planted by Gayle and the other visionaries. But mostly I miss the possibility of friendship that might have stretched over the years. Thankfully, I have it now.

The outside thermometer reads zero; cold, but virtually no snow this early winter. I offer a prayer for Marc Stewart this morning, who today seeks the blessing of his new congregation in Grand Rapids, Michigan.

I was in the throes of a terrible dream before the alarm clock jarred me awake. I was singing in a choir, doing warm-up exercises, when I realized that I had forgotten my music and concert attire. I knew that the director would notice, and that he had dismissed other choir members for lesser offenses. He was a slight man, but muscle-bound and snakelike, with a square jaw and steely eyes whose stare spits venom. Unhappily, he confronted me and we began to tussle; I was aware of a sword at his side and knew that he intended to run me through. I called frantically for the others, and with reluctance a few ambled to my aid; but to no avail, for the serpent man slithered around me and gained the upper hand. I wrested the sword from its sheath and carved his abdomen from xiphoid to pubis, disemboweling him with a single stroke. He gasped and died. I was much relieved, for often, in other anxiety dreams, the evil could be deterred but never disposed of. And I awoke to the alarm, exhausted but anxious to approach the journal, where I am safe and free of the terror. I wonder now: were the entrails those of Tammy's baby, who is recuperating from his surgery for gastroschisis at the Maine Medical Center? I will inquire after him tomorrow.

I received a note yesterday from Michael Doyle, who resolves this New Year to return all letters in a timely fashion. He discovered an unanswered letter of mine dated three years ago; in it I consoled him about a writer's block that was derailing his pursuit of a Ph.D. in American History. He intimates that he might visit this summer or next. It would be a welcome visit. He sends me, along with his warm greetings, a note card from his research on the lyceum movement, where he came across Barbara Hinds's 1949 M.A. thesis on the lyceum in Maine. He quotes: "Among other topics, the lyceum in Belfast, Maine in 1851–1852 sponsored lectures on astronomy, biology & physiology, the principles of geography, conversation, reading, the cultivation of memory, popular delusions concerning the Middle Ages, Iceland, the equality of the human condition, the domestic life of the Turks, the problem of the age, and the origin of letters."

He also sent a clipping from the *New York Times* dated 9 June 1992; it was a disturbing article on the "quiet exodus" of young folks from the midwestern family farm. Since 1980, the number of farmers under age twenty has fallen by half; the FFA (Future Farmers of America) has lost 20 percent of its membership, and only 25 percent of those who remain intend to farm. The pressures here, as everywhere, are to get big or get out. A beginning farmer must often invest over two hundred grand for the necessary equipment and leases. Says farm economist Terry Francl, "On a typical Midwestern crop farm today, you are going to need six to seven hundred acres to make enough money to sustain a family." A 1990 Congressional Budget Office report estimates that five hundred thousand farms must "leave the sector" to maintain the 1988 average net income. As the young leave, the average farm family shrinks in size, foreclosures add to the consolidation rate, and towns that supplied the agrarian economy slowly die. It is disheartening to hear of it from a distance, more painful to see it close up at each Iowa homecoming, and undoubtedly frightening for my friends who remain on their family farm, like high school classmate Jim Jordan in Atlantic, Iowa.

I went to Lindsay's day-long workshop yesterday, expecting no more than a chance to lend my support. She made a marvelous introduction, then quietly, and in her inimitable way, melted into the background. But the afternoon session on "The Special Grief of Children" by Bill Hemmens sent me reeling back to my father's death. Bill played a videotape of a twelve-year-old boy who shared his feelings about the death of his father, how it changed his life and that of his fourteen-year-old sister. These were our ages, my sister's and mine, when our father collapsed in his bedroom in Rolfe on that Sunday morning, Memorial Day weekend of 1965. The boy expressed worries and concerns that I have long repressed: the shadow, or a sense of impending doom, that hangs over the family and heightens your sense of global responsibility.

Lindsay's conference did me good if only for these few appreciations. And, with over ninety registrants, it was hugely successful and turned a tidy profit.

I talked with Tim yesterday at the conference's morning break. I related my disappointing conversation with Bruce Swarmi of two nights ago. Bruce is a third-year resident at the family practice program in Bangor. He had earlier expressed interest in joining our practice but now is leaning toward an offer by a multispecialty group in Bangor. The advantages there are considerable: it would mean no move, a higher salary, better benefits, and the opportunity to work with his best friend from training.

Clare is having difficulty as Lindsay's week-long Parisian vacation draws nigh. Her anxiety is manifested by dramatic displays of affection, soiling her pants, and difficulty sleeping. She cannot easily drift off despite her bedtime stories and the lateness of the hour, and so joins us belatedly in the Big Bed. And often she awakes, panic-stricken, in the middle of the night. Last evening, exhausted after missing her afternoon nap, she managed to fall asleep in her own bed but awoke later in sobs. Her bottom hurt, and she requested a bath to soak in. Lindsay obliged her at 1:30 A.M., and they both snuggled back in our bed afterwards. Perhaps, like her father, Clare will have more trouble with an anticipated loss than with its reality. We shall see in three short days.

It's the middle of the month, a "seasonably" cold day in January, zero degrees upon rising. The sand truck just ambled by at ten minutes before five o'clock. Yesterday we awoke to the first real snowfall of the season, a modest five inches.

We had our second St. Jude conference at the office, an hour-long group discussion of hopeless cases. It was again Scott-centered, with the four of us (Scott, Mary Beth, Tim, and I) attending. Two days ago, I had returned to the office at five o'clock, after a hospital staff meeting, to find Scott still wading through his schedule, nearly an hour and a half behind. He was counseling a young woman whose life was disintegrating. Bonnie approached me with the damage report: one patient pacing in an exam room, two others anxiously waiting, the last rescheduled to a slot on the evening panel. In a moment she came back to report that the pacer had fled; I agreed to see one patient; Scott emerged shortly thereafter to see the other. He had become overwhelmed, he later admitted, by the young woman's predicament, her woes, the depth of her suffering. I know this of Scott. He returns to his mother's kitchen with each vulnerable young woman and dissolves in their tears. We agreed to talk in group: what to do for the both of them?

Mary Beth led a fruitful discussion. We touched upon the doctor's sympathies and sense of duty that draw us to the patient's plight. Time, other patients, the schedule . . . cease to exist, and you pick up the patient's cross, wipe clean her brow, dab her tear-lined cheeks. But other patients *do* matter, even when in the last five minutes of a session, as so often happens, there is a revelation of incest, suicidal fear, or a life careening out of control. Setting limits is as important for the patient's sake as for the caregiver's; it must be modeled and respected, says Mary Beth. We learn, through our complementary angles on the case, that the young woman's plight is repeated in her sister. What light would a third sister's story shed? The men in the family are conspicuously absent: The husband died a year ago of cancer; the brother rooms with his ailing mother but is forever off larking; the boyfriend is kind but powerless to help. Men, in this family, are passive listeners who saddle the women with duty, guilt, and accusation, which they then pass back and forth bitterly between them.

Scott decides that he must muzzle his impulse to rescue. Otherwise, he risks becoming another sympathetic but ineffectual male. Mary Beth gives him a list of female counselors (not herself, as she is feeling depressed and overwhelmed and sets a limit of her own). And he will try to remember the patients who wait patiently as he falls behind and give them the courtesy of an explanation or the opportunity to reschedule—or, as I am more apt to do, conclude a difficult session and reschedule for a later time, perhaps with a therapist. Scott, our long history reminds me, is resistant to change. We will broach this topic again, but I leave it now feeling relieved for having made the effort.

Lindsay leaves today for Paris. She will call Sunday morning to confirm her safe arrival. I am anxious to get on with it after so much anticipation and worry. I'm looking forward to being top dog in Clare's life, to spending more time with her, and to deepening our relationship. She is watching *The Wizard of Oz* in the living room, unable to sleep, and I fluff her pillow on the sofa as I make my way to the kitchen coffeepot.

The frosty blue day begins to stretch at seven o'clock and twelve degrees. The land has a new comforter: six inches of freshly fallen snow. I hear the cars squeaking by on the snow-packed pavement. The far eastern horizon is rimmed in pink, and against the neighbor's towering black locust trees, snow feathers the charcoaled branches and brightens the pristine meadow beneath. A clear day hails the *bon voyage*.

Lindsay's departure was postponed by six hours as the result of a cracked windshield on the Belgium Airlines charter, so in the afternoon we all went sledding at Northport Country Club with the Stewarts, just back from their trip to Grand Rapids. Marc had been welcomed by a vote of the congregation, and he and Cheryl spent their hours looking at real estate. They are happy to have three or four good homes to choose from. Their timetable for leaving Belfast will be mid-March, with an April Fools starting date in Grand Rapids.

I believe they leave much the wiser. Young Protestant ministers brave a wilderness alone, without Rome's reinforcements or knowledge of the territory. Soon enough they find themselves at a Donner Pass, facing the elements with little rest or recourse. Good counsel and friendship can go a long way toward assuring one's survival, as I have discovered in my several years as Marc's friend. I hope that Marc can make the best of his next opportunity.

We drove Lindsay and her traveling companions to the Bangor International Airport in the evening. Clare was brave and saved her sobs for the car ride home: "Why can't we all go, like San Francisco?" she asked with an innocence that melts away reason. A stop at Dunkin' Donuts buoyed her spirits, as did a story about Peter Pan ("anything but Lobo; it's *too* scary, Dad") that put both of us to sleep. We had compiled a list of projects to complete while Lindsay is gone: see a movie in Bangor, build a snow fort, play on the Nautilus machines in the physical therapy room at the hospital, explore a new restaurant, visit the library, color pictures for Lindsay, swim at the high school pool. We have a dozen invitations for supper and play dates for Clare, which are appreciated but (I think now) unnecessary. I want my time with Clare, my day as Daddy, some growth in our relationship. Can I take a rain check, I ask?

So far, I'm enjoying the time. Last evening, after waking from her nap, Clare began to clutch her abdomen and call for Mom. Why doesn't she come home? Why can't we call her? But after the gas settled and the spaghetti was served, Clare felt better and we were best of buddies again. Lindsay called around lunchtime with news of her safe arrival and a skeleton report of her itinerary.

Clare and I took a bath together yesterday morning. As I wriggled into my swimming trunks, my daughter objected. "I won't laugh, Daddy. You see my bottom so I won't mind seeing yours."

Then it was off to Mass, stocked with such spiritual aids as a *Beauty and the Beast* coloring book, Etch a Sketch, and a dinosaur pop-up book. Clare contented herself by coloring on the kneeler, studying the stained glass windows, and humming piously to herself. When we returned home, I called a friend of hers and arranged a play date for 2:00. They played "dogs" (I was the prowling wolf), Cinderella, house, and computer. They made ice cream out of chocolate pudding and strawberry yogurt and, much to my surprise, ate it! An hour later, they dragged an infant walker, a comforter, blankets and pillows, and half of Clare's battalion of stuffed animals downstairs to make a fort. It was a well-behaved two hours, but I was ready for Hilly to leave and had high hopes for a return invitation.

Late yesterday afternoon, after retrieving Clare from day care, I tucked her in a blanket on the sofa and stuck in a favorite video ("the yellow one with black letters"). In the few minutes that it took me to prepare tortellini, apple slices, chips, and milk, Clare had dozed off. I made a futile effort to revive her, then changed her into a nightgown and bedded her down for the night. The evening stretched before me unencumbered.

I ate what I had prepared, all of it, then scooted my chair next to the computer and contemplated some long overdue letters. Ah, solitude, a frothy-headed beer, and the cozy confines of my lamplit den. And now, as I listen to my thoughts, I hear the comforting sounds of the old house: computer whirring, refrigerator humming, furnace clunking in fits and starts, dishwasher rattling at full tilt. My top priority is to reply to Wally Lim's Christmas newsletter, in which he reports receipt of this year's Special Recognition Award from the family practice residency where he teaches (and where I taught for a year).

I next write to our friends Rob and Cathy in Hilton Head, with the silliness we have always enjoyed about each other: "Lindsay is cavorting about Paris on a week-long lark, touring museums and sipping espresso in sidewalk cafes and speaking French with abandon. She got a budget ticket on a Brussels charter, $195.00 round trip, and she and Heather took off to escape the dark and cold of a New England winter. Cheaper than antidepressants. So I am Doctor Mom, and Clare and I are surviving nicely, thank you. The hardest part has been picking out Clare's clothes in the morning. She insists on the tutu (the temperature at daybreak was two degrees) or the party dress that specifies 'dry-cleaning only.' So we compromise: I let her wear the party dress."

Women, I say to Cathy in the office today, are engineered to raise children. They are capable of finesse and compromise; they steer clear of ultimatums and open declarations of war; they leash their ego. But males lumber toward conflict with a brute mentality, a sorry singlemindedness, and all the strategy of a battering ram. A kid will call our bluff, and taunt us until we become raging lunatics. We are putty in their hands, and soon enough find ourselves in a lose-lose proposition. I am learning this week to think like my wife, do as Lindsay might do, give slack on issues of dress in exchange for firmness where values or safety matter, and where not simply my *authority* is at stake. The week is racing by. I only have tomorrow's date with my daughter, and Friday's sleepover with Tim's daughter, Rozy, before Lindsay returns triumphant, Queen for a Day.

I recently wrote to one of my medical school professors, a national leader in family practice, chair of a major department, editor of a major text, member of every important committee. He replied that he was delighted to hear I was living and practicing in Maine. He had recently sailed our coastal waters during his sabbatical ("the first in twenty-four years") and thought it one of the most beautiful spots in the world.

If I were his native guide, I would have turned his expedition inland, taken him past Harveytown and Liberty Tool and Tranquility Grange, over the length of the long run, deep into the heart of the county where stark beauty is revealed in the furrows of indigenous faces and in the eyes of people who have survived both the Maine winter and the rock-hard, threadbare economy—survived through sheer force of will, through tenacity and grit and canniness and, no doubt, that much maligned spirit of Yankee independence. I would let Scott Bailly show him a face or two, the ingrained and inbred who scavenge the aisles of Mickey Marden's Discount Barn, Al Salvatore's Ya-low Garage, Caswell's Liquidation Center, and L. Ray's Packing Company (where locals buy sardines wholesale in cans sorted into "fats" and "slits," while the outsiders pay full fare).

The latest issue of *JABFP* had arrived yesterday, and, with it, my essay "The Watch." Perhaps in the flush of publication, I was strengthened to be able to level with my professor: "We didn't see eye to eye fifteen years ago, when you were the powerful Chair and I was a rebel without a cause. Some of the rub, I know, was my issue with authority; some was our differing views on family practice. I respect all that you have done to legitimize and advance our specialty. And I realize that my own meager contributions are important, too: those of a foot soldier in the front lines, the generalist who bears the heart, not the brains, of family practice. Someday I hope we can speak about these differences face to face."

Yesterday at the office, I sat with an obese patient as she chattered along, clackity-clack, vocalizing her anxieties without direction or aim like a string of cans behind a newlyweds' car. The nurse ahead of me, who had only attempted to record the vital signs, had been trapped for fifteen minutes. Yes, I nodded intently, your chest pressure, your insomnia, the diffuse achiness and night sweats and fluttering of the heart *could* be due to chronic fatigue syndrome, *could* be due to allergies or menopause, but, taken as a whole, they are probably symptoms of anxiety.

End discussion. My job, under the circumstances, is to separate the wheat from the chaff, establish a diagnosis, tailor a strategy, and bail out within the allotted time. I may not help her *today,* but I cannot risk my other obligations trying. I accept these limits without bitterness or resignation. Doctors often rob Peter to pay Paul, scrimp on sore throats and hypertensives to linger a while longer with depressives and lonely hearts. Today I didn't uncover her needs, let alone determine if I could meet them. But I was *certain* of the dangers of being caught in her whirling anxieties, and struggled to hold my ground. There will be other visits and other opportunities.

Yesterday was pleasurably replete with errands and activities. At EmBee Cleaners, I discovered that the broken zipper on my eight-year-old coat needed only a pinch from a pair of pliers. "Saved ya ten bucks," smiled the young man behind the counter, proud father of an infant I recently delivered. He could have saved me eighty if I had come to him before buying a new coat at L. L. Bean. A surprise at the Fertile Mind Bookstore: Tolstoy was in, *The Death of Ivan Ilych, and Other Stories;* and on the shelf of new releases was *Dakota: A Spiritual Geography* by Kathleen Norris. I bought both and, while on a roll, ordered *A Home for Everyone: The Greek Revival Movement in Maine.* My only disappointment was that Patricia Hampl's *Virgin Time* is not yet in paperback.

Last night Clare and I dined at the Stewarts', who are madly packing for their April departure to Grand Rapids. They had just encountered that monstrous injustice, closing costs, amounting to 10 percent of the cost of their downpayment. We feasted on roast chicken, mashed potatoes, mixed vegetables, and a good homebrew of Marc's (well-hopped and spicy) to wash it down. The conversation seemed clipped and chaotic in the face of stiff competition from our daughter, their sons, the cats, and my impending departure for choir practice. I skipped the last hour of rehearsal and returned for apple pie and ice cream, but Clare was deliriously tired and staged an imperative exit. It was good to see these dear people, befriend them, reassure them that they leave deep roots and many friends in Belfast, the birthplace of their three children.

My dream last night: I was scheduled to perform a double hernia repair in the office. I was sure I could do it, having previously assisted on many, and recalling several I had performed solo during my residency training. But this patient, with whom I had always enjoyed good rapport, kept probing me with her unsettling questions and whittled away at my time and self-confidence.

I suggested that we repair only *one* side today. "And have me come back?" asked the patient incredulously. "Are you saying you can't do it, that you are masquerading as a surgeon? Listen, Loxterkamp, I'll tell all my friends about you, who will tell their friends, and you'll have no practice in this town." She stormed out, but I was greatly relieved to have postponed the operation, realizing now that I had no training in hernia repairs after all, having confused it with the excision of a sebaceous cyst.

The dream anxiety may have come from several sources. One, most certainly, was from my encounter yesterday. I saw a woman who had complained of tiny "bunches" popping out beneath her arm and all over her body in the last several months. She had seen several doctors—a surgeon, a dermatologist, a neurologist. Her husband had "fired" her previous family physician because "she just wasn't doing anything." No one knew what caused the bunches, although a local surgeon had taken a biopsy, and a Portland dermatologist attributed them to the use of phenytoin, an anticonvulsant drug. One bunch, near the medial condyle of the right elbow, had reddened the overlying skin; I suggested we might remove it to avoid infection and relieve pain. But on palpation, it felt rubbery, elongated, possibly attached to underlying structures and not freely mobile under the skin like a lipoma or sebaceous cyst. My mind raced to the patient whose neck I had opened several years ago, only to realize, as I stared into the wound, that the lump was odd and atypical. Head and neck surgeons later diagnosed it to be a malignant schwannoma; even they could not eradicate it despite bold and radical attempts. I cared for that patient as he died a slow, painful, disfiguring death in a local nursing home.

So what do you wish of me today? I asked without words. I can coordinate your consultations, perform your annual physical, care for your incidental illnesses. But let's leave the lumps alone until the biopsy report returns and you've had a drug holiday from the phenytoin.

Another insecurity has been brewing these last several months. The number of new prenatal patients has fallen sharply, due in large part to the arrival of the new obstetrician. Yesterday I learned that one of our prenatals is electing an early termination; another transferred to a Bangor obstetrician. Will we be able to maintain? In many areas, women cannot find an obstetrician, especially if they are on state aid; in others, family doctors are deserting OB in droves. But here in Waldo County, population twenty five thousand, five family doctors and one obstetrician perform deliveries, and, for the most part, do it well. I have less insecurity about my skills than disappointment in not being chosen to exercise them more often.

Yesterday was the eve of Lindsay's return. Clare was tearful at nursery school, and our separation time doubled. During the day, I avoided the one goal I had set for myself: to write for several hours on my dad's death. But the air was not right (balmy and wet and extremely un-January-like), my legs were restless, and I roamed about the house looking for distractions. They were strewn everywhere, easy to locate: I organized my correspondence, cleaned the guest room, finished the laundry and the dishes, and attended to errands downtown (irises for the table, quilts to the cleaners, clothes to Salvation Army).

Last evening, Rozy Hughes came for a sleepover. Together we chose a video, gobbled bow-tie pasta and fruit for supper, ate dessert while we watched the Children's Theatre Company production of *Alice in Wonderland,* and read stories in bed. An exhausted Clare held out for fifteen minutes after "lights out" but gave up the ghost with loud snores in the still of the winter's night.

At 2:00 A.M. I heard Clare's whimpers in the other room and went to fetch her. Tummy hurting again, as the day care worker had earlier reported. I brought Clare into the big bed, and she flipped and flopped until bright beams of light rose on the western wall, car doors thunked, and I rose with Clare in my arms to investigate the commotion. Lindsay was home! Quick hugs all around, a retreat to bed, and flipping throughout the night. It will take a while to return to the normal household routine.

Since Lindsay's return, there has been loss of order and growing chaos. Chores in the common domain—Clare's mess, laundry, dishes—are left partially complete. Parental authority is divided. Errands go unattended. I have become testy at compromises and second opinions. As a single parent, I harbored a perpetual and overwhelming sense of responsibility, but without any of the tug-of-war of temperaments, habits, and values that couples must face. It will take us a few days to find our stride and reassume our complementary roles.

We held our retreat yesterday morning, Tim, Mary Beth, and I, at Cathy Rispoli's oceanfront home. She offered it to us for our experiment: three hours set aside to talk instead of Thursday morning's usual one. A fire crackled in the Jötul stove, wind chimes tinkled on the back porch, and the Bay danced in an angular light. The pewter gray sky reminded me of Iowa and the land's foreboding, especially after harvest when the ground is stripped bare and the sky is as colorless as the day my father died.

Tim came by kayak across the inlet of Belfast Bay. He had packed freshly ground coffee in his backpack and was now brewing it. Mary Beth had just baked a coffee cake from a Susan Loomis recipe and was slicing it in the kitchen. I fiddled with tapes of Aled Jones and Christopher Parkening and William Byrd at the tape deck. All of these preparatory tasks before we could sit together and break the silence.

Tim wanted to delineate, in these few hours together, the past and future direction of our Thursday morning group. Mary Beth was just happy to be here. I wanted, more than anything else, to avoid running my mouth. But Tim was now hurting from the wounds of a marital spat (on this and recent mornings); he was feeling vulnerable and conflicted and confused. I told him how difficult it was for me to see him this way, but how I suffered, too, when he spoke of his honeymoon marriage. My own marriage often seemed empty and distant by comparison. I could not bring my feelings to group for the shame and sense of inadequacy they caused me. I see now that I was depressed, living on a lifeboat plunged in fog, propelled solely by the passage of time. But connected still, by a thread of hope and my faith in God.

I mentioned how proud I felt when our practice volunteered at the Stone Soup Kitchen. We cooked and served over thirty noontime meals. As many as sixty are served on any given day in that cramped space above the naval recruiting station. Many of the guests are our patients. The kitchen supervisor confessed how odd it felt "giving orders to her doctor." Our practice has fostered a sense of camaraderie and purpose in the lives of our employees, more than I would ever have imagined. We have gone through a lot together: many hard days and crisis situations and mean-spirited patients, and too many deaths for any one of us to handle alone. There is a collective feeling that we have brought something of value into the world, as much for each other as for our patients.

I often come to Thursday morning group seeking refuge. I come to sit in a place free of scrutiny or agenda, to sit among friends, to celebrate and probe and embrace my life in its web of joy and frustration. I come to give thanks for what God has given me, and I, in turn, have learned to love. Where will it lead me? To death, eventually, which is all the more reason to cherish it now.

A warm front has moved through, bringing fifty-degree weather and an early thaw. The ground is brown, almost green in places, and littered with leafy detritus. The sky at sunrise is pale gold with puffy violaceous clouds skipping over the Bay. This makes for a dismal January, one betwixt and between the seasons. I hope for a quick return to the enamel white and bitter cold of winter before that inevitable penance we call Mud Season.

Driving home from work two nights ago, I saw the new moon smiling like a Cheshire Cat. The Evening Star lay to its side, gleaming like a pearl in the western sky.

This hospital week has been unrelenting. Tuesday began at 7:30 with a nurse's call; a patient had died unexpectedly with a profusion of sweat, a gasp, and a glazed stare. Peace, finally, after the night's long struggle. Fortunately we had just clarified her resuscitation status, and she told me "No, let me go if the Lord is bidding." In Maternity, a mother had brought along her husband and five children for her Pitocin induction. On the floor, the general surgeon had requested a medical consultation on a patient with possible bowel obstruction. In the ER, a woman arrived by ambulance after she had been found unresponsive by her neighbor. They are both octogenarians and cling to their independent living by a morning ritual of checking to see if the other is still alive. My patient suffered an apparent stroke. While I was writing admission orders, her breathing ceased and the nurses rushed to alert me. "Bag her, but no full code," I advised cautiously. Then I called the office to verify her living will. Yes, it was there. And bagging was sufficient; the patient's tongue had occluded the airway, but she now breathed easily with head support and a nasal airway. We would treat her "expectantly" over the next twenty-four hours, allowing her the chance to survive or fail according to the severity of her stroke and her willingness to be treated.

At the IDT meeting, we discussed a patient on the Hospice Wing for whom we had no mechanism to notify the family after death. It was a woman who had let her hoarseness go for over a year before allowing a biopsy of her laryngeal carcinoma. Now what to do for this old, crippled, and sofa-bound rheumatic? Radiation therapy stood a 40 percent chance of cure. But it also would require daily trips to Bangor for a month, and would cause a sore throat sure to further compromise her nutritional status. Without treatment, the cancer could kill her within a year and likely require a tracheostomy or feeding tube before it obstructed her completely or eroded her esophagus. But the cancer would likely do this anyway, and what quality of life would treatment preserve? This is for our patient to decide. My partner will present the facts, mired in all their uncertainty, to the patient and her family at next week's meeting.

You might conclude from my writing that doctors attend only deaths and deliveries. These mark the territory; they are the polar extremes. Sometimes I fear that, if I let go of OB, I would be plunged into hospice like a child deserted on a teeter-totter. Yet, after talking to family doctors who have quit OB, I learn that their lives are the better for it.

At yesterday's conference I remarked to Tim how lonely it felt on the front lines. There is a familiar dynamic, alternating weekly, whereby the hospital doctor faces the dragons of clinical practice, takes his licks, empties his reserves, and enters the dark realm of self-doubt, despair, and personal neglect. But yesterday, the tide of battle turned in my favor.

Tim and I agreed to meet for lunch at 90 Main; we would talk about obstetrics and recruiting, and simply share a meal. In the morning I was able to round, dictate three discharge summaries, insert prostaglandin gel in an OB patient, pick up a book on interlibrary loan at the Belfast Free Library, and sort through mail at home. I received a letter from a reader of "The Watch," just published in *JABFP*. He was a family doctor who had practiced across the Bay in Blue Hill before I moved to Maine and now teaches in a residency program near Lancaster, Pennsylvania. Yesterday's office schedule was a blessing: nickels and dimes, prenatals and physicals, headaches and stomachaches and social visits for the worried well. I ran a little behind but apportioned my time equitably and allowed my office notes to reflect the attentiveness and thoughfulness of my day. Last night Lindsay and I enjoyed marvelous Indian cuisine at a friend's birthday party, ate much too much, and suffered dreams seasoned with curry and pickled mango.

I regret to have neglected our ten-year anniversary. It recalls not the wedding date but Lindsay's and my first meeting at Jimmy's Bar and Grill in Hyde Park, Chicago. Lindsay remembered, and that night left a lovely card on my pillow with this poetic verse:

> T is for the telegram you sent me;
> E is for your eyes that afternoon.
> N is for the night-train journey eastward;
>
> Y is for our youth that hot hot June.
> E is for the Eugene I deserted;
> A is for adventures in your car.
> R's for Rolfe, Rosemary and a romance
> S started in that darkened Jimmy's Bar.

We shared a Sammy Smith's Nut Brown Ale and thumbed through pictures of Paris with Lindsay's running commentary. Then we drifted to sleep, only to find ourselves entwined in each other's arms at midnight. As the moment dissipated, the telephone rang with expected news: the kidneys of one of our patients had finally failed him.

The coldest night of winter arrived on January's tail. All afternoon and evening, northwesterly gales blew an Arctic air mass over New England. Our outside thermometer stalled at minus ten. Yesterday, as I drove across the Memorial Bridge, the Bay gave up its heat in great wisps of steam like a boiling caldron. Ice crystalized on the shoreline trees, giving their black branches a shimmering sheen. Plumes of smoke rose from every chimney, and the whole harbor seemed cast in an ethereal spell. When I drove to the emergency room last evening, the Jetta slugged along, moaning with every turn of the wheel and creaking at the slightest pressure from the brake pedal. Our furnace churned all night long, baseboard registers rattled, and deep swirls of frost etched our window panes. Clare couldn't sleep, not because of the nocturnal clatter but because of her stuffy, crusted nose; she and Lindsay slipped downstairs and propped themselves upright on the sofa and played lullaby tunes.

Yesterday morning I met a new resident at the Bradbury Nursing Home. She is a nonagenarian of French Canadian descent, an Old World Catholic from St. Agathe up in the County.* Over the past year, she had lost her only daughter to cancer, fallen twice at home (bruising her ribs badly), and suffered a heart attack. The granddaughter, who now had power-of-attorney, felt she would be safest in a nursing home.

The patient's hearing was gone, but her eyes remained as clear as her memory. I scribbled questions to her on a yellow tablet, and she responded eagerly. When asked about the sacraments—was she up to date?—she burst into tears and related how she had learned her prayers in French at her mother's knee. I then asked about St. Agathe; did she know the story? No. So I vowed to surprise her at my next visit with a description from Chambers's *Lives*. The revelation that I was German Catholic was greeted with shrieks of "Oh, my angel, I've been sent an angel." And when I asked if I could examine her, she replied as innocently as a saint, "Do you mean my conscience?" "No, with this," I replied, raising a stethoscope to her chest. But she deflected me: "What kind of a scapular do you carry there?"

* Aroostook, where the wasteland ends.

FEBRUARY

The abbot must take care, with diligence and cautious
practical wisdom, not to lose any of his flock.
He must remember that he has undertaken the care
of sick souls, not the repression of healthy ones.

☀

The Rule of St. Benedict

Three degrees. A powdery blanket of fresh snow shimmers under the street-lights. In the past week the weather has become more seasonal: lows hovering either side of naught, bitter northern breezes, and snow. We are all groaning: people and cars and furnaces alike.

Yesterday was unsettled by my conversation with the obstetrician. I had referred a patient with twins to her, wanting specialist to meet mother before the onset of labor. The hospital requires (and common sense dictates) that a specialist attend every twin birth in case one or both babies are breech. The obstetrician seemed irritated by my desire to participate. No matter that I had cared for this patient throughout all of this pregnancy (and the last). The suggestion of working together seemed a nusiance or an insult. "Give up the patient in the first trimester, or, if you feel confident, deliver her on your own," she put it flatly. When I approached her again, later, she would only add indignantly, "What do you want from me?" I tried to explain but she cut me off, explaining "I have two patients waiting. Bring this up at the Perinatal meeting, and we'll see how the others feel." Water in oil; no meeting of the minds.

This alone was worth stewing about, but yesterday would embroil us in another crisis. A patient of mine began labor at 9:00 A.M. The fetal heart rate began low at one hundred ten beats per minute, and occasionally fell below that with a contraction. I admitted her to the hospital, and by 11:00 A.M. the membranes ruptured, initiating hard labor. By 1:00 P.M., the cervix was fully dilated but the baseline fetal heart rate crept lower. For the next forty minutes my patient pushed steadily as we watched the baseline fetal heart rate fall to one hundred, with decelerations to eighty and seventy beats per minute with each contraction. Oxygen and frequent position changes could not free what we had conjectured to be a pinched umbilical cord.

I called the obstetrician in the hope that the application of forceps might deliver us from our predicament. She arrived quickly and determined that the head was too high for forceps. C-section, crash. Thirty-one minutes later we were circling the OR table, the obstetrician, myself as first surgical assistant, and a pediatrician waiting in the wings. All was going well; the fetal heart rate, especially, had improved to one hundred twenty beats. As we entered the uterus with a low transverse incision, we were greeted by the umbilical cord. The obstetrician reached low with her hand to disengage the head and deliver it, but it would not budge. It would neither rotate nor flex. A minute of gentle manipulation went by, with reinsertions of the hand and changes to the opposite side of the table. Her voice grew uncertain, with a note of panic. "This has never happened to me before. I don't know what's wrong, I don't know how to free the head. It's too tight." She glanced at the anesthesiologist, but he assured her that the patient's abdominal muscles were fully relaxed. I suggested that I insert my hand in the patient's vagina and push the fetal head upward, or that she enlarge the surgical wound. She chose to widen the incision, cutting vertically through the skin, muscle, peritoneum.

Still the head would not budge. "Get a surgeon. Get him here now," she instructed the circulating nurse. At the prompting of the scrub nurse, I went to the foot of the operating table and pushed with my hand through the vagina, lifting the fetal head into the uterus, but still the infant would not be delivered abdominally. Moments later the general surgeon appeared, unscrubbed but in gown and gloves. He inserted his hand through the uterine incision, groped in the pelvis, and retrieved the head. The rest of the baby followed promptly, and it cried faintly before flying away in the arms of the pediatrician. He would later report that the baby needed only blow-by oxygen and a brisk rub to revive it. The infant boy weighed a meager five pounds, six ounces. Our estimation of a due date, ten days hence, had been ironclad, with good dates and confirmation by ultrasound, but mother was a cigarette smoker who admitted to a pack-a-day habit.

Baby was fine, mother was happy, but what had gone wrong? Why the fetal distress and the difficult delivery? I was more concerned now about political repercussions. Would the obstetrician feel less inclined to allow family doctors to assist at C-section? Would she feel more vulnerable, more exposed? Would she question my handling of the labor, my reaction to the falling fetal heart rate? I don't know why, but I called her office and left a message of thanks for helping me today.

Last evening, by the end of work, I felt chilly, sickened, exhausted. I drove to the hospital to visit mother and baby and review my documentation of the day's events. I dictated a delivery note that summarized my observations. After arriving home, the muscles in my neck tightened like a vice, and neither a pale ale nor acetaminophen nor naproxen could relieve it. I could not eat supper or think about choir, so went to bed with Lindsay and Clare at 7:30 P.M. Lindsay had been on the couch all day with a stomach virus, and Clare had collapsed for the night without a daytime nap.

Yesterday was a stressful end to a stressful week. I was awakened at midnight by OB. "We have a lady here in active labor, six centimeters dilated, no doctor and no prenatal care and I don't feel head. Could you come in?"

Of course I could, and sailed to meet my young patient as she writhed with another contraction. Her mom and dad stood anxiously by her side, having learned only an hour earlier that they would become grandparents. The family was from Stockton—our neck of the woods—and they assured me that they "would have chosen us for their doctor had we known about it earlier."

Judy appeared to be a plain, pimple-faced twenty-one-year-old girl. She stopped moaning long enough for me to examine her vaginally. My hand palpated a spongy dome pressing through a partially dilated cervix. Too firm for a bag of waters, no hint of anus or leg to suggest frank breech, and, with firm pressure, I could almost trace the outline of the fontanelles. Yet I had no knowledge of this baby, only an approximate due date (it was now forty weeks from the date of conception) and a hint that the baby was good-sized, judging by the mountain of an abdomen that tossed on the birthing bed. I ordered an ultrasound.

"Tell me all you can about this baby," I urged the X-ray technician. He studied the screen, combed the abdomen with his transducer, and in a moment replied, matter of factly, "Eight pounds, adequate fluid, no obvious birth defects."

So I let her labor, ordered prenatal labs, studied the tracings, and documented her rapid progression to full cervical dilatation. But thereafter, no further progress, no descent. An hour plodded by, then two, with intensified sporadic decelerations (to sixty) of the fetal heart rate, which resolved with oxygen and repositioning of the patient. I now fretted over how long Judy had been in labor (she complained of having a "stomach flu" for the last three days), the prolonged rupture of membranes (as much as twenty-four hours), and the plummeting heart rate of this spongy-headed baby.

2:30 A.M. I decided to call the obstetrician for a C-section; she agreed that "the troops" should be summoned. We delivered a healthy eight-pound, four-ounce baby with incredible cranial moulding and a boggy scalp, but cute as a bug.

In the meantime, another OB had presented with a history of ruptured membranes. I evaluated her before the C-section; waters intact, and I saw only an occasional contraction on the monitor. Even though she had delivered her five previous children in less than an hour, I felt confident this one would wait, and excused myself to assist with the section.

When I returned, there was still no active labor, only an intermittant blip on the monitor strip. So I nicked her membranes and started pitocin, all of us anxious (after a week of false starts) to get on with the delivery. By 6:00 A.M., she had gushed a river of clear yellow amniotic fluid, and her labor was strong and regular. The head nurse asked that I place an internal electrode because our external fetal heart rate signal was weak. I did, and returned to the safe and cozy confines of Room 224 to watch snow blow furiously in the streetlights and pile in deepening drifts.

At 7:30 A.M. I hustled down to the cafeteria, ordered scrambled eggs, and waited for Tim. It was Monday morning: the passing of the torch. After exchanging the beeper, I could sign out from my hospital charge and sign off on this dreadful week. "Dr. Loxterkamp, call OB," announced the page operator overhead. So I scurried up two flights to Maternity and found my patient pushing mightily. "Time?" asked the husband, and I nodded. Within minutes, a parade of children entered the birthing room and lined up behind me, quietly, patiently, looking for all the world like the Von Trapp family from the *Sound of Music*. Five minutes later a new baby boy, coated in vernix and dashed with blood, was born. Mike, the oldest son, could only ask, with mouth agape, "How will you ever get the blood off those sheets!" My partner, who peeked in the door just moments before the birth of Baby, was handed a camera by the father and took the portrait, a vintage Norman Rockwell pose.

Home and shower and goodbye to my Lindsay and Clare. We had a skeleton crew at the office to handle the few brave souls who would venture out in the snowstorm. It would be a relaxed and easy morning. I approached the paperwork on my desk and gradually began to make out gray countertop. "Do I think so and so is a good enough mother?" the forms demanded to know. At nineteen, single, pregnant with her third, how could anyone be? But in whose eyes, by what standards, and with what degree of certainty should I reply? "Do I think so and so is ready to return to work following his injury?" I had examined him only once, several months ago now, for a sinus infection. Disability reports and abnormal tests and trouble with medication; a half-dozen telephone calls to wade through before disappearing at noon for the Perinatal Meeting.

I was nervous about it. Three weeks ago I had been asked to review charts.

Four seemed appropriate for discussion and raised interesting questions, so I summarized them for the committee's review. Our discussion was lively, the opinions frank. I took issue with a colleague who had deviated from protocol with a new drug for postpartum hemorrhage. By his nature, Bob is more aggressive than I and leans toward the dramatic resolution sooner than I would. But that is not at issue here, only his reasons for taking this course of action. The committee concluded, wisely, that there is more than one way to skin a cat.

I knew the review had gone reasonably well by the remarks of a colleague. "Seems like Perinatal is becoming more educational these days," he offered during our stroll to the parking lot. "We've gotten more comfortable around each other and can differ without arguing." Comfortable, indeed. There is a fine art, and no mean amount of courage, needed for doctors to begin learning from each other, so that dialogue develops, ties are strengthened, education becomes a shared proposition. It happens rarely in Perinatal Committee, and probably nowhere else in the hospital. We doctors defend our bad habits, rationalize our mistakes, and relegate them to a cursory discussion of "complications." Who would have done it differently under these circumstances, with *this* sort of patient, given the lawyers and DRGs and the limitation of a small hospital. All the while we chant the physician's mantra in silence: "There but for the grace of God go I."

We all blunder; that is not the point. But I believe there is a professional obligation for us to face our mistakes together, with kindness and honesty and our patients' best interests in mind. Conspiracies of silence, this minding of our own business, will never do. In five months I must again lead a chart review; will I do it with edges?

The obstetrician was conspicuously absent from today's meeting, so what does that mean for the group? I know it is threatening to have one's conduct or outcomes scrutinized. Is she defensive, or was she busy, or did she simply forget?

Under the pressure of the week, my poor cheeks were mauled by nervous chewing. They are healing now, and I'm settling into a quiet winter's week.

I have not settled in, really. My uneasiness and restlessness and chest tightness did not roll away as expected. Will I be ready in three short days when hospital week returns?

Two days ago I entered the room of a woman who had come for her annual pap and pelvic. This much I knew; it was indicated on the schedule. She is not a person who volunteers more. Today she sat expressionless on the examination table, two hundred pounds of ballast and blank stares. "So how are you?" I ventured. "Any problems since your last visit?"

"Not really," she mumbled. "I've been waking up nights with tingling hands. A pause, an averted gaze, the intimation of a smile, then nothing. With prodding, I discover that the dizzy spells, chest discomfort, lack of energy, and weight gain all began after the delivery of her last child. I learn that the biological father has been pressing for paternity testing. The baby was conceived out of wedlock, during their separation, in the midst of an affair. Surprisingly, her marriage held and her husband accepted her two conditions before their reconciliation: this new daughter, and marriage counseling. But in therapy my patient began to recover an abused past. "Sexually?" I probe, as if I had the time and wherewithall to pursue her answers. She nods. "Your father?" Her eyes bore a hole through the floor and she nods again. "Are you having active memories; do you recall the circumstances?"

My patient remembers nothing particular, only the growing sense that she had been molested. "All the evidence points to it," she whispers from her round, sad face. "I feel nervous around my father. And growing up, I can hardly remember him."

I note in the record that she is depressed, overweight, and making little progress in therapy. Is this "history" of sexual abuse a therapist's working hypothesis or an example of "false memory" that is so much the topic of debate? I go no further, resist any comment, wrestle with my own doubts and disbeliefs. My patient seems neither disappointed nor relieved that I have turned to the perfunctory elements of the H&P. Before leaving, I offer the usual advice. "Take some time for yourself, away from the kids. Try to exercise regularly; it would help you lose weight, and might lift your spirits. And if your therapist is not helping you, consider another. I am not recommending that you switch, only that you consider it. It's your decision, your life. As a doctor, I've learned that it's impossible to help everyone with every problem."

I have no delusions that she will ever find the perfect therapist, the right drug, or the whole truth about her molestation. What key might unlock the mystery, melt away the pounds, or lead her to a place of forgiveness and healing?

I mentioned my mixed emotions to Scott after morning hours. "People need a ticket into a group," he stated matter-of-factly, "a place where they belong, a group that will listen to them and accept them. Which ticket, which name for the disease, doesn't really matter much. But *everyone* needs a group." Scott became—at this precise moment—acutely aware of the contradiction in his position. We have badgered him for months to join our Thursday morning group. Just a week ago, Mary Beth invited him again and nearly hooked him. "But I love the morning routine of grinding coffee, filling the humidifier, feeding the birds, and stoking a fire in the woodstove," came the reply. "And if I arrived at 8:00, I would have an hour free before appointments at ten. And I couldn't come tomorrow morning because my pipes are frozen and need thawing . . ." Exposed, Scott sheepishly ackowledged, "I know, I know, groups are good for everyone but me."

"No," I objected, "groups are hard for us all." Later, as I gathered my coat and belongings to leave, I saw Scott at the front desk rearranging his schedule to accommodate the Thursday morning meeting.

My last patient of the day was another in need of a group. She had made her appointment to discuss allergy testing, but we got to talking. New in town, Ann had retired here with her husband. A few months later, he died abruptly while they were vacationing in California. Now all of the decisions and responsibilities fell to her: fix the car, make the repairs, file the taxes, manage the estate. And she had no circle of friends to support her.

She still could not mention his name, recount their adventures, touch her fond memories without dissolving in tears. That was the hardest. Why was she stuck? In the course of taking a family history, it emerged that her mother and father had both died suddenly, before there was a chance to say goodbye. "Are you grieving," I suggested, "for both your husband and your parents?" I once again heard ice cracking beneath my feet and asked Ann to think about a bereavement support group that my wife helps to facilitate. "It will be starting in March. You might benefit from talking about your husband without being a burden to your friends. Others have gone through similar pain; sharing it can lift everyone a little higher." We all need a community to absorb our grief.

A silver moon floods my western window like a lamp in the star-speckled sky. It is bitterly cold, the coldest night of the winter. Minus fifteen. Earlier, as I opened the back door, crystallized vapor from the mud room was sucked out of doors by the temperature gradient, like in the wind-tunnel experiments you see on TV. The furnace has been moaning since I awoke, and (I presume) has done so throughout the night.

Bruce Swarmi called yesterday to decline our partnership offer. Though he initially mentioned money as a motive, he later alluded to his opportunity to work with a fellow resident, and to the convenience of staying put. One doesn't strike camp and move on unless there is a driving, a hunger, some unspoken need. Moving takes a leap of faith, and if you are reasonably content where you are, why bother?

Bruce had called me because he couldn't reach Tim. Tim was out attending the coroner's case of a twenty-one-year-old male in the High Street Apartments. Apparent suicide by gunshot wound. I was glad they nabbed Tim and not me. That section of town, the seat of so much of Belfast's poverty and misery and hopelessness, makes me nervous. I don't want to face another fifteen-year-old mother clutching her underclad infant, or another dingy room littered with beer cans and butt-filled ashtrays, mattresses on the floor, and dirty dishes moldering in the sink. Where are the parents? Do these kids matter to anyone but the police?

We are a small town. How can we not regard these children as our own: truant from our schools, regulars at our soup kitchen, fixtures in the downtown doorways and on every corner? These are *our* kids being booked for petty larceny, filling the maternity ward, and aspiring to nothing higher than a life on the public dole. I know through my work as a medical examiner that their fortunes can go lower, so tonight I am thankful to have been spared.

I have had a wonderful weekend. On Friday morning, Lindsay and I packed Clare's suitcase for her big adventure, then dropped her off at day care, from which she would go to spend the night with a friend. Lindsay and I fled for Portland in anticipation of Thai dining and bookstore browsing and the sheer thrill of escape. Upon our return that evening, we rented *Europa, Europa,* a German movie about Solomon Perel, a Jewish boy who had successively survived the Warsaw Ghetto, a Russian orphanage, Hitler Youth Camp, and the Russian liberation. We have not watched an adult video in so long that we savored even the movie's deep sorrow. After such an unfettered and romantic day with Lindsay, I feel rejuvenated. Now I am hospital doctor for the next two weeks while the Hugheses fly to California.

At 6:30 A.M., the thermometer has not budged. A thick mat of steam rises from the Bay, every chimney sports a plume, and the moon has slipped from the midnight sky.

A light salting of snow sprinkles through the glow of streetlights. The temperature reads a comfortable twenty degrees, but inside we feel the desiccating effects of a prolonged cold snap.

I could have brewed beer this morning but decided against adding yet another project to an overflowing weekend. My belly is bursting from last night's feast on Susan Loomis's cajun cookin' at Darby's Restaurant. I also tried Andrew's Brown Ale on draught. It is a local beer from Lincolnville that recently made its debut. Though I applaud the effort, I find the beer lacking. The hops seem dusty and cloying to the palate, masking whatever sweetness you expect from an amber ale. It also seemed thin, but that may reflect the English fashion of undercarbonating their draught ales.

Scott's birthday is two days off, according to Lindsay's calendar of events. I have been thinking about him in the context of St. Luke's story of the prodigal son (15:11–32). In this beautiful parable, the youngest son asks his father for his inheritance. The father obliges, and the boy flees the country with his fortune in hand. But after squandering it on a life of debauchery, the son comes to his senses. He makes his way home to beg for his father's mercy. "Father, I have sinned against heaven and against you; I no longer deserve to be called your son; treat me as one of your paid servants."

My favorite lines of the parable are these: "While he was still a long way off, *the father saw him and was moved with pity.*" He runs to his younger son, hugs him, and kisses him tenderly. Afterward, confronted by the older, obedient son, he replies, "My son, you are with me always *and all I have is yours.* But it is only right that we should celebrate and rejoice, because your brother was dead and has come to life; he was lost and is found."

These lines illuminate the difference between justice and mercy. The word "prodigal" comes from the Latin *prodigus,* which means lavish or recklessly wasteful; it could also describe someone endowed with surprising qualities and gifts, or a wanderer who has at last returned home.

The father's joy is my own, for Scott has joined our group. It was my selfish wish. Scott is endowed with surprising qualities and gifts, and I see in his return the chance for deeper friendship. But I don't want my joy to reflect poorly on Tim and Mary Beth, who are my faithful family.

The first day back on hospital duty, and I am exhausted. In the morning I saw three patients in the emergency room and four on the floor: The most interesting was a pregnant girl with flank pain. She had a slight fever, increasing abdominal pain, and a falling white blood cell count (17.6 to 12.6 thousand in four hours). The consulting surgeon poked and jabbed the girl and decided to operate. We entered at McBurney's point, that mythical pole halfway between umbilicus and the anterior superior iliac crest. Bingo. The first slice yielded a well of straw-colored serous fluid, suggesting hidden inflammation but not rupture. The odorless liquid was cultured, and the surgeon dislodged the swollen sausagelike tip of vermiform appendix, with omentum matted about. We irrigated, found cloudy liquid in the hepatic gutter, and placed a drain to avoid a postsurgical abscess.

I asked about the falling incidence of appendicitis, but the surgeon was unsure. I remember reading in the rural weekly newspapers—the Rolfe *Arrow* and Kremmling *Times*—frequent reports about one child or another recovering from an appendectomy. These were the years—circa 1948 or 1949—when Ernest Ceriani and my father settled into their rural practices. The major surgical texts support my suspicion, noting a significant decline in the number of appendectomies worldwide over the last four decades. The fall (40 percent in the 1940s, 25 percent in the 1970s, 15 percent currently) may be due in part to fewer diagnostic errors, but this doesn't account for it entirely. The texts do not speculate on why, but a recent article does. Finnish authors have found that proximity of pigs significantly increases one's risk of acute appendicitis. Pigs harbor Yersinia organisms, which may be the causative agent in 30 percent of cases. The declining rate of appendicitis may reflect the dwindling farm population in developed countries.

Office hours in the afternoon were a nightmare. Fifteen patients were scheduled and everyone came, each overflowing his or her time slot. Fifteen minutes for a postpartum depression, an insomniac teenager, a "walk-in" with unstable angina, an unexpected pregnancy. Fifteen minutes for an HIV-positive patient whose psychosocial issues alone could absorb twice the limit (and did). After finishing late, I arrived home with ten charts yet to complete.

I am thankful for the images on the walls around me—Erasmus, my father's portrait, the Angel Gabriel, Lev Tolstoy, Our Lady of Guadalupe, and St. Dominic. And for the artists whose inspired hands created them. For Handel, whose *Carmelite Vespers* have become my morning fare, and for Kathleen Norris, whose *Dakota: A Spiritual Geography* merges with my sleep. And for Lindsay and Clare whom I take too often for granted as they sleep snugly beyond the stairs.

I am reminded, on the eve of Scott's forty-seventh birthday, that we are all destined to die. Even with generous allowances, Scott has exhausted half his life. The rest pours through the hourglass in grains of frustration, sorrow, and pain. Scott clearly savors these moments, every one of them, which offers me hope.

The last two days have reaped rewards at the going rate: bone-grinding exhaustion; niggling worry. The office continues to surprise me. I innocently inquired about a young woman's weight, but she anwered with sudden sobbing. Her husband no longer loves her, he announced two months ago; he wants out; he wants no part of "working at things." She is my age, her marriage also the same age as mine. We met through the community chorus. She has brought her tears to me because there is nowhere else to turn, save to her friends who are also facing divorce.

I saw a sweet sixteen-year-old, pretty and shy and pregnant, who was joined today by her mother. The boyfriend fled when he heard the news, Mother mutters under her breath. His parents have contacted hers; they will pay for an abortion. But my patient's father will hear none of it. What nerve! What rights do they have, anyway?

"A lot of nerve but no rights," I reassure him. I mention other sixteen-year-olds in my practice who had become pregnant and still made something of their lives.

There was a sprinkling of earaches, pregnant bellies, postpartum checks, blood pressure readings, blessings for a benign mole, and balm for a lame hip. Then I sat down to a peculiar man, a *big* man who was "all stove up." He related the story of his artificial hip, the sling around his left arm, his bag of pills, and how he squandered an $80,000 disability settlement. But I do note his weight and scold him for straining his loaner hip. He agrees with me. He mimics the gruff voice of his orthopedist, who would cross his arms and curse and walk out in disgust at his excessive weight. He takes the words from my mouth (or rather *puts* them there) with a thrust of his good arm. "Jerry," he says to himself, "how do you expect me to help you if you refuse to help yourself? Why should I try when you've given up? Every month you return fatter and lazier and whinier than the last. You know what you need to do; you've got all the answers. Well, if you're gonna throw in the towel, throw in the towel."

Enjoying his soliloquy, I cut him short. I haven't given up, I reassure him. I want him to lose a pound a week and see me in two months. And if the neck, back, and hip pain are worse because of the weight, I threaten to send him back to his orthopedist.

Last night I sang Bruckner, Handel, and Mendelssohn at community choir practice and forgot about Jerry and the others. The new day rolled me out of bed early for the delivery of Evan Tyde Moody, born with a single push at 12:23 A.M., the third in a series of Moodies that I have personally delivered. They want a fourth, and I agree to stay for the fireworks.

The Thursday group today was altogether different with Tim absent and Scott present. I shared my thoughts on the prodigal son and drew the parallels: I rejoice, like the father moved to pity, that Scott has taken a step closer, but my sympathies lie also with the obedient son, who is jealous of the plans for his brother's homecoming. I welcomed Scott, this man of many talents and much love.

We talked superficially, but I learned more about Scott's intense disdain of winter: cold floors, creaking wood, long nights, endless drudgery, starvation for the animals stranded outside. For Scott, the yawning doors of the woodstove reveal his blackened interior and the faceless form of death. He wonders if Mary Beth and I ever become depressed. I reassure him that I do; it is a bridge between us all, the composers I listen to each morning, our clientele, and those of us who provide for their care.

The dark hood of night still cloaks the eastern sky, but I can now see a thread of orange branching into pale yellow and then into violet-gray. The dawn intensifies over Blue Hill, then dips into the waters of Penobscot Bay and becomes luminescent in the snow outside my window. I savor the last remaining moments before I must rise to the day's demands. The ER just called; a patient who was threatening to miscarry has made good on her claim. She will arrive soon by ambulance, so I'll pop off my Macintosh and rush to get dressed.

The miscarriage was the beginning of a twelve-hour stretch of quirks and surprises. No sooner had I completed the D&E than Bonnie called from the office. An Italian sailor, just off the boat, was in the emergency room complaining of abdominal pain. No interpreter; he spoke only enough English to order a meal or find a bathroom, and he needed neither. There was no one at the hospital who spoke Italian, so I called Lindsay, who had mentioned to me an advertisement in the window of the Belfast Travel Agency for Italian lessons. The agency retrieved a name and number, and by good fortune Enzo Palmeri was home and agreed to come quickly.

The sailor, a twenty-nine-year-old Sicilian, lay apprehensively on his cot. He was a small man, unshaven but fine featured, and "in no apparent distress" from what I could tell by the lively conversation he carried on with the first mate. Enzo learned that the sailor had been diagnosed with an ulcer five weeks ago and placed on medication. But he stopped taking it once he felt better. Now the pain had returned, stools were black, food nauseated him, and he got lightheaded every afternoon when he lugged beef quarters to the kitchen.

The sailor had been a pastry chef in Italy, but shipside he assumed the duties of a chef's assistant and was assigned the most strenuous tasks. He hated his job and the boat and desperately longed to be home in Sicily. Enzo could collect no family history because the sailor was an orphan. After the rape of his mother, he was abandoned on the steps of the local church. His surname, which in Italian means "thorn," was given to him, he explains with a shrug of his shoulders, "by the Virgin Mary."

Bleeding ulcer was, of course, at the top of our list of diagnostic possibilities, but why was movement of his right leg causing such a piercing pain? And why, also, flank pain? An examination of the patient's leg, abdomen, and urine revealed no clues. X-rays ruled out peptic ulcer perforation; ultrasound found an empty gall bag, an unobstructed ureter, and no evidence of abdominal abscess. Moreover, the patient was afebrile and his normal white blood count argued against infection. Enzo, who is Italian-born, sensed an emotional overlay—the combination of homesickness and native temperament—that might explain our confusion. But I consulted a surgeon anyway, who concurred. Enzo agreed to be available by telephone, and would return at 9:00 the next morning for an updated report.

Somehow we marched eighteen patients through a chaotic afternoon schedule. With Tim gone, there is no slack, no space for emergencies. We learned that a nurse of ours had ruptured her bag of waters at thirty-two weeks gestation and was rushed to Eastern Maine Medical Center for an impending delivery. I was home in time for pizza, and braced for the gathering storm. Snow, turning to rain: a heartache in midwinter.

Fourteen degrees and snow are forecast for the afternoon and evening. If the storm materializes, tonight's office hours will be curtailed. Rose-colored streaks in an otherwise blanketed morning sky, so the forecasters may be right. At this magical moment—ten past six—the first morning light gives our snowy lawn a perfect sheen.

Miraculously, I am back at the computer. I was on call for family practice over the long weekend and swamped by hospital admissions and the incessant ringing of the telephone. The sailor left the hospital yesterday, Italy-bound with no more than an upset stomach and homesickness. We didn't complete the workup with an endoscopy, although the patient agreed to have it if necessary. "If I can do thirty," he explained in colloquial Italian, "I can do thirty-one." Enzo drew a blank on the origins of the expression. Perhaps it is similar to our own "the whole nine yards," which always seemed curiously short of a first down.

Lindsay made a marvelous dish for Valentine's Day—chicken in a vegetable cream sauce, served in a heart-shaped pastry shell. We had invited Mary Beth and her family, but their son, Evan, developed a stomachache so severe that he required IV rehydration. Lindsay presented me with a box of Godiva chocolates (which I could share) and I reciprocated with a bit of verse:

> I call to mind your dainty feet
> that keep a Sandy Nelson beat.
> Once, that danced a disco floor
> Now patter to our daughter's door.
>
> I see your cherry lips impressed
> on napkins, envelopes, and the rest . . .
> These perfect loaves, their ruby hue,
> Fuel my lasting flame for you.
>
> Fingers tiny, features fair,
> The glanced, discrete, and stolen stare.
> The perfect poundage, not too slim,
> "Just two, two-and-a-half to trim."
>
> On Valentine's, like mating birds,
> I find the object for these words
> And bow to say, *tres musical,*
> "Yours, and not another's, gal."*

She would have preferred something more romantic, more serious, but my poetry doesn't run that way. I borrowed the reference to mating birds from the Chambers *Encyclopedia of Saints,* which cites the ancient belief (dating from Chaucer) that birds begin to choose their mates on Valentine's feast, the very beginning of spring.

In the hospital this morning, a young, asplenic child is being treated for pyelonephritis. The rest are old: pneumonias, end-stage emphysema, congestive

* A paraphrase and translation of the words Lindsay had engraved on my wedding ring, "toi et nul autre."

heart failure, and a recovering heart attack. I will hasten through my rounds, attend the IDT meeting, and attempt a few errands today before 1:00 P.M., when office hours begin in earnest.

After three hospital admissions yesterday, we have reached the high-water mark. Our rubbish collector came in during last night's snowstorm with severe cramps and bloody stools. A prenatal patient was admitted with *hyperemesis gravidarum* and treated with *hypervolemia intravenum*. And a lung cancer patient rolled in with the "dwindles"—probably an admixture of dizziness, diabetes, constipation, and too many birthdays. Her admission is all gristle and fat, the kind Medicare hopes to cut, the kind that earns the rural physician his sullied reputation. So be it. Add these to the six others. And Noble.

I was called away early yesterday morning with the news of Noble's passing. It was, as we often say, a blessing. I remember his comment the day before, "These have been hard days, Reverend, but getting harder." Only sixty-nine years old, his lungs were like bubble packing, full of tiny, useless air sacs. The nurses found him dead at 7:18 A.M., called his wife (no answer), then found me. By the time I arrived, they were "right wild" with the thought of his wife appearing unforewarned. And she did, as I was reviewing a fresh EKG on the heart patient in the ICU. The supervisor danced me into the hallway to intercept the Mrs. "Could I walk you to the room," I volunteered.

"Has Noble turned?" she asked pointedly. Without answering directly, I recalled how Noble had said his goodbyes yesterday, as if he knew, as if to ready himself for the journey. We were in his room now, accompanied by the unsettling silence, so different from the usual pants and groans and the "hi, doc" that Noble could muster no matter how deep his oxygen debt. In the room with us, sitting beside Noble, was an old friend whom the wife credits (along with half of Waldo County, at one time or another) with saving her life. Her tears flowed freely, so uncharacteristic of these preceding months. I would have stayed, been the attentive hospice physician, had my heart patient not needed me now. I hugged the Mrs. and left her for the urgency of the ICU.

Before choir rehearsal last night I went to "the viewing," what Catholics call the wake, where we find the souvenir prayer cards (with a litho of a popular saint on the back), recite the rosary, and shake hands with family on the receiving line. A good funeral home is a Victorian one, and Rackliffe's is architecturally among the best. In the front hallway I met the assistant director, who had dropped by the office with Noble's death certificate earilier today. We chatted about music, compared birthdates (1949 and 1953), and talked about war, Vietnam and Desert Storm and the factional fighting in the former Yugoslavia, smeared with reports of ethnic cleansing that recall the Holocaust.

In the next room congregated the green, decorated caps of the American Legion and VFW; both were worn in the leadership roles that Noble and his wife asssumed for years. I sidestepped their covey and went directly to the Mrs. She was sitting beside the casket in the front row. I squatted down and introduced myself to the family. But soon the wife was engaged in other handshakes, and I was left with the Legionnaires. There was no choice but to wedge myself into their conversation. One had served in Vietnam, two in Korea, and another was "career" with a double dip into America's armed conflicts. We cleared the air about "what's wrong with the country," figured how much money we all might be making elsewhere, and tapped the general vein of apprehension about our president. I nodded and bided my time. I know how little sympathy there is for Mr. Clinton in these parts, even on issues of the deficit and health care.

Those of us who live here make a choice, and a good one, I'll wager, about what we value most. The green caps nodded attentively, with thumbs tucked in their front pants pockets. They piped in, one by one, each offering a personal testimony. How odd it is, in this small town, to be banding together in such an unlikely group. We share so little in common, or do we? That is the magic of politics: building consensus, drawing divergent groups together, mobilizing folks around mutual concerns. In a small town, it is easy to find your enemy or a kindred spirit in the same person, depending on the time or topic.

This morning I met Don in the ER. I had seen him in the office three days ago and suggested that, if he wasn't any better, we should meet here for tests. He is *never* any better, always refuses to get well, and I should accept this. Yet I pull out my hair every time.

Don is my age, perhaps a little younger, and a linesman for the local district. Likable, laughable, an easygoing sort of guy. Underneath our pleasantries simmers a tension, some unspoken conflict, even palpable anger. I feel pressured by the implicit bargain: if he follows my orders, I will make him better. So when illness lingers, who's to blame? Is it the result of my incompetency, my dishonesty, or my total disregard for his time and money?

Last winter, after a particularly slow recovery from a virus, I asked Don to see my partner for a second opinion. It amazed me when Tim, after his examination and review of the records, told him flatly, "I don't know. I don't know what's wrong with you, but I think you'll get better. Keep doing what your doctor ordered."

Come on, Tim, what are you doing for this guy? He's sick and you turn your back? Toss him limp reassurances and walk away? Well, it was sufficient. Don did not leave in a huff, transfer his care, assassinate the doctor, or die at home with a stash of pills and our knowing reassurances. And Tim, meanwhile, seemed oblivious to the dangers.

I don't remember how I first got tangled in the web, but I've seemed stuck from the start. There was a time—several years ago now—when I thought I had beaten it. Don had been hospitalized for "walking pneumonia" after several weeks of outpatient treatment. In and out of the hospital, we swapped one antibiotic for another. Finally I consulted a psychiatrist, who started him on antidepressants, and the pneumonia improved. But what worked for the psychiatrist, or for my partner, has failed me miserably.

I have seen it often enough now, the ebb and flow of his afflictions. I have wrestled with the tides of anger, his brooding and impatience. We play a game of doctor-over-the-barrel, where he gets no better and I run out of new ideas. It is as if the shield of objectivity had evaporated and I stood defenseless against his claims, his unmet needs. There is something familial going on here. Does it parallel my relationship to my sister, where she is a victim and I the success, and I am somehow responsible? I am to see Don in the ER this morning. What then?

The beeper went off as Scott, Mary Beth, and I closed our meeting. "Don," I pronounced, having devoted the last ten minutes of the meeting to the matter. The ER's extension "123" flashed on the beeper screen, and the receptionist confirmed that he had just arrived.

I entered the ER by the rear entrance and picked up Don's chart at the nurses' station. Out of the corner of my eye I spied him in Bay 6, behind the curtain, sitting quietly on a gurney and hunched in the department's pale blue johnnie. The nurse had collected a new set of symptoms since our last visit: episodes of morning vomiting; transient spells of substernal chest pressure; pills that have stopped working. His normal body temperature argued against a systemic infection; pulse and blood pressure reassured me that he was not in acute distress. I gripped the chart and ducked into his curtained stall.

And as I did, Don crossed his bulky arms, grinned, and needled me, "You're a hard man to get ahold of." I offered a lame apology and began my own line of questioning. "Does exercise, certain food, time of day, or position bring on the pain . . . Is it sharp or dull . . . Does it catch your breath or leave you short-winded . . . Does it make you nauseous or lightheaded or bring on a sweat? My barrage only delayed the moment of truth.

Symptoms pointed to the esophagus. Perhaps they are related to his Crohn's disease, now unattended for over a year. Don had acknowledged a regular showing of blood and cramps and fistular drainage. So here was a handle, an approach, and Tim's strategy flashed in my mind. "Here's what I think, Don, but I can't guarantee it. You probably have acid in your esophagus, and medicine will help it in time. It won't heal quickly because your body is fighting on two fronts.

I recommend some tests that will tell us if you are infected or anemic. And I'd like to ask a surgeon to see you. He can provide a second opinion about your chest pain and recommend treatment for your Crohn's."

Don agreed, and I let out my breath. Things were falling too neatly into place. I had seen the general surgeon moments earlier in X-ray and knew he was available for a consultation if I so desired. The blood test was normal. Don was on his way.

I know that things will not remain neatly in place. He will not get better, even if the surgeon and I agree on the diagnosis and Don follows our recommendation to the letter. But now I will have another colleague to fall back on, endoscopy to offer, a treatment to encourage.

In any chronic disease, including those that infect the doctor-patient relationship, it is crucial to know your limits, anticipate the next turn, observe yourself in action, refrain from making impossible promises, and—most importantly—share the burden. I need help with Don. He draws me in, snags me at every turn, and I can't say why. Do I hear my sister's voice? Do I recognize the family dance, where the sick never grow well, and seem to worsen with age and each intercession?

I know that I am not responsible for Don's illness—either its cause or its cure—and that, as a professional, I am accountable only for my own actions. But we have gone beyond that, Don and I. We share some strange, unexplained sympathy. I *feel* responsible for his pain. And like a gambler who's in over his head, I hang on every minor success to signal a change in our fortunes. But the game is rigged against us. Don has a chronic disease from which he will never recover, and my choice to participate in it carries a personal risk.

I know that we are both here for the long haul and that, as a consequence, there is still hope.

The end of a pair of weeks on call. Yesterday—a Saturday when otherwise I might have signed out—was spent on hospital rounds in the morning and deliveries in the afternoon. While waiting, I dictated discharge summaries and watched medical videos. Lindsay kept the home fires burning, attending our feverish daughter who was sickened by "the bug going around."

It has been bitterly cold all week, minus eight at sunrise. So cold that I crept to the compost heap entirely on the crust of our last wet snowfall, which glistened in the severe light of the morning sun, a quilt of ripples and dimples where concealed subterranean rivers once ran. A new snow gently falls at 8:00 A.M., and the Tercel has turned over, to my delight, purring proudly. We hobble out of the drive, shifting gears with a strong shove, and run an ice-caked course to work.

It is snowing briskly outside, a typical Nor'easter. A bank of Arctic air is barring this southern front from fizzling into rain. It will force it over the Atlantic Ocean where it can pick up moisture and fold back onto itself. At least this is how I understand the process from "The Weather School" on Channel 5. The temperature held at fourteen degrees all night, and I couldn't sleep, my brain idling high with anticipation.

I am brewing beer this morning for the first time in over a year. A strong ale, perhaps the equivalent of a German doppelbock: two pounds of an amber Bierkeller malt extract, four pounds of a light Mountmellick malt extract, four gallons of water, Hallertauer hops (a pinch for the wort and a half cup for the fermentation), Whitbread Ale yeast, and a dash of Irish Moss (a clarifier) for the end of the boil. It is a simple process that fills the kitchen with sweet maltiness for hours after the brew. But I have not achieved, cannot master, the perfection of the premium commercial beers, the likes of St. Ambroise of Montreal, Maine's own Geary's Hampshire Ale, or the Belgian Trappist line.

After moving to Maine, I attempted to bake bread as a means of self-expression, and failed. Maine brings it out in you, this need to be crafting with your hands. Most newcomers try their luck: we become writers, carpenters, boat builders, entrepreneurs in this or that alongside our primary profession, those of us lucky enough to have one. What might a full-blooded German consider? Brewing, naturally. And so I quickly found the necessary paraphernalia and encouragement. Waldo County is a haven for home brewers. Soon after, I entered a John Bull doppelbock in the Common Ground Fair and won "first in category." I was also given a maroon "Judges Award" for second place overall. My head swelled beyond my abilities, and thereafter I suffered through a spate of average beers, stronger than what you might buy in the store, better than you might imagine, but not spectacular, not anything I would pay money for.

Ash Wednesday and sixteen degrees. I hope to get smudged today at Mass, though feel the conflict it creates. It will require that I trim my morning with Lindsay and Clare (on the day following her bumpectomy,* which I could not attend) and arrive late at my business meeting with Tim and Cathy. All of this for a sign of Catholic solidarity. I have resurrected another Lenten observation from my childhood: real Catholics don't eat meat, at least not on Ash Wednesday or the Fridays of Lent.

Yesterday Maine Public Radio reported a February snowfall of thirty-three inches; more is forecast for the weekend. One must go back twenty years to find a snowier February.

---

* Clare had a pilomatrixoma removed from her neck.

Last evening, as I left for RENEW, James Kennedy called. I have been trying to reach him for four months. Jim and his family moved to Kremmling, Colorado, in the fall of 1973 to film a documentary on the life and practice of Ernest Ceriani. In 1976, Jim returned alone to complete the project. When I initially called him, he was recuperating from a bout with hepatitis C. Now he is interested in my plans and has agreed to help me find a copy of *Doctoring* in its uncut ninety-minute version. To make the telephone call worth his while, I pass along a tip about Glenn Willumson's recent critique of Gene Smith's photo essays,* which contains fascinating details about Smith's trip to Kremmling in 1948 and *Life's* agenda behind the shooting. Curiously, and unknown to either, both Kennedy and Willumson live in Santa Monica, California.

The primary fermenter is burping every five seconds through its air lock. If I listen carefully, I hear that reassuring sound behind the closed door where the beer lies incubating. We are now forty-eight hours into fermentation, and everything is going well. I knew that I could count on this yeast when, after pitching it, the most unbelievable fruity aroma filled my nose. This is a time of great optimism, following a successful boil and a vigorous fermentation. But what will it taste like, and will the secondary fermentation (so-called "bottle-conditioning") finish it properly? I am eight weeks from an answer.

Eight people returned to RENEW, in a shuffle that included one new entry and three dropouts. It is a solid group. There was much laughter and serious talk from all participants, and I suspect we are forming some bonds. Last night's topic was "risk"; and one of the selected scripture passages troubled me again. "Follow me, and let the dead bury the dead," Jesus cautioned a disciple who was in need of burying his father. It seems such a hard line for so worthy a task. I suppose we don't have the whole story; indeed, we have thirty-one words. The RENEW exegetes see it as the rebuke of a procrastinator. Would we be willing to risk everything to follow Jesus, or would we, like the dutiful son, beg for a little more time to attend to our worthy causes, our prior obligations, our special circumstances?

The question was raised, "Of whom does our faith demand more—the monk or the missionary or the suburbanite, whose Christian values must compete with every possible distraction?" The comparison seems a trap. We each have our careers and responsibilities, so the goal should be to execute them in fidelity to God and our true selves, and by this means "pray without ceasing."

I underestimated the stress of my daughter's bumpectomy. Clare has been obstinate, sassy, physically combative, and just plain *angry* since she and Lindsay went to the surgeon two days ago. Lindsay felt abused by Clare and deserted by me,

---

* *W. Eugene Smith and the Photographic Essay* (Cambridge: Cambridge University Press, 1992).

for I attended an hour of RENEW on the night of the bumpectomy. It proved to Lindsay how far down on the list of my priorities our family had fallen.

Out of a sense of guilt I bought Clare a Little Mermaid puzzle and a "Courtney Cheer-Leader" doll. Not to buy her affection, I say to myself, but to show her that I understand how badly she feels. I had reserved Wednesday afternoon for projects, but, as Lindsay and Clare prepared to leave on a shopping junket, Clare stalled at the door. She wouldn't tell us what was wrong; she wouldn't open her mouth or look at us; large crocodile tears flowed down her cheeks as she clung to the knob, halfway in, halfway out. Finally I whispered, "Would you like Daddy to go, too?" And, with her almost imperceptible nod, I shifted gears and joined in the spree.

Clare has not been able to talk about the operation. But yesterday afternoon she showed me the scar for the first time and reported it to be painless.

Last evening, after we returned from Shop 'n Save, had a snack, and played Barbies with "Courtney," Clare collapsed on the couch and slept through the night. I took the opportunity to attend Ash Wednesday Mass. The altar was dressed in royal purple, the liturgical color of penance and expiation. Catholics have little occasion these days to set themselves apart from the great wash of mainline protestantism, fundamentalism, secular humanism, eastern philosophy, and twelve-step recovery. After Vatican II confined the Friday meat ban to a Lenten observance, the smudge of ashes—a mere thumbprint on the forehead—survives as our most distinguishing sign. There is cult value here, and high ritual, and a chance to accrue plenary indulgences, which are like green stamps for heaven. Catholics line up for it in droves. On the Feast of St. Blaise, we are marked by an invisible sign, the blessing of our throats. But later comes the true test, when the wood of the cross is presented at the Good Friday veneration. I expect that kissing the crucifix makes even the most stalwart Catholic cringe.

At RENEW the other night, I brought up the idea of community, and how this Lenten season has called me closer to it. Two recent readings have complemented this growing appreciation. The first was Henri Nouwen's meditation on icons, *Behold the Beauty of the Lord.* He begins his reflection on "The Descent of the Holy Spirit," a fifteenth-century Russian icon, by saying:

> God reveals the fullness of divine love first of all in community . . . Community is first and foremost a gift of the Holy Spirit, not built upon mutual compatibility, shared affection or common interests, but upon having received the same divine breath, having been given a heart set aflame by the same divine fire and having been embraced by the same divine love. It is the God-within who brings us into communion with each other and makes us one. (pp. 60 and 65)

A few days after reading those words, I happened across a review of Stanley Hauerwas's new book, *Naming the Silences.* * He questions why the experience of illness and death should seem so inexplicable and unnatural for most Americans. He wonders if the notion of suffering has run aground on the shoals of liberalism, "the Enlightenment assumption that we are most fully ourselves when we are free of all traditions other than those we have chosen from the position of complete autonomy." Americans who strive to become self-sufficient and self-satisfied end up living their lives in isolation, fragmentation, and doubt.

When God is absent, "the best we can do is comfort each other in the loneliness and the silences created by our suffering." Hauerwas contends that what drives modern medicine is the fear of abandonment in the face of suffering. He sees the need for communities to shoulder the pain. Medicine—at its very best—responds with a personal presence in the company of those who suffer.

Yesterday was consumed by the computer. My mind was full of the Ernest Ceriani story, which seems such an overwhelming project for this hack historian.

It did not help, either, that I received an acceptance letter for "A Good Death" in yesterday's mail, along with demands for an immediate revision. They would prefer fewer commas, obscure analogies, and incomplete sentences. I'll ask Lindsay for help, knowing how ruthless is her editorial eye.

Medical practice paces one so strenuously, and with such clear objectives (the needs of the patient), that it is hard for doctors to cope with "free" time. I approach it like a kid in a candy store. I hurl myself toward the nearest project without any thought of selection or ordering of priorities. Today there will be no manuscript revision or work on the *Life* magazine story. I am attending Mass, sledding with Clare, and calling Mom a day after her birthday.

* Edwin R. Dubose, *Second Opinion* (July 1991).

MARCH

February's snowfall—a lush two-foot snowpack—has assured us a genuine winter. The snow crests around our garden statuary, reaching the folded arms of Francis and the armpits of our putti. Temperatures fluctuate between zero at night and twenty during the day. Our fuel bill will keep the memories of this cold snap fresh.

Yesterday we made the quintessential family outing to the Northport Golf Club. Its steep hill provides the best sledding in town. We were the first to arrive. Cathy appeared momentarily. Our Bumpertubes carried us with speed and cushioning down the long slope. But then the Hugheses arrived . . . with the Rocket.

Their Snotube is a baby-blue-and-white, flimsier rendition of the Bumpertube, the kind of innertube you might bring to a wading pool. It lacks the substantial textured vinyl of the Bumpertube, and as a result, you can s-a-i-l on its smooth skin. Then Bonnie, Joe, and the kids arrived, and we experimented with stacking the tubes vertically, or stringing them together in long trains.

It was a glorious day, with no serious mishaps, a small crowd (eighteen of us), firmly packed snow, and sunny skies. Ideal conditions, and hot cocoa to warm the gullet. Clare frolicked for two solid hours before collapsing in a whining heap. Later, we enjoyed a quiet afternoon of reading and putzing while Clare napped on the sofa.

Mass readings in Lent always seem to carry a punch. After Jesus fasted for forty days and nights, he entered the wilderness to face the devil (Matt. 4:1–11). "If you are the Son of God, turn these stones into bread." From the dome of the temple, the devil taunted him again, "If you are the Son of God, throw yourself down and let your angels protect you." At last, the devil took him to a mountain top and tempted him with the splendor of earthly realms. "I will give you these," said the devil, "if you fall at my feet and worship me." Jesus replied "Be off, Satan. For Scripture says: you must worship the Lord your God, and serve him alone [Deut. 6:13]. Then the devil left, and angels appeared to look after him."

This is powerful scripture about the showdown between righteousness and evil. It weaves the Old Testament into the New for the sake of authority, strength, and continuity. I don't handle temptation well; I lack the ready retorts. But I am learning to avoid it where it lurks, and to recognize it for what it is.

Clare had her stitches out yesterday. She refused my services, so we took her back to her surgeon. It was a wise decision: a suture had become embedded in the skin margins and bled upon its release. Clare was a little trooper, though; she whimpered but otherwise lay still beneath the surgeon's nimble fingers. Afterward, she pouted for an hour, but the hurricane winds of last week died today before breaching land.

The pathological diagnosis was pilomatrixoma, an oddity that acts like a sebaceous cyst. If left alone, it can grow larger and become infected. But our reason for removing it was that it resembled the more troublesome branchial cleft cyst. I wonder if it was worth it, really, for a bump that was benign, or might have been excised at a later age. Parental anxiety expiated at our daughter's expense. We can never win at this guessing game. We do our best, learn from our mistakes, and provide our kids with as much love and support as we can muster. After the doctor's appointment, Clare and I went to Shop 'n Save for a popsicle reward.

I bottled my beer yesterday and got premonitions of a good batch. The yeast was caked at the bottom of the food bucket like pudding. Another innovation: I sterilized the bottles in the dishwasher using liquified B-Brite detergent. There is much to be learned from an early tasting: the smell is clean, slightly fruity, not overly hopped; the color is rich caramel, but the taste is not as sweet as I had hoped. The aging process may still temper the bitters and clarify a lingering haze. Another week in the toasty *incubatio* (a closet under the stairway where I keep the fermenter), then I will lug it down cellar for a month or two before it reaches peak potability.

Twenty degrees at 4:30 A.M. February's glacier is receding from the roads, ponds, and rooftops. A Charpentier Mass springs lamblike into this new morning.

Yesterday, with its abundance, brings me to a familiar crossroads: too much to record in too little time. I spent two hours on the computer, dashed for donuts with Lindsay and Clare, then bid them adieu at 8:00. The business meeting with Tim and Cathy was followed by ten patients in the morning, a staff meeting for lunch, a dozen patients in the afternoon, and messages to return at day's end. I raced from work to buy a bottle of wine, then hauled Lindsay and Clare to Marc Stewart's for a surprise potluck birthday party. The recurrent theme in the office yesterday was mother-daughter relations. A school guidance counselor called me about a patient whom I have seen twice for headaches, fatigue, and poor appetite. I remember her well, her sulking, moody, obstinate, lackadaisical attitude that seemed, well, "normal" for a teenager. What did her mother expect? All my haranguing on the mother's behalf would not budge the child from her lousy diet and late bedtime. This was a family problem.

The school counselor had referred the girl to an addiction therapist, suspecting that "food issues" were involved. Would I check her electrolytes, she wondered. Have they gone over the edge?

I am annoyed by the contemporary urge to treat all bad behavior as an addiction. I don't understand the motives of an adolescent, but it seems likely that food is often a symptom, just another fault line for splitting parental authority. The important thing is not to remove the addiction but to change the family's focus.

In the afternoon, two school physicals were scheduled back-to-back: teenage sisters. Mother came along with questions about knee pain and scoliosis and poor posture. The oldest daughter was sixteen, fair-skinned, pretty in a fashion after her mother, hair thickly drawn into a ponytail. I noted that her cuticles were gnawed to the bone; she fidgeted on the exam table, sitting with stooped shoulders. My examination uncovered only a laxity in her quadriceps tendon and symmetrically brisk reflexes. I advised an exercise program, to which the mother enjoined, "Listen to the doctor! I've been telling you this for months."

Oh, the doctor's dread: parents who appropriate our authority. I am not a psychologist, but I could see the outlines of the rebellion. Mom is a dance and fitness instructor. Her eldest daughter, so similar in appearance and temperament, is struggling to find her identity and independence. A formula for conflict unless mother lets go. I declined my opportunity to join their struggle. Perhaps it might have worked, my partner suggested later, if mother had sought my collaboration earlier, and in privacy. But I couldn't enter into maternal alliances now without jeopardizing the daughter's trust. I offered an olive branch on mother's way out. "My daughter is only four years old, but can I call you for answers in a dozen years?"

I left Marc Stewart's birthday party early and arrived late at RENEW. Two of the old crew had wandered back. The readings again sparked conversation. In Matthew 22, Jesus is baited by the Pharisees: What is the greatest commandment of the Law? they ask. Jesus replies, "You must love the Lord your God with all your heart, with all your soul, and with all your mind. This is the greatest and the first commandment; the second resembles it: You must love your neighbor as yourself. On these two commandments hang the whole Law, and the prophets also."

Matthew 25 speaks of the last judgment, when God will separate the good from the evil, the sheep from the goats. All hinges on good works, one could argue—our willingness to provide for the hungry, thirsty, lonely, naked, or imprisoned as if attending to Jesus himself. "I tell you solemnly, in so far as you neglected to do this for one of the least of these, you neglected to do it for me." This is solid Catholic social teaching. But one participant shook her head, "I'm having a reaction to that old Catholic guilt trip, just when it seemed the Church had changed. Never enough, always more for the poor and starving and unhappy souls of the world."

I took her side, as much as I wanted to avoid it, for God's judgment is veiled to us all. Jesus replied to Satan's temptation, "Man does not live by bread alone, but by *every* word from the mouth of God"—not just scripture that can be used for the sake of an argument. We are asked to read the whole of the Bible, take account of God's hand in our lives, listen to the faith-sharing and testimony and friendship of all His followers. The human animal craves reassurance, especially around matters as critical as one's salvation. And the Church, as a pastoral institution, responds with a checklist. Good works reassure us about where we stand. But they are also a public expression of our faith in God and love of neighbor. On this the whole law hangs.

One of my favorite patients returned today following a recent hospitalization. His complaints are unchanged: "I'm winded, doc, all played out after just a few steps." Ever since his stroke six years ago, he has been on a downhill slide for reasons variously attributed to pneumonia, congestive heart failure, and emphysema. I have treated him with antibiotics, heart stimulants, bronchodilators, and home oxygen. Nothing helps. In the middle of yesterday's chaos and calamity, I had no patience to consider every unturned stone, or to provide an illusory ray of hope. So I asked him to see my partner in two weeks, realizing that my eyes have grown accustomed to his condition.

And the Enigma returned with her husband. Overcoming her embarrassment, she let me feel her tumors, a dozen or more firm growths scattered on the inside of her right arm, left thigh, and buttocks. Most were half-dollar size, tender, and fixed to the underlying structures. The overlying skin was inflamed, purplish-pink, thickened, and, in some cases, ulcerating. I stared at the biopsy reports from a general surgeon and dermatologist. But she has brought her problems back to me.

The biopsies suggested obscure disease: syphilis, or viral lymphadenopathy, or systemic fungus, or some strange pseudolymphomas caused by the phenytoin the patient takes for epilepsy. The phenytoin hypothesis was scrapped after she stopped the drug and the tumors worsened. The test for syphilis was negative. It *could* be fungus, blastomycosis, or sporotrichosis, and, of course, these are all treatable. The nodules followed the lymphatic chain from their origin below the right elbow to the proximal mid-arm. I called a dermatologist in Bangor who agreed to see the patient "in a few days." Wouldn't it be nice to find a curable cause and to participate in its diagnosis? Seldom does a family doctor get to unravel a case after the specialists become involved. I had purchased a car from the patient's husband when we first moved to town, so he trusted me. I explained that I was only a family doctor but would do my best to find an answer, if one is to be had.

Great news yesterday for the "Larger than *Life*" story. James Kennedy's documentary about Ernest Ceriani arrived in the mail. And I received a telephone call from Ernest's son, Philip, who is an orthopedic surgeon living in Salt Lake City. We had intended a leisurely chat yesterday afternoon, but Philip was detained at the hospital. He will try again tonight, or on the weekend. And my order arrived at the Fertile Mind Bookstore, Gary Wills's *Lincoln at Gettysburg*. It has nothing to do with doctoring, but will likely grow in my imagination and emerge in some written form. A wonderful expression in the first few pages: Wills's depiction of the battlefield, where horseflesh and manflesh "deliquesced in the July sun." The word does not quite work, for bodies decompose by bacterial action, not through the absorption of water vapor. Nevertheless, a beautiful word where the choices are thorny.

Yesterday I ran again for the first time in a month. A warm front lifted the afternoon temperature into the forties, and the misty breeze, melting snow, and my mounting anxiety conspired to draw me onto the asphalt. The run was not enjoyable, but the freedom was, as was the thought of taking a first few steps toward the spring campaign. When Lindsay asked what I wanted for my birthday, I immediately thought of running shoes. My current pair is two years old. Though they are still comfortable and wearing well, there is nothing like the bounce of new shoes for an old stride. What will be pushed aside when running once again consumes three hours of my week?

Twelve degrees, and a surprise Nor'easter has just dumped eight inches of snow across the state. Spring has been thrown back, the snow cover replenished. Perhaps today will bring another round of sledding at Northport Country Club.

The office and its concerns are a distant but advancing worry. Tomorrow I resume command of the hospital. I know that Tim's full house has experienced some recent attrition with a discharge and the death of a hospice patient on Friday. The office troubles began around closing time Thursday, when a patient called to request that his prescriptions be transferred to another pharmacy. Such requests are routinely reviewed by a nurse before we honor them. She noted that it had been over a year since his last appointment, and he had failed to heed Scott's advice for a "follow-up in two weeks' time." The nurse had no choice but to deny the request and encourage him to schedule an appointment.

He mulled over her remarks and redialed. "What's this shit about a physical?" he demanded. The receptionist quickly clicked the "hold" button and signaled for a nurse to pick up the line. He again disgorged his foul mouth while the nurse defended our office policy. Unappeased, his anger was passed to Scott, who had been apprised of the situation. Now the mood changed. Forceful but not belligerent, the patient pleaded with Scott for another three months of medication and promised to come in "when I can afford it." Scott patiently reiterated office policy but could not deter him from his mission.

Overhearing parts of the conversation, and aware of the escalating conflict, I stayed afterward to discuss matters with Scott. He was perturbed, but what could he do? The man was deranged, and Scott wanted to avoid the possibility of violent repercussion. But I emphasized the need to defend our staff, who keep *our* policies and don't deserve the abuse. I reassured Scott that our policies need not be justified; the patient was free to take his medical care anywhere else if he was bothered by our rules. And I strongly advised Scott to write down whatever limits he had set over the telephone, and stick to them, for surely the caller will test him again. Our job is hard enough when people are well-intentioned, appreciative, conscientious. But people are people, and when they face an incapacitating illness, or feel the pinch of its expense, they can be manipulative, rude, and irresponsible. Caregivers, it seems to me, must let anger roll off their backs as much as possible, and stick to the rules the best we can. Ultimately, the patient may be right about the ambiguity or excessiveness of a test, but we must live with the consequences, and it is better for us to err on our own terms.

I had lunch with Marc Stewart on Friday, a nice chat at Darby's Restaurant. Marc was just interviewed by the *Republican Journal*. The only controversial quote, taken in summary of Marc's controversial ministry, appeared at the close of the article. "I believe there are angels looking over the church. In particular, there is one who is probably an old sea captain. He's kind of stingy, but he loves this church. It is God's gift to Belfast." The First Church, to this

Catholic outsider, has always struggled with *precisely* those issues that confront and divide our wider community: stinginess (the reluctance of wealthy new arrivals to help the native poor) and inflexibility (the refusal of oldtimers to welcome change). That church, as the oldest and largest in Belfast, simply constellates the community-wide conflict.

Clare cried yesterday when she realized that Gabriel, her long and devoted friend, and the eldest of the Stewart children, will be leaving for good. I will miss Marc, too, his struggle, the ideals he stood for, and the odd and tentative relationship that had formed between us. Though I sometimes felt myself to be in the role of mentor, I loved our friendship, the hearty laughs, the parallels between our lives of ministry, and long chats where we expounded upon, railed against, and shouldered each other's burdens in the service of this small town. As a going-away present, I have ordered him *Dakota: A Spiritual Geography*, which speaks directly to the role of secrecy in preserving a small town's myths, and of the enormous challenge faced by professionals (especially ministers) who seek the truth and challenge complacency. Our social circle contracts, and Lindsay and I must fight to expand it, to stay open to new friendship, and to preserve that binding arc of love that leads now to Grand Rapids. Our four-year tradition of Christmas dinner with the Stewarts is now over.

Five o'clock A.M., thirty-two degrees, and just back from the hospital. I had been asked to see (and decided to admit) an eighteen-year-old with active ulcerative colitis—her fourth admission since her diagnosis five years ago. This morning, severe lower abdominal cramps and profound anemia canceled her discharge. I applied a "bandaid" to tide her over the three hours until her attending arrives: intravenous fluids, hydrocortisone, a blood transfusion, and medicine for pain and nausea.

The roads are soppy wet with snow, which is expected to fall throughout the day. Another storm is forecast for Friday, and it is predicted to be the winter's worst. We are longing for our trip to Washington, D.C., at month's end.

I had a feast with James Kennedy's *Doctoring*, a ninety-minute film on the rural practice of Ernest Ceriani. It was shot on location in Kremmling, Colorado, in the spring of 1973 and winter of 1977. By then, Doc was an institution (not just a *Life* legend) as the town's physician for over a quarter century. It was exhilarating to finally meet him, hear his voice, observe his gestures, see him in action. Film is able to capture far more than the written or photographic essay, filling the senses with sound and movement.

I borrowed a projector from the local high school, invited my partners, and had a showing that night, during the middle of a snowstorm. I would later show it on my dining room wall several more times that weekend.

Doctoring is a well-crafted film. Kennedy splices Gene Smith's photographs and snapshots from the Ceriani family album effectively into his film. There are a few contrivances, notably the campfire scene at a hospital picnic where the employees gather around the campfire and sing "I've been working on the railroad." But Gene Smith was guilty of worse contrivances, often demanding precise staging and frequent retakes of his photographs. Smith, too, had the luxury of using a hand-held camera rather than the full complement of movie cameras, light boxes, and voice booms that Kennedy's film required.

During the first viewings, I was fascinated by Ceriani himself, the Ozzie Nelson voice, his loose frame (and the bedraggled way he carried himself), the Barry Goldwater glasses that masked baggy eyes set below his deeply furrowed brow. The villains of the story are evident: the young and restless Drs. Deagman and Zabielski and Hinz. On the other hand, Bryan Travis, a post-intern like the others, is refreshingly unpretentious, steadfastly refusing to blame Ceriani or Kremmling or medicine for his disappointments. What they all say bears wisdom. But in the end it is a partial truth, part of the ongoing saga of the country doctor. It is a story in need of a postscript, a perspective, a more inclusive cast, and deeper compassion on the part of the storyteller.

Phil Ceriani, Doc's son (and an orthopedic surgeon), ends the film with gloomy prophecy that echoes the earlier sentiments of Jeffrey Hinz: "I think the day of my father, frankly, is over. I think the day of the physician who does it all is gone. That's in an era passed, and I don't think that it will be repeated." Then a personal sadness: "Approaching the end seems to be suddenly filled with a lot of heartaches, perhaps a disintegrating family, a lot of bitterness on the part of people that my father has worked with for long periods of time. Now I really don't know what's going to happen." In the final scene, at dusk, an ambulance carries a sick infant off to the city specialists. We have seen this mother earlier in the film, receiving treatment in the emergency room after an automobile accident that claimed the lives of her fellow passengers, people Dr. Ceriani had known since the day he delivered them. *Her* child was delivered by the new guy on the block, Bryan Travis. But Bryan, we soon learn, has left Kremmling to study pathology.

Many are called, few are chosen. That is the lasting impression. But despite the pressure, isolation, and confinement of rural practice, the fledgling specialty of family medicine is attracting new recruits. Fifteen years later it is vigorous and strong and fit to carry the banner proudly into the twenty-first century. Perhaps old Doc Ceriani, a laggard in medicine's rush to become a race of urban specialists, did not die in vain.

James Kennedy's documentary is about the changing of the guard, the passing of a generation, a shift in culture twenty-five years after the shooting of W. Eugene Smith's "Country Doctor." His subject is someone we thought we knew when "we" were all of postwar America scanning the pages of *Life* magazine.

Ernest Ceriani had become a favorite of the journalists. They would flock to Kremmling for the nostalgia, or because of Doc's enduring popularity, or for the smell and touch of success (Smith's and Ceriani's alike). We conflated the man with the iconography that Smith, a master of the photographic essay, so ably crafted, and that Ernest Ceriani brought to life.

Over the years, an endless flow of patients came to Doc for "just a minute of my time." They brought their aches, miseries, despair; their lives pregnant with hope and possibility; their collective successes and failures. They waited expectantly in his office, on emergency room gurneys, in hospital beds and parlors, on the banks of trout streams, or wherever they could find him. It was a brand of medicine he loved, which he spoke of as being "intense and personal." How did Dr. Ceriani change as a result of it? What allowed him to survive?

"He was never one to tell you much, no matter what it was," his mother once remarked. He sought his restitution in solitude more than in the intimacy of friends. As his mother remembers, "On his half-days or days off, he takes off by himself and he goes. I don't know where he goes, just wants to be alone. He may have things to think over, to get straightened out in his mind, or . . . I don't know, he doesn't say much. He just goes, and when he comes back he's a different person."

Solitude is the necessary antidote to an "intense and personal" life with your patients. My partner escapes in his sea kayak, on cross-country skis, or with a backpack; I write in the early morning hours and flee on a long-distance run. We each seek seclusion somewhere within our lives of public service; we find a time and place for brooding, an outlet where we can disparage or disown or in some way distance ourselves from all the injustice and misery that parade past us on a daily basis.

Over the years Doc began to see his role differently: "I think some things can become too sophisticated, really, to the detriment of society. Using the cancer victim as an example, we encounter them down here, at this level. We do what we can. We know, pretty well, that things are pretty grim, the outlook is pretty hopeless. Yet, we feel we have to do something. We send Margaret out to the great cobalt bomb and out to the great chemotherapeutic center, and so forth. But those people come home to die. And here we have them. And we have to take care of them, we have to console them. We have to keep them comfortable. We have to console the family. We have to answer a lot of questions that we have no answers for. Again, I think we play one against a thousand when it comes to direct patient care. One cobalt bomb would build our hospital."

The older Ceriani slowed down, listened more to his patients, responded to their social needs. His son, Phil, reports proudly that "I know people who have come from sixty or a hundred miles to see my father. I know people that have come from Arizona. And you ask 'em, 'Well, why did you come all this way just to see Dr. Ceriani?' He says, "Well, you know I've got a disease I'm going to die from,' or 'you know I've got asthma and it's not going to go away, but I just enjoy talking to your old dad for fifteen or twenty minutes, and somehow I feel better when I go away."

In Kennedy's film, we witness the death of general practice and the birth struggle of its successor. The tragedy is that Ernest Ceriani could not pass the torch before it was wrested from him by the march of time, or before its brightness had been dimmed by his own pride, stubborness, and emotional insularity. We are often blind—and all of us vulnerable—to these afflictions, but especially the doctor-hero. Doc Ceriani could not escape his era, his upbringing, his fame, or his flaws. His full and accomplished career was the deep well from which he drew a sense of pride and purpose, and in which he drowned his failings and missed opportunities. Later in his life he acknowledged some of the trade-offs and complexities and perhaps weighed them in the balance, but always he accepted responsibility for the outcome, as he had done for his patients over a lifetime.

We are nearing the fiftieth anniversary of Doc Ceriani's arrival in Kremmling (1947) and the publication of Smith's famous photo essay (1948). Perhaps the jubilee might spark some discussion of his legacy, without nostalgia or a rush to judgment. Have we, the heirs of general practice, identified the enemy, heeded the warnings, changed or adjusted to the harsh conditions? What is the moral to the story? How surely have we grasped it? How self-evident are these truths? Ernest Ceriani and Gene Smith were strong men of enormous talent, fighting a changing enemy as well as the demons within. What can we say about them, finally, in fairness, and gratitude, and love for their labor?

Two nights ago I fell asleep on the far side of the bed. So when the telephone rang at 3:30 A.M., rousing me from deep sleep, it took me three turns around the bedroom to locate it. It was the hospital, requesting my presence for the birth of Twin B. The obstetrician had not yet arrived, a colleague had just delivered the first, and they needed a second pair of hands for the second. Without questioning the logic, I scrambled for some suitable clothes, located my glasses and keys and billfold, and dashed into the snowy night.

It was slippery; already three or four inches of snow had accumulated in these thirty-two degrees. The obstetrician must have been delayed by the weather. But who were the twins? I rushed into the birthing room as the second twin popped out. My colleague was beaming widely, but it was *my* patient, I could now see, propped upright on the birthing bed and looking tired, proud, and jubilant. The obstetrician, who walked in behind me, now surveyed the action approvingly, pleased that things had gone well in her stead. I asked the nurses, "who would be the babies' doctor?" The pediatrician, they thought . . . or were pretty sure . . .

but they would check again with Mother. I walked into the hallway to sort things out. Wasn't this the patient I had referred to the obstetrician two months ago, who now had been fortuitously delivered by my colleague, and for whom I had been called for want of a pediatrician? One of the nurses scooted by, and I pulled her out of the flow of traffic for an explanation.

It all happened rather precipitously, she explained. The patient had come in for a morning induction, went into spontaneous labor during the night, was dilated to six centimeters by 2:30 A.M., and was pushing within an hour. My colleague had been sleeping in the call room while a patient of his labored, so the nurses grabbed him in the heat of the moment when it was clear that birth was imminent. Dr. Hughes had been called earlier (I later learned) and referred the call to me. I was called, well, because the pediatrician was not available, and I was the doctor of record on the call schedule. Another nurse approached us with the news that the mother had chosen me, after all, to be the babies' doctor. Why hadn't the nurses just asked her in the first place?

I was steaming, and hid it poorly. The hour was too early, my bones were too tired, the circumstances seemed too bizarre. By now, the obstetrician had come out of the birthing room and saw my long face. "Loxterkamp, why are you unhappy?" she asked, boring her gaze right through me. "The babies are well, mother is elated, everything turned out fine. I missed the delivery, too. So why this unhappiness?"

"Because I wasn't called," I blurted. "I would have preferred to have been notified, included in some way, that's all." Deep down, I was feeling snubbed, left out, called as a mere afterthought to satisfy a hospital policy.

"You should be happy. I don't understand," is all she said, and we parted in that busy hallway outside the nursery, so full of congratulatory grandparents with their Instamatic cameras and beaming smiles.

I completed my cursory examination of the newborns, healthy and pink and good-sized for twins, born mature in the thirty-eighth week. They would pose no problems. As I finished their charts, the obstetrician walked into the nurses' station. It was otherwise deserted. So rather than brood, backbite, or swallow my anger, I spoke with a candor rare to me. "I would just like to have been called. I know the twins came quickly, but if my name had been somewhere on the chart, the nurses could have summoned me for the last of the labor."

"No, no, no, she is my patient," she retorted. "Loxterkamp, it disturbs me, it disturbs me *profoundly,* that you think only of missing the delivery and not of the patient. I don't know what it is. It is greediness, it is unethical behavior. I have seen it too many times, and it bothers me profoundly."

"It is *not* greediness," I insisted, my voice trembling, "but a matter of professional courtesy, a wish to be included, a desire to be shown respect."

"Don't," she shot back, "just *don't* refer to me in the future. Send your patients to someone else, if this is what you want. How much do you care about your patients when you can't even remember their due date?"

"But listen, I would like to refer my patients to you! I only request that you include me somehow in the process." These were my last words. The room was now refilling, but nothing had penetrated, and I would be bothered by our interaction all day. It would trouble me as I slept, and taint every brush I would have with her hereafter. Who needs it, this stress, her goddamn attitude, when the work alone creates it in abundance? But, as I later told Tim, I don't want to leave OB on my knees, slinking from a fight. I am proud of what I said, the attempts I made. Yes, of course, the timing was wrong: 4:00 A.M., both of us exhausted. But once my anger surfaced, the cat was out of the bag. I tried to express myself clearly, defend my point, find a common ground. Perhaps if I had hidden my disappointment and swallowed my pride, our surface relations would, after a time, have "normalized." Now I carry with me her charges of greed and unethical behavior, and her annoyance with me that has blossomed into "profound" disdain. I hate to miss deliveries, and part of it, I will admit, is the remuneration that comes from the service. Not a larger part—I must quickly add—than it is for other doctors. But that is not the issue. The question about who would deliver the twins was settled two months ago; in my mind, the matter was closed. What burned me was that I had become the doctor of last resort; neglected; an afterthought . . . after six months of caring for the patient, in a practice where I care for most of her family.

I hate this crap. Perhaps, for whatever reason, it is my cross to bear. And, no doubt here, buried from my sight, is a mess half of my own making. I don't want to be left holding this emotional bag and would be happy to pitch it. Thank God that, when another prenatal patient of ours went into labor that morning, all went well and there was no need for an obstetrician. My week away from the hospital will pass too quickly.

The lawn statuary has disappeared again into the snows. The temperature fell overnight to ten degrees, and ice crystals glitter in the uppermost crust, creating a brilliant luster. Another large winter storm is approaching the New England coast, full of Gulf moisture and on a collision course with our stationary Arctic high. These are the ingredients for a genuine Nor'easter, or so the computer models say. If the cold mass can hold, we have the potential for a massive snowfall. I relish the possibilities, and brace myself.

I spoke with Scott briefly before he left on his Cajun vacation. He spoke of desertion, feeling as if he were leaving his friends in the lurch. This is winter, Lent, a time of scarcity and sacrifice, and Scott is leaving for the sunny south and two weeks of respite. Three nights before he left—I am happy to report—Scott returned a call to his hostile patient and laid down the law: His behavior the other day had been rude, demanding, unacceptable, and deserving of an apology to the nurses. If he were not willing to do that, he should seek his medical care elsewhere. Before Scott could finish, the patient boasted that he had already quit the practice, and slammed the receiver. Scott wrote him a polite, perfunctory note to document their understanding.

Doctors need not martyr themselves to the few angry, abusive, and manipulative patients who populate our practices. We must set a proper example. How many of our patients, too, feel powerless in an abusive relationship? If we suffer gladly the excrement of that rare but insufferable patient (or colleague), what example do we set for others who must learn to free themselves?

Five degrees. Five A.M. on the morning of "the blizzard of the century." Too much hype for one storm. I've noticed a pattern: our hospital workload has paralleled the snowfall this winter, with light amounts in December and January, and a heavy load in February and March. I will face a charge of eleven when I creak into the hospital this morning: pneumonia, influenza, congestive heart failure, "rule-out" heart attacks, prostatitis, twins. And a social admission for a staunch old Democrat who fell in her home and crawled to her telephone to summon the ambulance.

As the crew rolled her into the emergency department, her first words were "I need a shot of insulin, two Darvocet, and a cup of coffee." She is legendary, this grande dame of the Maine Democrats. At eighty-eight, she is mentally sharp but physically broken, and here's the rub: She turns away Meals on Wheels, remembers her insulin but forgets to eat, and gropes about her tiny apartment in a sensory brownout, falling frequently. Visiting nurses report an untouched hoard of food in her icebox and pills in her medicine cabinet. But she rules the roost and has kept her children, state agencies, and the visiting nurses at bay. After an ultimatum by her son last fall, she agreed to be admitted to the Camden Health Care Facility. But she didn't last among the bare walls and rattling beds and demented cries in the night. One day she picked up the telephone and "made the necessary arrangements" to bail herself out, and her life more or less resumed where she left off.

She has backed herself into the health care system once again, and if all goes well, she will be placed in a nursing home. It will not happen against her will: her sons will not force the issue. And she has a tight ring of supporters, including most of us at the hospital, who champion the independent elderly who retain their wits and a semblance of self-sufficiency. But her stubbornness has caused no end of worry for those closest to her, which is the price exacted of our Yankee-spirited aging parents.

In the main intersection on the hospital's second floor sits a familiar figure, a legless old man in his trusty chariot. I heard yesterday, while rounding at the nursing home, that he and one of my stroke patients are a "unit." So that accounts for the rebound in her condition over the last few months: flowers and hugs.

No more fallout from my confrontation with the obstetrician. To my great relief, she was not in OB when I made my rounds. I still feel maimed and numb but not hurting.

Clear skies, biting breath, crunchy snow, and a perfectly halved moon to the south. Only four degrees at 6:00 A.M.: winter drags on. I have just returned from delivering my third baby in twenty-four hours, all healthy and normal and vaginal. The worst part was worrying about the need for obstetrical backup.

Last night's delivery was the closest call. The nurse called at 7:00 to report swelling of the cervix, molding of the baby's head, and no change in cervical dilatation for better than three hours. When I arrived, the monitor strip revealed absence of beat-to-beat variability, and my cervical exam confirmed a five-centimeter rim of cervix. Though the patient had ruptured her bag of waters, the bag was now bulging, and I easily nicked it. Meconium-stained fluid flowed, and I decided to attach an electrode to the baby's scalp to obtain a more reliable tracing of the fetal heartbeat. The pattern was now reassuring. With intensifying labor came rapid cervical dilatation, and by 8:30 she was complete and ready to push. She handled it perfectly, and by 9:11 I laid a sopping pink bambino on her lap. What great satisfaction!

Yesterday, on the morning after the blizzard, Mass was nearly empty. I knew almost everyone there: nurses, patients, a fellow tenor in the Pen Bay Singers, two hospice volunteers at the organ and lectern, and my neighbors who distributed communion. Familiar faces, all. There was another gospel account about Samaritans, but I cannot remember the sermon, only some phrases and Father's Godly tones.

The blizzard dumped another foot of snow onto an already treacherously deep cushion. Francis and Angel are now hopelessly buried; not even a ripple betrays their wintry den. Yesterday, as I was pulling Clare and a friend on a sled, my legs sunk to midthigh, well over my Wellington Boots. I worry less about the snowfall than the snowplow, which, with each determined pass, creates an insurmountable bank at the foot of our drive.

OB called at 2:00 A.M. yesterday morning to say that a prenatal patient was five centimeters dilated. It was her second baby, but I knew it was a big one and that her labor should move slowly. Just in case, I would shovel the drive. So I donned my boots and coat and my insulated overcoat and set out with shovel in hand. After fifteen minutes of scooping and heaving, I abandoned the effort and trudged to the hospital on foot. Scattered pickup trucks with mounted steel plows were roaming the streets. I passed a pedestrian who tried to bum a cigarette. Why are you out? I asked instead. "Insomniac. On my way to the all-night market for a cup of coffee." The hospital was battened down and staffed by leftovers from the previous shift. I checked my patient, slept for an hour, checked her again. And at 5:12 A.M., little Lucy was born a-bawling. She was named for her mother's friend who had been diagnosed a year ago with ALS.

When I came downstairs this morning, a car, visible only by its yellow parking lights, was poised at the mouth of Condon Street. At precisely 4:43, it pulled onto Northport Avenue and headed south toward the hospital, with a thick slab of snow frosting its roof. Does he notice my kitchen light burning, and the shadowy figure who darts behind it? We share this small part of the morning, perhaps in casual awareness of each other, before parting to go our separate ways.

It is five degrees, too cold for too long. But this may be the last bitter pill of winter. A warming trend is in the forecast, and spring waits in the wings. These are the last days to enjoy our abundant blanket of snow.

Ten degrees at 5:00 A.M. Yesterday the temperature topped forty, and melting waters cascaded down Salmond Street to swell the storm sewers. But last night a Canadian wind howled and several inches of new snow fell to replace the old. Our poor cars are covered again, snow on ice on snow. This is getting to be a bit much, even for us enthusiasts.

Marc and Cheryl Stewart will be leaving tomorrow for their new home in Grand Rapids. We invited them over for homemade pizza last Saturday night in the thick of the blizzard. Two nights later, we shuffled into Belfast's First Church for a going-away service. The program was called "Times of Passage: Ending an Authorized Ministry."

My contribution to the memorial service was joining Cris (Tim's wife) and Cheryl (Marc's wife) in a rousing rendition of "How Can I Keep from Singing?" My guitar did me in: the strap pulled loose as I walked to the front of the church, and the E and B strings flatted as the guitar warmed in the ovenlike hall. One more glaring imperfection, one more clumsy try, for the glory of God and the love of us all.

Two degrees, and the eastern sky lightens at 5:00 in salmon hues. This is the Feast Day of St. Joseph; the swallows will return to Capistrano, and I turn forty today.

I have not given it much thought or anticipation. I am still healthy and get away with too many lazy and dangerous moves. I still sport a respectable mop of hair and need only a single lens to perfect my vision. Over the past week I have pondered the fates of Ernest Ceriani and Marc Stewart, and examined my own considerable weaknesses. Still I am convinced, like the Old Style Beer boys around their campfire, that it doesn't get any better than this: my life in this community. But the opposite is equally true: it won't get any easier. At every age, at every turn, an unexpected nemesis will appear. It may take the form of the "young Turks" who pompously arrive and plunder my reputation in the twilight of my career; or a "wiener dog" (masquerading as a dragon) that exposes my weakness, or a marital spat that brings me back to an appreciation of the one person who sustains my life with love.

Tim, at morning meeting, repeated the words of his mother on his fortieth birthday: "It's not the end of the line but you can see it from here." What is most visible at forty is the end of the parental line. Parents often serve as a kind of barrier reef, a buffer between ourselves and the eternal beyond. As long as they survive, *memento mori*—all those daily events that would remind us of our mortality—never quite personally apply. Yet they do, and at forty the realization begins to sink home.

It is a welcome day off. I have already committed it to errands, hospital dictation, and helping the Stewarts pack. But it began with an hour's quiet, in coffeed conversation with Lindsay at the dining room table. Moments like these happen too infrequently, given Lindsay's need to sleep and mine to write. As we spoke, the yellow ball of sun rose over the blue-white tundra outside our window; in two days, we will greet the first day of spring.

From here, the day will yield two, perhaps three, hours of writing or scheming or leisurely reading. My planned absence from work today forced an early birthday party for me yesterday at the office. Cathy posted signs that alternately warned "It's all downhill at forty" and celebrated "Life begins at forty." Take your pick. After seeing the posters, a patient ordered black helium balloons for the occasion. Cathy baked two cakes, a poppy seed and an angel food. Both were a penance for the chef, who is trying to adhere to a grapefruit diet. The staff also presented me with a large box, gift-wrapped, that concealed a case of Quaker Oats caramel-flavored popcorn cakes. I enjoyed them all the more by slathering Ben and Jerry's Cherry Garcia ice cream between two cakes to create a sandwich. I hope for a smooth day, unruffled, unhurried, steady, punctual, and home by 5:30 P.M.

Two nice telephone calls last evening. Pete Kerndt called from L.A., hoping to make final arrangements for an upcoming visit and to proffer again his standing invitation for me to relocate to his hometown of Lansing, Iowa. Then Wayne Bigelow of Anchorage, Alaska, left word on my answering service. He is a retired physician and now a pastor who had read "The Watch" on a flight back from California and called to express his appreciation.

March 21, the Feast Day of St. Benedict, as cited in the Pius X Breviary, Confraternity Version, which is printed "Word for Word as read from the Pulpit." It is a feast I have committed to memory, along with Patrick's on the 17th, Joseph's on the 19th, and Cuthbert's on the 20th. Benedict's day is now officially July 11, the day he died in 547 at the monastery of Monte Casino while "in prayer, having taken communion, supported upright by his brethren before the altar."* Benedict is said to have foreseen his death and directed the digging of his grave six days prior. Because of his foreknowledge and calm acceptance, he is invoked by the terminally ill. His famous Rule, the cornerstone of Western monasticism, fuses prayer and labor with community life. It proscribed individual asceticism and gave due respect to manual labor as both a productive and a dignified means of serving God. Two days ago, Lindsay and I discussed the possibility of my taking a monastic retreat, and she consented. I am hoping for Gethsemane—for romantic reasons, I admit, more than spiritual ones—but if not there, then at some Benedictine or (probably) Trappist monastery, St. Joseph or New Melleray or Genesee.

A bountiful weekend. I missed the journal yesterday morning when, for unknown reasons, Clare awoke at 5:30 A.M., tiptoed downstairs, and scurried onto my lap. Was it because of the Stewarts leaving, or the commotion of my birthday? Friday evening Mary Beth and Mac came over, bearing "bianca" pizza and presents. I received a box of icon cards and a beautiful icon of the Virgin of Vladimir. Lindsay presented me with running shoes (Saucony, made in Maine) and *Bridges of Madison County*. It is dedicated "for the peregrines," among whom I belong.† Lindsay baked a tasty cake basted with butter cream frosting; what a treat! I received a telephone call from Bill DeMars, a note from my nephew Gabe, and a Cajun postcard from Scott and Debbie. I went for a modest jog with Sam Mitchell (inaugurating my new shoes); and last night I attended a baby shower for Carol (one of our office nurses) at Darby's Restaurant. I suspect we will be dining with the Hugheses tonight, because of words I overheard between Lindsay and a babysitter, and because we traditionally share these high holidays.

All is right with the world: I can account for my belongings—my beret, my gloves, my watch, my replacement wedding ring. And this morning I tasted the homebrew that has been fermenting "down cella" these past several weeks. It was evenly carbonated, wonderfully "nosed," sparkling clear, and without aftertaste. What will a month more bring?

Depression hung over me like yesterday's low-lying clouds. The sky spritzed all afternoon. I jogged on slushy gravel at the shoulder's edge, running past pocked and filthy piles of snow, high-stepping puddles and dodging the splash of motorists, pondering the long heaviness of the day. Depression is the word.

---

* "Saints," Chambers Encyclopedic Guides, p. 46.
† From the Latin *peregre* (*per* through, plus *ager*, territory).

It flared before Mass when Lindsay and I quibbled over the problem of Clare's fecal soiling. "The problem" started three weeks ago, after Clare's operation. Now it is complicated by the secrecy, lies, and embarrassment it has engendered. Even when we spot her crouching in the corner, we cannot change the outcome. She has already yielded to the urge and stained her pants, and she has made up her mind to reject the potty no matter how much we try to bribe or coerce her. Lindsay broke down in tears, one more worry among the many: hospice events, birthday plans, the trip to Washington, D.C. She would prefer to take Clare to a play therapist (at $65.00 an hour); I want to ask around, believing that the problem is a self-limited one, understandable and natural as a response to stress. I will make a few calls today to see if an intervention, or simply more time, is advised. Lindsay agrees.

My depression deepened at Mass today when I reached into my wallet for a collection offering and came up empty-handed. It was just my luck that our hospital administrator was passing the collection basket. And there was a second collection to boot. Then at Communion, some guy in a ponytail, tweed jacket, blue jeans, and cowboy boots sang "Kumbayah," swaying and wagging his head and singin' 'cause the spirit said "sing." Voices in the congregation joined in slowly, but swelled to a chorus that became anthemlike. At the close of Mass, Father thanked the guitarist, and the parish applauded. Ugh. Are we so desperate for a familiar tune and easy lyrics that we'll accept anything in the name of "liturgy"? Kumbayah is emblematic of a Vatican II fervor that led to sanctuaries everywhere being stripped of their dead wood—Latin and communion rails, incense and benediction. We sanitized the Mass of its organic mystery, its sacramentality, its individuality. It became a mass of the people, and poor baby Jesus was cast out with the Holy Water.

To make matters worse, our music director called last night to discuss the possibility of organizing a folk group replete with electric bass, drums, brass, and the whole nine yards. Croak. Yet I know that my opinion is one among many. I will help, I agreed, but please reconsider the drums. The sound of them at Mass would disturb me more than at a men's group.

I could not muster the motivation to write Gayle Stephens or call the Abbey of the Genesee or work on any of the projects at the top of my list. Genesee has become a candidate for the retreat ever since my rediscovery of Henri Nouwen. I have just finished reading his small book *Behold the Beautiful,* and thoroughly enjoyed the description of his extended retreat in *Genesee Diary.* But the telephone intimidated me all day.

Last night's supper with the Hugheses was a gustatory delight; we enjoyed Thai cooking by a guest chef at Darby's Restaurant. But somehow our small group lacked a feeling of intimacy, closeness, warmth. It's still the depression, I wager, and will lift in time.

Last night, as I headed out the door for the grocery store, I got a call from OB. "Are you on tonight? The obstetrician wants you to come see a floppy baby." So I changed my itinerary to stop by the hospital first. The infant was tiny, born at term, and seemed severely stressed by the pregnancy. Mother had smoked two packs of cigarettes a day, developed preeclampsia, and was on a Pitocin and magnesium sulfate drip throughout most her labor. Baby had weathered it well, displaying not a single deceleration of her heart rate. But after delivery she would not breathe, lay limp on the apron of the birthing bed, and sent a ripple of panic through the nursing staff. By the time I arrived, of course, the child was pink. Her purple hands and feet retracted with adequate muscle tone, and she waved a Moro reflex. The only hint of that initial drama was the slight tugging at the ribs as she breathed. I reassured the mother and spoke briefly afterward with the obstetrician.

She thanked me for coming. We agreed that magnesium was the source of the hypotonia and discussed possible causes for the baby's small size. She stepped into the nurses' station as I dictated my consultation report, and we spoke pleasantries. I relaxed a little, opened up, welcomed the thaw in our relations. We were both groping for a conversation. She tried to recall a patient of mine who was booked for tomorrow's D&C; darn, she had intended to call me, and will definitely do so after the pathology report returns. I asked her about the new Bethesda system for reporting pap smear results. We exchanged patient stories and chatted longer than I could afford. But I savored the opportunity, felt in it almost a quality of tenderness, and hoped that our tensions might finally ease. We both seemed to be trying in our awkward ways.

A patient of mine died on his way home from the Hospice Wing yesterday. The death certificate recorded the time as 11:30 P.M., but the fatal insult occurred twelve hours earlier. He had collapsed on the top step of his trailer, and the ambulance crew raced him back to the hospital. But it was no use. Blood pressure hovered at sixty systolic despite a continuous flow of IV fluids. Tests provided a flicker of hope, but his extremities remained edematous and icy, and his mind drifted aimlessly among old fears, imaginary guests, and urgent tasks that required his immediate action. He would die on the wing that he had dreaded to leave, and (in hindsight) should not have left.

James had metastatic lung cancer, diagnosed eighteen months ago in Portland and treated with surgery, radiation, and chemotherapy. In recent weeks his condition had deteriorated rapidly, forcing him to give up the walk to his clipping service (where his obligations were mostly social). After that he never left his tiny trailer. "Call him a loner," his ex-wife volunteered; their cordial relations were maintained only for the daughter's sake. The last two weeks in the hospital were a godsend. He enjoyed the flow of company, especially as his death tiptoed closer. No one had expected him to live this long.

Yet how could I justify his continued hospital stay? He was eating and showering and tottering to the commode by himself. We expected his shortness of breath because his lung cancer was growing and created a malignant effusion. Though he was anxious about the prospects of going home, he agreed to try it. As the appointed day approached, he began to doubt and tried to delay our decision. "I'll try it, Doc, whatever you say," he assured me, "but not now. Maybe tomorrow. Can we see how it goes?" Finally we set a nonnegotiable date and braced ourselves.

The discharge was fortified by a ring of support services: visiting nurses, home health aides, the oxygen company, Meals on Wheels, Lifeline, and my promise to visit him at home on a weekly basis, more often if necessary. He was frightened that morning, but had resigned himself to his eviction. His drooping face, bulging eyes, bent frame, potbelly, and swollen legs made him look worse at the time of discharge than most patients appear when they arrive. But nothing more could be done in the hospital than what might be provided at home.

Dressed in civilian clothes, and now scarcely panting, he echoed the staff's sentiment that he would be happiest at home. Before signing the discharge order, I made a cursory examination of his heart and lungs, noted the vital signs and pulse oximetry readings, and squatted to press my thumbs into James's spongy shins. Then I rose quickly and declared without hesitation, "Let's give it a try. You can come back whenever you need. These next few weeks will be hard no matter where you are. But we'll help as much as we can." He nodded with a doubting, daunted look and allowed me to scurry off to my hospital rounds.

What happened next is a matter of conjecture. Did he suffer heart damage or a blood clot to the lungs, or did the tumor erode through a pulmonary vessel? Or did he simply cross that tenuous line that separates the living from the active process of dying. We can sometimes mark the juncture by a subtle change in breathing, or a shift in fluid balance, or the rise of serum calcium. But such studies are set aside when a patient becomes "hospice," when we agree that death is no longer the enemy, that it will inevitably come, and that the path should be made clear. All I really know is that James collapsed on the threshold of his trailer and was whisked back here to die.

All afternoon the patient floated in and out of consciousness; his mind was muddled, his speech unintelligible. The receptionist canceled my last hour of patients so that I could attend his bedside (or rather be there for the ex-wife and family). As I opened the double doors of the Hospice Wing, I found James's twelve-year-old daughter hovering outside his room. "Please, come in," I insisted, and made a place for her beside me, moving the oxygen tubing, trays, and

IV poles. I tried to convey the seriousness of his sudden turn, and encouraged her to remain as long as she liked.

But there were competing interests. Grandmother was downstairs on an emergency room gurney, awaiting my admission. She was bedbound with rheumatoid arthritis and toxic from digitalis. The twelve-year-old was doing her best to cope with a dying father and morbid grandmother, and the two of us swapped death beds several times during the course of our long evening together.

On my last trip to the wing before leaving the hospital, I found James unusually clear, despite no appreciable change in his blood pressure or oxygenation. Before matters deteriorated, I asked if he would like to receive Last Rites, and he agreed. Father came bearing the holy oils, and within two hours the patient was dead.

I would learn the next day that he had been the hospice client of our office nurse, Bonnie. She was shocked by his sudden reversal, disappointed at missing the final drama, saddened by that lost opportunity. Bonnie's daughter is also twelve; her faith, too, is Catholic. And her hospice work with James had just begun. Unbeknownst to me, she had been spending her lunch hours visiting him in the hospital. She knew of his planned discharge and had smoothed his fears surrounding it. How nice it might have been had we all joined together in the anointing, instead of leaving it to the last, a few mumbled words over a withered corpse.

Spring

IN THE MIDST OF DEATH

It was toward the close of Mass on the Second Sunday of Lent. Twenty screeching voices and three clanging guitars were barreling down the home stretch of the finale, "He's Got the Whole World in His Hands." From the rise of the altar where I directed the St. Francis Youth Choir, I could scan the whole congregation: below me, the smiling faces of the first-row regulars; high in back, balcony dwellers fidgeting through the final refrain; and to my far right, stragglers and families of unruly youngsters who took refuge behind the open doors of the adjoining Parish Hall.

Already parishioners were rising to leave by way of the south side aisle. Today they seemed unusually raucous, with bodies scurrying and arms waving and a crowd converging to a point several pews back. Suddenly I heard my name, "Dr. Loxterkamp, come quickly," as a young woman grabbed my guitar and another rushed me to a body sprawled on the carpet and wedged in the narrow passage. He made no motion or sound while all around me the crowd shouted, "He's a diabetic. Get him some sugar," and packets simultaneously appeared from a dozen different handbags. Others ushered the children toward their religion classes and urged lingering parishioners to exit at the rear of the church.

On further inspection I could see that the ashen man was our parish council president, only a few years my senior and in apparent good health. He was unconscious and could not be aroused. His skin was cool and mottled even though only a minute had passed since his collapse. Since he was not breathing, I propped his head, pinched his nose, and forced a full breath of air into his lungs. He gasped spontaneously, then again, now several times in obvious response to our urgent cries to "breathe, Greg, breathe."

But there was no pulse. I groped for the carotid and femoral arteries and pressed my ear to his chest. Where was it? *Surely* it was there, for hadn't he just sighed and turned his head; wasn't he merely suffering from a drop in blood sugar? Reluctantly, disbelievingly, we began CPR, I and the three nurses who now huddled around him. With glacial speed I pondered the conflicting evidence: A young man was having an insulin reaction. How could he be unresponsive and pulseless! I heard Father softly intoning what sounded like the prayers of the Sacrament of the Sick. Someone assured me that an ambulance had been called; another instructed the onlookers to "give them air," followed soon by the clunk of double doors swinging ajar and a blast of cold air reaching us from the rear of church.

Without any tools—a stethoscope or blood pressure cuff, a bag-and-mask or IV line—I felt astonishingly naked and helpless. Yet we labored on, doctor and nurses, priest and parishioners, through the unpardonable delays of the ambulance crew. When it finally arrived, the wall clock recorded—to my astonishment—a lapse of only eight minutes. The crew and I hoisted Greg to the back of the church where we attached the defibrillator leads. It confirmed the presence of ventricular fibrillation, and with two jolts from the paddles we converted our patient to a normal sinus rhythm. But still no pulse, still a stillness in that bared chest and heavy mottled limbs.

The hospital was only a half mile away, and there we continued the rescue efforts for well over an hour. Thankfully, a colleague of mine took charge, though he allowed little hope for a reversible outcome. Despite the march of regular beats across the monitor screen, our patient and friend and fellow parishioner lay moribund on the cot, having died instantly in the side aisle of the church during his unbroken fall to the floor.

I accompanied the attending physician to the small office where Greg's wife was waiting. As we entered, the younger daughter arrived and embraced her Mother, weeping, "I knew something was wrong, something had to be wrong." My throat tightened as a wound reopened inside me: memories of a Memorial Day Weekend in 1966 when I returned from a canoe trip to learn of my father's fatal heart attack. He was a year older than Greg; I was the same age as Betsy when we heard the dreaded news.

I reviewed the morning's details with Greg's wife and daughter, who had been absent from the 8:30 Mass. I assured them that we had done everything possible, and felt terrible that we hadn't done enough. And I found myself repeating these words over and over during the ensuing days, to acquaintances of the deceased and nurses who assisted me and office staff who comforted me in a genuine show of concern. I confessed to one of the nurses that this was my first resuscitation outside of the hospital. "Mine, too," she replied sheepishly, "Do you think we did all right?"

"The best we could," was all that I could muster.

It was a week of strange conjunctions. I would turn forty in a few days, and birthdays are a treacherous time for me to plumb the mysteries of mortality. Even though I am in good heath and free of the niggling ills that, after a certain age, badger us into believing we have hit the downward slide, I am also adopted and—therefore, in my wife's opinion—a walking genetic time bomb.

I recently heard from a social worker friend that April is the peak month for suicide. In the season so redolent with rebirth and awakening, hope and renewal, perhaps the contrast with one's own despair can be utterly overwhelming. So the words hit me hard, those of John Rutter's *Requiem* that we had been rehearsing in our community chorus. During the "Agnus Dei," Rutter writes a sobering chant in the bass clef where the men maintain a monotone, "in the midst of life, we are in death." This notion is what makes the "Lamb of God" the Good Friday of the Catholic Mass: As unbelievable as it may seem, we beseech the very Lamb whom the Father had forsaken to grant mercy on our mortal souls. So saturated were these words with the memory of Greg and my father and my own tenuous circumstance that tears flooded my eyes as I sang.

A doctor's life is a continuous *memento mori*, a reminder of death and of life's unfairness, fragility, and the speed with which all good things pass. Everyday we console families in their struggles with disabled children, untimely deaths, or the decline of aging parents. Why are *we* spared? When will our trials begin?

On Monday evening I attended the wake with my fellow parishioners, patients, acquaintances—all of us connected to Greg Maguire by the Appleton School or the Catholic Church, Democratic politics or Greg's video business. As we passed through the receiving line, I suddenly came to Greg's daughters and squatted low to grip their hands and whisper, "I was at your father's side when he died. I just wanted you to know how much I liked and respected him. Even though my father died, too, when I was your age, I have felt him beside me my whole life."

Indeed, I thought, his death had changed me forever, kindling an interest in hospice care, attracting me to my wife, who had also lost her mother in adolescence, driving me to seek out the Spirit abiding in every death. For it has been the Spirit I have sought ever since. In the midst of death, *we are in life . . .* I recall now how the *Requiem* tide turns, and our voices swell with the Easter refrain, "whom soever liveth and believeth in me shall never die."

Easter, the time when catechumens traditionally enter the Catholic Church, is more than a witness to faith. It is about a community of faithful. It is about how communities respond in good times and in bad. I could now view our rescue efforts in something other than a medical light. It was not just a failed attempt. It was not just an exercise in moral or professional obligation. What mattered was the privilege we all felt as we rushed to Greg's side on that Sunday morning, trusting that he would have been there for us, knowing we may be called upon again.

After a time, this small community has brought me to an understanding that pilgrims often reach on their road to a religious shrine, or that anthropologists absorb in their studies of exotic tribes: that I am like my neighbor, and part of my neighbor is in me. I am the lucky one. I had the necessary training, a role to play, the means to express my love for my neighbor, and a way to exercise my belonging in the community.

I have learned by living here that we are all part of the same family. The baby I delivered for the mother who sings with me at church is married to my auto mechanic whose father brokered the purchase of my home. Anger and frustration in my practice often stem from an injured or empty place in my own heart that my patients help me to see and that, because of its exposure, can now begin to heal.

Without a sense of community, Greg's tragedy might seem an imposition or intrusion into the privacy of my prayers. Without community, I would forfeit the support of my fellow parishioners. Without community, I might have choked in my grief instead of dispersing it through words of sorrow and sympathy and thanksgiving. Without community, I could not rebuke the claim made against all of God's creation, at every moment and with every turn: that in the midst of life, we are in death.

Tuesday brought the Funeral Mass and the return of the St. Francis Youth Choir. We gathered in the chapel to rehearse our songs before Mass. I was surprised to see all twenty members in attendance, plus four more who had asked to come along, maybe out of a need to say goodbye or bring closure to the terror and confusion of Sunday's ordeal. The family had chosen "He's Got the Whole World in His Hands," the last words Greg had heard before he died. But I was having doubts about it now and meant to assuage them, or at least address them, in front of the children. Twenty-four intent, frightened, innocent pairs of eyes fixed upon me as I rose to speak.

I told them, in words as straight as possible, what I had lately come to know: that Greg had been sick for a long time and knew—better than the rest of us— that his end was near. His wife had asked us to sing, but that was only part of the reason we were here today. Singing is also a way to say "thank you" for all that Greg did for the children of the parish: for the religion classes he taught, the parish outings he organized, the interests of kids he defended as council president. We were here, too, to finish what had been left unfinished: the song we were singing on Sunday; our lives, which God had chosen for us to continue.

A tiny hand shot up and wiggled from the second row, "But why do we have to sing the same song? It feels a little creepy."

"To me, too," I agreed. "But when we sing the words, remember not only Greg, but all your relatives who have gone before us, and 'you and me, brother,' believers all."

A wide swath of community had collected that morning for the Rite of Christian Burial. We were Catholics and Protestants, the young and the old, saints and sinners, the living among the dead, all lining the wooden pews like the fingers of a folded hand. We had come to honor a soft-spoken man who labored a lifetime for his community and for our greater awareness of an unseen Hand.

By the sheer strength of our numbers, we can believe that, in the midst of death, we are in life. Living among friends, and in my line of work, that is the only faith you need.

APRIL

That is what people are like in this district. Always expecting
the impossible from the doctor. They have lost their ancient
beliefs; the parson sits at home and unravels his vestments,
one after another; but the doctor is supposed to be omnipo-
tent with his merciful surgeon's hand. Well, as it pleases them
... if they use me for sacred purposes, I let that happen, too.

FRANZ KAFKA

A Country Doctor

After our week's vacation in Washington, D.C., we have driven back, pelted by snow, to find six inches of it frosting the land. A bit of April Foolishness, this snowfall. It is twenty degrees. Out my east window, the view is anything but vernal, looking more like late November than the third week of spring.

The closing days of the holiday were a disappointment, tainted by my failed rendezvous with Robert Coles. Without a firm time and meeting place, he could not be located on the Harvard campus.

His letter to me dated February 16 had said simply, "Thanks for yours. Yes, I'd be delighted to meet with you at the end of March. How about the 31st, Wednesday, in the late morning? I look forward to meeting you." I had jotted a confirmatory postcard on the eve of our departure and assumed that the particulars might be worked out through his secretary when I arrived in Boston. I could be flexible, having two days to negotiate a brief encounter.

But his return address—Harvard University Health Services—is only a sub-basement mailbox. The woman at the information desk confessed that she had never met the man, though may have spied him once, fleetingly, as he disappeared around a corner. The telephone directory provided little help; I reached a recorded message to write or fax Dr. Coles at this address. I wandered down the two flights to his mailbox in hope of stumbling upon the professor, but of course never did. Then left a message with Betty at the front desk, who promised to drop it in campus mail. "Sorry we could not meet," I began. "If you have time in the next twenty-four hours, please call me at this number, where I am staying with friends. Otherwise, we can try again when the particulars have been settled in advance. Warmly . . ."

It was my fault, this aborted introduction. His note to me was merely an overture, a green light to schedule an appointment with his secretary. But I had been too scattered before my vacation to plan it. Now my disappointment was obvious and unshakable, and challenged me to question my original motives. Was I seeking some direction and encouragement for my writing, or just the chance to rub shoulders with a famous writer? When I undertook the journal, I pledged it to my patients. It is they who feature in the ordinary affairs of the country doctor. It is they who test our fine conceptions, cobble the road of self-scrutiny, push us to the very limit. We know them by the smell of their breath, the feel of their skin, and the answers they expect in calculated but not uncertain terms. A writer can fabricate pretty prose. A doctor can dictate an airtight H&P. But it is the actual practice of doctoring, day-in and day-out, with all of the interruptions, demands, plain affections, obvious mistakes, eventual declines, and the converging goals of doctor and patient that keep you on the even keel.

In the early years, the worry about my clientele nearly undid me. I had hoped for a certain cleverness about them, a high social standing, respect and gratitude for my services. This would reflect favorably on the new doctor. Of course, part of my concern was financial: welfare work was not well reimbursed, and the uninsured could afford even less. Part of my concern was social: new doctors in town always attract the deadbeats, social outcasts, and hopeless cases that peel away from the established practices. I wanted patients whom I *deserved*, as if one's self-worth hinged upon an exit poll at the office, or a ledger at the bank.

To say that it has all changed would be a lie. But at least I am aware of it now and occasionally manage to stare it down, this attitude toward the poor, the foul, the unwashed specimens of humanity who fill my examining rooms with their social disorder. How did they end up here, the Medicaid recipients with their scrawny, runny-nosed kids who scrap for a healthy meal and a decent future, their parents who angle for an "easier" life on food stamps and disability? Easier than what? I ask.

Writing is one way for me to scrutinize the value of a human being, a value present before there was someone to acknowledge it. It is a way to recognize, in each unfortunate soul, Christ come a-calling. Is one of them, after all, my orphaned twin, who but for some divine miscalculation landed in a tar paper shack instead of on the doctor's doorstep in my hometown of Rolfe, Iowa? The poor magnify my blessings and humble me by their unruffled dignity and indomitable spirit.

It is Palm Sunday, the 25th anniversary of Martin Luther King's assassination, and Cris Hughes's birthday all rolled into one. I am too busy preparing for an upcoming AIDS talk to ponder the significance. On the 14th, I travel to Portland to address a group of home health nurses who want to hear how a family doctor approaches AIDS. The week promises to be rugged: a RENEW potluck supper tonight, Clare's birthday party on Wednesday, Lindsay's bereavement group on Thursday, Good Friday services, Saturday night's Seder meal with the Bakers, an Easter Sunday folk Mass, and—wedged in somewhere—a family meeting with the Moultons. I hope the hospital behaves itself.

The switch to daylight savings time has erased whatever serious gains the sun had made in its hour of rising. Now dawn pales my east window at half past five. It is still cold: twenty-two degrees at dawn, and a half foot of snow on the ground. I will stay in good cheer as long as there is *no more snow.*

A C-section this morning with the obstetrician; afterward she thanked me and complimented me on a fine assist. I sense a warming trend, but weather in Maine is treacherous and unpredictable, and obstetrics is practiced on the open terrain.

Last night was the RENEW potluck at Phil Carthage's home. And, even on the Monday of Holy Week, everybody came. Phil gave us tours of his mid-nineteenth century Greek Revival home, built "squarely" in the tradition, with a curved staircase and high ceilings but no cupola or columned porch. We had a social hour, then a fine meal of a pasta and Greek salad and New England baked beans and white rolls. With my plate piled high, I wandered into a room of women who were discussing issues of education. Mostly I listened. Only when a fork dropped (its burden of sauce staining Phil's white carpet) did I speak, and then to tell the story of my visit to the Doctors Ott in Stuttgart, Germany. They were friends of Lindsay's parents, who met while on sabbatical at the National Institutes of Health. We had accepted their gracious invitation to stay with them during our European vacation five years ago. I tried not to embarrass Lindsay with my unrefined manner. But on the day of our departure, I accidentally dropped a sausage in my wine glass, spattering their immaculate linen with lakes of red wine. "Never mind, never mind," they insisted, "it's not as bad as when the parson came to visit."

The Otts were in the habit of keeping *vogels*—bullfinches, to be exact—as house pets. Since the bullfinch is a protected bird in Germany, the practice has been outlawed, but the Otts were allowed to keep their one remaining specimen. One Sunday the parson, a much-liked and well-respected friend of the family, came to dinner. While they socialized over cheese and sausage, dark bread and wine, the Otts let their regal pet flit happily about the room, as was their custom. Unfortunately, it came to rest under the parson's feet. As he rose to assume a place of honor at the dinner table, a wee "snap" was heard, and the poor *vogel* lay limp on the living room carpet. The Doctors Ott, of course, made a valiant attempt at resuscitation, but could not undo a broken neck. No amount of lively banter at the dinner table could lift the party's downcast spirits, or the parson's embarrassment at having squashed the family pet.

While we finished dessert, I heard the telephone ring and the sound of Phil's voice, murmuring briefly, quietly, then with intensity. Within a few moments he collected us into the dining room and asked for our attention. First, he offered an impromptu prayer in thanksgiving for the blessings that RENEW had brought our lives. Then he dropped a bombshell: Father Michael would be leaving, effective immediately. The bishop called our parish council president, who had just now relayed the message to Phil. The bishop used the word "resign," but quickly revised it to a "leave of absence for personal reasons." Nothing more. So sudden, a lightning bolt in the middle of Holy Week. It was impossible not to speak, each of us with our nervous, tearful, aimless musings—some of it gossip, some speculation, all rising out of our sense of wrenching loss and our deep concern for Father Mike. Some spoke of Father's discontent, his recent remarks about a lack of commitment from the parish, his slight but noticeable rise of anger that morning over the petty bickering of a parishioner about "the kids running wild at Mass." Others spoke of the hardship imposed by his vocation, the relentless strain, the isolation and lack of support, the rigid expectations and ceaseless criticism. I passed over other possibilities in my mind: a nervous breakdown, an ailing parent, an allegation of impropriety. The latter would be the most crippling for the parish. We were promised more information at an emergency parish council meeting scheduled for Wednesday, the evening of Clare's birthday party.

I spoke aloud, as a family doctor who knows the burden of belonging to a healing ministry. I expressed my own regret at not giving Father Mike more support. I suggested that we reach out to him now, not as a people grieving the loss of our spiritual leader, but as one Christian neighbor to another. Several of us drove past the rectory on our way home. The lights were on, and two strange cars were parked out front, but there was no answer at the door. His Siamese cat was perched on the dining room table, studying us, providing nary a clue. We went home to our separate beds, wondering what had gone wrong and what would happen next.

I was called to the Moultons Tuesday morning before office hours began. Elena is in the last stage of ALS, lately choking on pureed food and even her own secretions, which flow heavily from her mouth and nose. I hoped my visit would carry them through the busy week ahead. I would be surprised not to find her close to suffocation or pneumonia.

I knocked on the side door and poked my head inside, catching the glint of her eyes. Harry greeted me and gestured me to sit at Elena's side. Clear mucous coursed from her nostrils, and she choked with a repetitive, whimpering cough. Her eyes seemed glassy, pleading in a way I had not seen since the early days of her diagnosis. I drew my stethoscope to her back and listened intently; the lungs seemed remarkably clear, but I knew that only the most fulminant process could make itself known through her shallow movement of air. She reported no fever or pain or difficulty sleeping, nor was she obviously choking. I prescribed an antihistamine syrup to dry her nasal secretions, and encouraged Harry to call me if he felt hospitalization would be of benefit.

I knew they would make a strong attempt to hold out until Easter, until after Elena's brother Roger had visited. I had expressed an interest in meeting him, shaking his hand, supporting him through the ordeal. Given his anticipated arrival that afternoon, and the suddenness of Elena's decline, I thought that we could arrange a family meeting for 5:00 P.M. I knew that Lindsay would not be happy, with so much preparation still needed for Clare's birthday party tomorrow. But it is Holy Week, a time for faith and compassion, and I knew in my heart it was the right thing to do.

When I pulled in the drive around 6:00 P.M., I noticed the strange car, undoubtedly Roger's Lincoln Continental with the New York plates. He was the first to greet me at the door, and introduced me to his wife. Harry, as is his usual fashion, drew a chair to Elena's side and sat me down. I looked around for signs of hospitality—a tray of drinks, a plate of cookies, fresh cut flowers on the table—but these were gentilities far beyond Elena's means or Harry's grasp. I sat quietly in the plain room filled with plain people but marveled, all the while, at this extraordinary gathering!

Around the circle, beginning at my far left, was Elena's brother Billy, a mildly retarded achondroplastic dwarf; sitting next to him on the sofa was John, the Moulton's adopted son, who is also mentally retarded. Across the room was Roger, Elena's youngest brother, and, next to him, his wife. She was a stocky woman, in appearance fifteen years his senior, who spoke with a thick Eastern European accent reflecting her Estonian childhood and German education. She sat silently and without expression, arms folded on her lap, guarded, it seemed, against any gesture of concern or pleasure or encouragement. Roger explained that she fell on the ice a year ago and struck her head, resulting in a subdural hematoma that required surgical evacuation. On the mend, she inexplicably awoke one morning without use of her left side. Eventually she recovered from the stroke, but the surgery and the stroke and a resultant seizure disorder had aged her beyond her years.

And then there was Harry, deaf as a board, who absorbed only a fraction of the conversation even when I shouted it into his ear. Elena sat drooling in her chair, propped by strips of bed sheeting and heavily sedated by antihistamines. Surprisingly, the conversation moved briskly, pivoting around two key issues: should Elena get a second opinion from a Boston neurologist? And should she go to the nursing home for fifteen days so that her home health care could be paid for by insurance? Elena spelled out her desires clearly on the message board: she wanted to learn more about new treatments for ALS ("t-e-l-l d-r w-h-a-t") that Roger had reported to her earlier. And she also had made up her mind about the nursing home ("i d-e-c-i-d-e-d n-u-r-s-i-n-g h-o-m-e") for its financial advantage.

Harry would hear none of it (even if he had not heard all of it); the nursing home could never care for Elena properly; they didn't know her, her needs, the little quirks of her care, her special positioning, her meal preferences. Both parties wanted to sacrifice for the other. But Elena had nothing else to give Harry; nothing was within her capacity to give except her very life and death. I explained this to Harry, loud and clear. The decision to go to Boston should be Elena's, even if the trip would be exhausting, disappointing, and void of any real solutions. Elena needn't decide now, not in these two or three minutes, I assured him. But I could see sparks of hope flickering in the moist eyes of the patient by my side.

At the meeting I learned that Elena was a bit of an upstart, a second child and only daughter, the "brightest of the lot," who had met Harry while looking for land in Maine. The Rouge family had passed through Waldo County on a Maritime vacation, and Elena had fallen in love with the land and sea and, suddenly, this solidly built, painfully shy mill worker who would later elope with her to Virginia. "They had no waiting period there," Harry explained to me, "so she picked me up in her car after work one day and off we went to be married." Elena's parents later moved from Maryland to Maine, heartsick over the loss of their defiant daughter.

I made a point of praising Harry for his love and devotion; Elena's illness had made for a long, uncertain, and trying time since the diagnosis was established eighteen months ago. I encouraged Roger to return again, and offered to do whatever I could to make his visits easier.

Clare's fifth birthday. The celebration is planned for 5:00 this evening; seven kids are expected, though Lindsay tells me that our daughter invited her entire nursery school class. We have already unveiled the parental gift, a Huffy 16–inch bicycle with training wheels, which Clare has been tirelessly riding up and down the hallway.

I was glum all day as I carried around the troubling news of Father Mike's departure. Midday I telephoned the Chancery office, and my call was directed to Father Hanschel, who had spoken with Mike that morning. My purpose in calling, I assured him, was not to pry or meddle, but to offer my services wherever they might be needed, and to express the concern and sadness that all of us felt at St. Francis. I scribbled down the address of the Chancery with the intent to distribute it at tonight's emergency parish council meeting.

It was a day of dialogue with fellow Catholics, neighbors, pastoral colleagues of Mike's, and concerned staff and patients at the office. We needed to talk and to grieve. The Church—in its haste to appear "responsible," to stand for the rights of the victim as well as the perpetrator, to take seriously every allegation and charge?—seems to have ignored the grief of the parish. The Chancery carried out an abduction. Mike has become a missing person. But the parish has lost a friend and a shepherd. Just tell us, dear Bishop, what happened (generally, please, if you cannot speak in specifics). We can handle the news; we can take it like adults. To suggest that "Father was feeling the pressure of personal problems and requested a leave of absence" is to make his departure seem impulsive and irresponsible. Leaving without so much as a goodbye on the Monday of Holy Week? Allegations of misconduct (which is everyone's suspicion) are the scourge of the Church, and our trust is only eroded further by each evasive report.

After today's contacts, I feel a little better, eased of the burden, knowing in faith that the parish will survive. But there are duties to execute, and a responsibility owed to Father Mike and to the next parish priest, who will need us far more than he suspects.

Clare's birthday began with a furious attack on the presents Lindsay had labored so hard to choose, buy, and wrap—only to learn, to her deep dismay, that "I really wanted a playhouse." Five-year-olds can pull that line off with such refreshing candor, then go on to enjoy whatever it is they have been given; but the parent is left devastated. Lindsay was stressed by the approaching festivities and asked that I be home by 5:00. It would mean switching the last two patients of the day to the beginning. It would mean asking Tim to cover OB during the critical two hours prior to the party. We often ask each other for the sacrifice, never expecting it to materialize. On the way to the office, I slipped home to finish clues for the treasure hunt and string a rope across the driveway for the piñata. A note on the dining room table confirmed that Lindsay had arranged for a pizza delivery at 5:30 P.M.; the cake was baked and decorated with Beast, Belle, and Lumiere; the birthday table was aglow with party plates, napkins, hats, and helium balloons tied to each chair. All the ducks were lined up.

At 4:15 P.M., on schedule and with charts complete, OB called to say that my laboring patient was eight centimeters. Would I come now to avoid the last-second rush? She was a primigravida who had been laboring for nineteen hours, hospitalized for seven. I knew that there would be plenty of time to call Tim for the delivery, even if she was complete when I arrived. It was a big baby, overdue by ten days, and unlikely to be birthed with a single push.

But on examination, the patient was only six centimeters, the same diameter she had been at noon. The head was molding, which suggested a hard labor encountering an obstruction. Her contractions had remained two minutes apart all afternoon; they were strong, and lasted seventy seconds. Judging by her concentration, and the redness in her eyes, the pains were "adequate" and would not require an intrauterine pressure catheter to prove it. Things were not going well. Should I allow her to labor another two hours before calling for a section? The fetus was healthy. Mother had emotional support from her mother and husband. Should I call for surgery now and avoid what seems now to be needless suffering?

The obstetrician had arrived on the floor to check two of her own patients, and so I discussed the case with her. Upon repeat cervical exam, she concurred with my assessment and suggested sectioning her now. "Sure," I said, but explained my predicament and proceeded to call Tim. He was gone, off shopping, but Cris expected him home soon. I was stuck after all! It was 4:45 P.M. and I was held hostage by the decision to section. I could not leave the obstetrician in the lurch. During the wait for surgery, I explained our decision, and my imminent replacement by Dr. Hughes, to the patient and her family. Their weary, beaded brows wrinkled agreement. Then, at a minute before 5:00, I got word that Tim was on his way.

I picked up Clare and her friends at day care and whisked them home. They bounced and yapped in the back seat like puppies. Gradually all seven guests trickled in. I whipped up a bit of frenzy with my makeshift pirate suit, all part of the treasure hunt scheduled for later. Around 5:30 we began to seat them for pizza. Several declared that they would prefer macaroni and cheese (including the birthday girl), and so Lindsay put herself to that task. I poured drinks, sliced watermelon, displayed the cake, and kept the peace. Still no pizza. I telephoned the pizza house and was reassured that the delivery boy was on his way. At 6:00 there was still no pizza. Lindsay dialed again and discovered they had made a terrible mistake; all this time, the pizzas were boxed and warming on top of the oven. They arrived at 6:15 and were instantly consumed. But the bulk of the party loomed before us with only forty-five minutes left before parents arrived.

Group photo on the sofa, then on to the treasure hunt. The search went well, though Clare and Lucy got into a tussle, and Clare objected to going last (even if it positioned her to find the biggest treasure). The treasure was a piñata hidden in the garage. They would beat mercilessly until a seam exploded and candy, peanuts, feathers, and trinkets showered onto the driveway. Then back inside for cake, singing, and free time with a gaggle of Barbies. At last, tearful goodbyes, and all was over for another year.

I rushed off to the emergency session of the parish council and found a seat at the table despite a full house. A letter had been photocopied and distributed, the one read aloud at the penitential service two nights earlier. It said, in part, that "On Monday, April 5, your pastor, Fr. Michael, met with Bishop Gerry at the chancery in Portland. Father has lately been experiencing a great deal of stress and felt the need for a personal leave of absence. Bishop Joseph accepted Father's resignation as pastor of St. Francis Parish and granted him leave for as long as Father feels it is necessary."

Few believed it. Rumors of sexual misconduct had circulated for over a year, and the circumstances of his departure seemed so much out of character. Father had not appeared overly distraught; had not breathed a word of a possible or impending resignation to his confidants; had earned a reputation as a fastidious planner, one who took his responsibilities seriously and would never bail out during Holy Week. But more to the heart was the absence of a goodbye.

Those who trusted and loved Father Mike found this to be incomprehensible. Betrayal, loss, abandonment were the operative words, along with anger at the diocesan office for mishandling the affair. The council moved and approved that a letter be issued to the Chancery, and I was nominated to draft it. We needed accurate and complete information about Father Mike and requested a face-to-face meeting with the Chancery. The only dissenting vote came from a council member who believed that silence was Father's wish and the kindest of mercies.

Good Friday is a Catholic high holy day. I am always moved by the reading of the Passion, transfixed by the Way of the Cross, and embarrassed at the "Veneration of the Cross," which translates into the kissing of Christ's feet on the crucifix. The collective guilt of our religious heritage emanates from the twelfth station,* where Jesus dies on the Cross. The celebrant reads "It is now about the sixth hour, and there was darkness over the whole land until the ninth hour. And the sun was darkened, and the curtain of the temple was torn in the middle. Jesus cried out with a loud voice and said, 'It is finished. Father, into your hands I commend my spirit.' Then, bowing his head, he died."

The congregation replies, speaking rhetorically for the obedient Jesus, and for

---

* The 3:00 P.M. service, for (all over the world) Christ was crucified at 3:00 P.M.

his Father, "My people, what have I done to you, or in what way have I offended you? Answer me. What more should I have done and did not do? I led you out of the land of Egypt, and you prepared a cross for me. I opened the Red Sea before you, and you opened my side with a lance. I gave you a royal sceptre, and you have given me a crown of thorns. With great power I lifted you up, and you have hung me on a cross. My people, what have I done to you, or in what way have I offended you? Answer me!"

The convergence of Passover and Holy Week is a logical and historical one. Jesus' Last Supper was a Seder feast. The symbol of the Redemptive Christ as a Paschal Lamb originates in the Passover story, where lambs' blood was used to mark the doors of God's chosen people during their exile in Egypt, thereby sparing their firstborn males from God's vengeance. The Latin word *pasch* is applied to the celebrations of both Passover and Easter, and is taken from the Greek and Aramaic *paskha,* similar to the Hebrew *pesakh.* Jesus is, for Christians, the promised Messiah of the Old Testament prophets. So it is right and natural that I should feel, as I do, an overwhelming solidarity with Jews and Judaism at this time of year, at this singular moment. Lindsay, Clare, and I are privileged to attend our neighbor's Seder meal tomorrow evening.

Easter Sunday. Yesterday was one of the best Holy Saturdays I can remember. It began at 4:30 A.M. Instead of meeting my computer, I enjoyed an intimate conversation with Lindsay over a long misty stroll around town, shared coffee, listened to public radio (a beautiful Taverner Mass, *The Crown of Thorns*), and scheduled our day. All of this was made possible by Clare's sleepover on Good Friday at Wee Care Day Care. The owners took the kids out for pizza, served them hot fudge sundaes when they returned, and circled sleeping bags on the rec room floor for bedtime stories. A good time was had by all, reported Clare on her return.

In the meantime, I made hospital rounds, finished two letters that had been hanging over my head, and selected music for the Easter Mass, where Scott and Jean and I will be singing. We cleaned the kitchen, turned compost, straightened the living room, and worked on our various projects. Mac Thomas called to reassure me that, according to reliable sources, Father Mike had simply burned out. In Father's own words, "I was burning the candle at both ends and ran out of wax." Good news (among the alternatives); Mike will get a well-deserved rest and a new start, and the diocese will not lose another priest. I feel petty and cheap for having assumed that the pedophilic rumors were true. But circumstances had allowed our imaginations to run wild, and it was somehow easier to cope with the thought of Father's forced exodus than with a voluntary one.

At 11:00 A.M., the phone rang and a tearful, trembly voice reported that she was ready to come home. "I'm lonely and bored," said Clare. "Everyone else left

. . . Could you *please* pick me up?" We were shocked! Hadn't we heard that the kids would be dropped off? Guilt-ridden, I raced to pick up Clare and discovered, happily, that she had now nearly forgotten this small snafu among her many positive memories from the sleepover. No fears at bedtime or crankiness in the morning.

Scott came over in the afternoon to practice songs for Sunday Mass. We spent the first hour coloring Clare's Easter eggs, after borrowing a quarter cup of white vinegar from our next-door neighbor to fix the dye. This was a fancy kit, Little Mermaid Glitter, complete with "sticky stuff" and glitter that went on after the coloring. Scott revealed his secret for telling a hard-boiled egg from a raw one. Spin them on the counter top; the hard-boiled egg will rotate more rapidly because its weight is uniform and solid. We also learned a lesson from the makers of the Little Mermaid Glitter kits. They provided us with a lot more sticky stuff than glitter, so that the first eggs got a disproportionate amount of glitter while the last were mostly sticky. As in life, glitter is wasted, and our lives get stickier as we go along.

Last evening we joined the Bakers for a Seder Feast on the fifth day of Passover. The table was set for Bernie and Laura and their two children; Doug Coffin, his wife, Kirsten, and their children, Harpswell and Sigrid; the three of us; and, of course, the prophet Elijah. We shared a lovely meal that kept holy the Sabbath and compared favorably with Seders past. We talked of many things, including tradition. Someone thought it important to create "new traditions" (an oxymoron, Lindsay later suggested) within our families, not borrowed or reshaped from the past, but totally fresh and imbued with personal meaning. I am too nostalgic for that, too Catholic, too lazy. Yet I see the problem: Traditions are the pack horse for family values. When homes are broken, or blended values clash, we must be willing to renegotiate the ritual. It is powerful medicine, and how we come to dispense it—our supper prayers, bedtime habits, television rules, the Christmas protocol, family vacation plans—matters immensely.

The conversation flowed toward small-town life. Bernie will be attending a conference at Cornell University in June, where twenty or so professors of history, sociology, American literature, and ethics will discuss curricula in rural culture. Bernie earned his ticket there by writing a Ph.D. dissertation on Wendell Berry. He asked my opinion about access to health care in rural areas, but I am frankly more concerned about the teachers and doctors and ministers who deliver care. How do they overcome the stress and isolation of rural living? How do we stimulate students and patients and parishioners to take charge of their own outcomes, or whatever they imagine their salvation to be?

Those of us who are part of rural culture are the least able to see it clearly. Level-headed observers need perspective, distance, and appropriate comparisons before they can begin to distinguish what belongs to their local culture from what is merely a parental or personal landmark. As with religion, I think that small-town life should be chosen only after you have left it for a decade. That has been my path, anyway; it is not a prescription for all.

I ran the "old long run" yesterday and did a respectable job of it. Down the deep descent, along the steamy Head of Tide road, past the osprey nest still clinging to the top of the utility pole. At the bridge, Passy Stream thundered through slate-ribbed rapids and boiled within its swollen banks. I climbed slowly up the mile-long grade, observing the signs "Speed Limit 40 MPH," padding steadily to the top. My legs were limber, my shoes broken in. And my lungs managed to recover on the downhill slope before the next incline. I had tried to avoid a mental agenda for the run but found my thoughts returning to tonight's parish council meeting and a presentation I will make in support of a memorial Mass for Father Mike.

I had asked a friend of mine to promote the idea at Worship and Spirituality Commission a week ago; they voted it down, citing the need by some parishioners to "put it all behind us." They disapproved of an invitation to the Chancery; they desired no undue attention to Father Mike. My friend was apologetic, but in the end his commission made a reasonable suggestion: float the idea before the parish council.

My point to the council was this: Had Father Mike left the parish when he first proposed, or even at his second request, he would have been feted in the parish hall. But now, under this cloud, he wouldn't get even a Hallmark card. Still, many of us need a venue in which to say goodbye, a chance to thank him and wish him well, to close the books on these unhappy times in order to welcome the new priest with a clear conscience and unburdened heart. To that end, we might gather as a community of faithful to celebrate a Mass of Special Intentions. A Mass would be the ideal vehicle: there is precedent for such a choice; it is bread for all Catholics; and, as ritual, it requires that nothing necessarily be said. Our feelings are, anyway, confused. No words come easily to express them. But at Mass, standing as a community, we can privately offer whatever we feel—thanksgiving or anger, fears or sadness—to the God of all sorrows, and expect a sacramental blessing in return.

Such a Mass must first be approved by the interim pastor, who would play a pivotal role as celebrant. Parishioners would be under no moral obligation to attend. Father Mike will be invited, but the Chancery need not be; this is, as it should be, an internal matter of the parish. The Mass should be delayed only until we can plan it and publicize it.

The proposal for a Mass of Special Intentions passed unanimously but without a list of volunteers. It was scheduled for the last Saturday of the month. Matters seemed well enough in hand until 2:00 this morning, when I awoke with a start and could not settle back to sleep. Only after a trip to the bathroom and a sip of milk could I go back upon the bed. The words of Julian of Norwich came to me like balm: "All will be well, and all will be well, and all manner of thing will be well."

I am beat. This morning I turned off the alarm at 4:30 A.M. and sat up again at 5:45, squinting as the broad daylight streamed through our bedroom window. Where had the moment gone, the hesitation as I squeezed off the alarm and paused under the warm weight of the covers? I had gone to bed at a reasonable hour, taken an afternoon nap, and run only a short run in the late afternoon mist. I had dreams of moving vans: driving them up steep hills, failing to make the snowy crest, and sliding backward along the slippery incline. Then I dreamed of dinner with Dr. John Rhodes, a colleague and friend of my father's, who was narrating a viewing of his home movies. One scene showed John and my father aspirating fluid from a patient's heart. Another had us bicycling along the country roads of Pocahontas County, searching for a particular house by a circuitous route.

The night before I had a dream about Bill Clinton. For some reason, I had pocketed his car keys and needed to return them. Several times during the day I tried calling the Oval Office, but the line was busy or no one was home or the secretary refused to connect me or I had misplaced the scrap of paper where the number had been scribbled. As the day wore on I became increasingly alarmed, for how otherwise could the President drive home? If I returned the keys today he would be grateful, but tomorrow, after all the inconvenience, what then? Thinking hard on the matter, I reasoned that our President could bum a ride; thereafter, the tension of the dream resolved.

My explanation: in the dream I was frustrated by the Administration, though I had a legitimate and urgent message for the President, as I have for the Bishop with regard to Father Mike. I may not hold the key to his homecoming, but I am willing to do whatever I can to prevent the *next* parish disaster.

Yesterday Tim handed me a letter from Robert Coles. "Dear Dr. Loxterkamp," it said, "We were waiting for you! We called your Maine office, but there was no way to reach you. I'm truly sorry. I'd be delighted to try to see you one of these days." Since I had been given no telephone number or street address or instructions on how to find him, what was I to do? Oh, frustration. Our meeting was not meant to be, but perhaps (with better planning) we will rendezvous one of these days.

I have recuperated. Last night, Clare collapsed on the sofa at 7:30 P.M., leaving Lindsay and me to our own devices until we finally drifted to sleep at a little past nine. An hour and a half can make all the difference. I worked on my AIDS talk and tailored the last third of it to the experience of being an "AIDS doctor" in a small town. My principal message is that we must all be "AIDS providers" so that the burden does not become sacrificial to the few.

Yesterday's AIDS talk went well, judging by the turnout (nearly two hundred, double the average attendance), my own sense of accomplishment, and the enthusiastic questions. But a speaker's evaluation will tell the truth: whether or not they liked it, and whether or not it satisfied their expectations and needs. Since the program was sponsored by the Pine Tree Chapter of the Intravenous Nurses' Association, the audience was nearly all women, nearly all nurses. They came from hospitals, home health agencies, hospice programs, nursing homes. The questions and comments showed an enormous compassion and concern, especially from one woman who worked in a state veterans hospital.

She had responded to my story about Terry, my only AIDS patient at the time, whom I had "deserted" in order to learn more about AIDS through a San Francisco mini-fellowship. He died while I was on sabbatical, but I felt little guilt because we had said goodbye, and I had left him in the capable hands of my partner and felt proud of the care he had received since his diagnosis four years ago. He died of wasting and mycobacterium avium complex, reaching the end of the line without crippling or painful opportunistic infections.

Doctors need assurances that we have done a good job, that we have performed up to snuff. Never mind that many of the longer AIDS survivors will die with profound wasting and diarrhea, with malignancies and dementia, long after their loved ones are buried or burned out or have left for other reasons. The V.A. nurse had just lost such a patient, and wondered what had been accomplished, what had been saved. At least, I reminded her, your patient did not die alone; you attended him these last several weeks. Such a scenario repeats itself frequently in the later decades of life; AIDS has simply introduced these issues to the younger generation. Doctors, with their merciful ministrations, their antibiotics and home oxygen and bypass grafts, routinely save the elderly, for what? If nothing else, for love, ours and theirs. The strategy is far from "productive." Whether or not it preserves human dignity or meets the unspoken need for love is up to those involved.

On the ride to Portland, I played a tape sent to me by a residency classmate. It was a selection of Bob Dylan's greatest hits, 1978–91. Chills ran down my spine during the brass opening to a chorus of "Is your love in vain." The first line hit home: "Do you love me, or are you just extending good will?" I would pose that question at the close of my AIDS talk. Do we care about our patients, get mixed up in their feelings, or offer them only a detached and sympathetic rendering of our clinical skill?

On the relaxing drive home, in the town of Damariscotta, the flash of brake lights suddenly riveted my attention. I slammed on my brakes. A van had stopped for a pedestrian in the crosswalk and I had narrowly missed his bumper. Suddenly there was a bang on my bumper as my car lunged forward and struck, with another loud bang, the van ahead of me. In the rearview mirror, I saw a pickup truck with an attached trailer that advertised City Power Wash.

We all converged in front of a delicatessen called Treats: the pedestrian from Hartford, the van driver, Mr. Power Wash, and I. Only my bumper was damaged; and only the pickup truck and my Jetta had actually collided. The town constable arrived momentarily, filed his report, facilitated an exchange of names and numbers, and ushered us back on our ways. Mr. Power Wash apologized by way of saying that this was his first motor vehicle accident, and that his dog had died last week, and that his wife had up and left him. I wish he'd left off the part about his wife and dog, for I began to doubt the accuracy of his insurance data. Well, the police knew how to find him, so I wished him well and we parted paths.

I didn't think that it had bothered me, such a little jolt, just a tiny bit of structural damage. But I missed my turnoff for Route 90, which forced me to backtrack ten miles. After arriving home, I got an estimate on the bumper damage: $1,055.92! Then a cleansing run around the perimeter of Belfast. More bizarre dreams last night, and several anxious jolts from my sleep. Dreams of Rolfe, old neighbors and high school classmates and my brother figuring prominently, each boasting some wild moneymaking scheme. Scenes of sexual tension, and threats of violence in a stranger's home. Was it, as Scrooge had said in *A Christmas Carol,* just "a bit of bad beef"? Or does the brain stew on these psychic blows, this jangling of the nerves, and regurgitate them in some altered form?

Yesterday threw me off balance. Everyone arrived fifteen minutes late for Thursday group, even the punctual Mary Beth. Scott complained that he just couldn't do it—be *expected* to do it—arrive on time when the morning is his worst time of day. He might get started late, then Debbie would describe a dream, or the neighbor would call to go running, or a bird song or the morning sun slanting through the trees just so would utterly captivate him. He feels like hiding. He wants to cancel all social obligations. Yet Scott wants to be here, too. He broods over his diffidence, his hesitation, his vacillation about making a commitment to the group. What does it mean? He wants to be here, he assures us, but time is the nemesis. And I know it's true. All our admonishments and maneuvers to get him to arrive punctually have proven futile. Yet I trust Scott and appreciate his conflict with time.

Today I had hoped to discuss a problem-patient of his, Margo Leach, whose chart I had recently cosigned. I had overheard patients complaining of their hour or more wait to see Scott after he had fallen behind with Margo. I read Scott's office note and discover that he is treating her headaches with sumatriptam. He believes them to be migraine; he knows how much they have exacted in terms of his emergency time, intramuscular narcotics, and endless worry. "If successful," he records optimistically, "we can taper back on the other meds."

Finally I screwed up my courage to ask, "so how is Margo?" Not good, not good, Scott admitted, and settled back into his chair to testify on his own behalf.

"We need to share these troublesome patients," Tim assured him, "as David and I do; we each need a reprieve, support, a little different perspective."

I agreed, but pressed the point. Scott is too kind, too self-abnegating, too pandering with Margo. Take back the control. Schedule her return visit in four weeks, not next, in order to give your treatment a sufficient trial. She holds the final trump; she decides when she is well or not. But *you* are the one who schedules the appointments and lays out the treatment plan and decides when you have reached your limit. I tried to help Scott identify some realistic goals. The sumatriptan *will not work,* or not for long. Then where do you go? All along, Scott has been unwilling to say bluntly "you need psychotherapy" or "I'm sorry, I can't help you; let's find you someone who can." He fears, as much as I do (though, oddly, more than Tim) the anger or rejection that might follow. He wants to help her, but worries that he has waded in too far, well over his head in time and expense and unfulfilled promises, handed himself over to her suffering and her distorted sense of reality. Stopping short of "the cure" would seem like desertion. With no escape, no end in sight, Scott has become a mere presence, a witness to her pain.

I cannot bring myself to address the havoc she wreaks on Scott's schedule; another sign of the power she wields.

Yesterday Lindsay's period came and dropped the bottom out of my day. How easy it was to get pregnant that first time around; easy nine months ago when we decided to try again. We have only been trying rigorously for four months, but I wonder, "what if it is no longer possible?" Lindsay and I had a good laugh the night before her period came, about the nature of the disappointment: how much less of an issue for us is childbirth than procreation.

Yesterday, at ten minutes before eleven o'clock, the husband of a patient of ours called from Arkansas. He wanted to know if I would fill his wife's prescription. He needed to know, even more earnestly, if I would still be her doctor. A telephone call on the ninth had left matters in doubt. We talked for five minutes and cleared up relations that had been muddled and strained for the past week, for which I was grateful.

Last week his wife had called to request a refill on Valium and Pepcid; could I call them into a Little Rock drug store? "Not," I said, "before you tell me why." The request had first circulated through the nurses, who caught the brunt of her fury. Hadn't I *promised* to help her in a pinch? Hadn't she suffered enough with her daughter's nervous breakdown, her husband's recent illness, and now *this* humiliation! I would eventually waste fifteen minutes of my time trying to make a point: I have no policy against long-distance refills, nor do I object in principle to Valium. But I had specifically ordered enough Valium to last the trip, and if she needed more, perhaps she should seek psychiatric help.

My patient would not be deterred. "My *reasons* are none of the nurses' business," she huffed. "I changed my pills from three a day to four; things are back to normal now, so would you kindly comply with my request?"

"OK," I relented, and did.

But the next day she was back on the telephone with a request for oxygen to assist her through a high-altitude flight. There was no mention of this in her old records; she had no sign of emphysema on her physical exam. I flatly refused! If such a need were acute and real, she should find a doctor in Arkansas to certify it. My message was relayed through the nurses, who one by one lost their patience with our formidable foe. They could neither express our concerns nor free themselves from the telephone. She insisted on calling back in an hour, and expected to talk to me. Meanwhile, I instructed my nurse to intercept the call, keep it short, and *stick to her guns*. If she wouldn't get off the telephone, threaten to hang up, and then do it! I returned to my afternoon of patients, only later reading the nursing note: "the patient became irrational, belligerent, and threatening when she heard the bottom line."

I sat down and wrote a letter to my patient in hope of laying down the law. We have enough aggravation in our lives, and too much to do, to put up with bad manners and unrealistic demands. I extended my sympathies for her recent hardships; I suggested she seek psychiatric help. And I remained specific and clear about what we considered to be inappropriate behavior. But no sooner had I received my letter back from the transcriptionist than I received the call from her husband.

It is sometimes easier just to send the troublemakers packing. They wander from the emergency room to the generalist, who tosses them to a specialist, who is never around at the time of crisis, so they find their way back to the ER. In the process they receive a thousand overpriced opinions, studies, treatments, and never get better—or, for that matter, never even get an honest answer. Perhaps my patient cannot be helped (I entertain that conclusion more as time passes). But if she were to stay with one practitioner, there is a chance he would, first, do no harm and, second, support the family who suffers alongside her. I will keep an open mind, try a little harder, persevere a little longer. As Dorothy Day has said, "What we avert our eyes from today can be borne tomorrow when we have learned a little more about love."

I missed the parish council meeting on Thursday night, when Sister from the

Chancery came to listen to our grievances. I might have been there, might have made it a priority, but this was Lindsay's first night of Bereavement Support Group, and I wanted to be with Clare. Or perhaps, even more strongly, I wished to evade the role of parish spokesman, no matter how flattering the offer. One member called later with the particulars. The meeting had been well attended, but subdued and polite and without controversy.

The only "news" *per se* was the report that Father Mike, as early as a year ago, had requested a transfer from St. Francis. The request had been denied by the bishop. Mike had hoped for an assignment closer to Portland, where he was needed for frequent meetings with the Chancery board as chaplain of the Boy Scouts of America. Two weeks ago, Mike had again initiated the same request; it was again refused. The Church blew it, admitted Sister. They did not see how little fuse remained. And they were not aware of the impact his leaving would have on the parish. In retrospect, someone should have delivered the message personally; if not Father Mike, then someone from the Chancery. Toward the end of the hour, one woman made a plea, formulated as a prayer, that we give our grief to God. Let it go. Ask no more of Father Mike or the Diocese but rather pray for the work before us, the healing and rebuilding that lie ahead. Her request held sway. And her words brought shame upon those of us who felt conflicted, as if these feelings were unjustified or petty or destructive. I wish I might have replied: We are all grieving now, each in our own way. Some prefer a closed casket, a few hurried rosaries, a Requiem Mass for the family and be done with it. Others have a different need. They need to touch the body, examine the wound, hear all the gory details, pore over the old photographs, and cling to every scribble in the scrapbook. Each of us has his own memory of Mike. He was more than a functionary, a replaceable part, the keeper of the Sacraments. To many of us he was a friend and spiritual father. Even at age forty-three, he represented the Church and the confraternity of priests. He symbolized Christ's presence and example among us.

So when it happens that a father walks out on his family, when he offers no goodbyes or any word of explanation, it is devastating to those who remain. We feel abandoned and betrayed; we feel his loss and the shame of his leaving. Presently, we are asked not to talk about it, to still our concerns, because it will make matters worse. Like a doctor who shields his patient from a terminal diagnosis, or the spouse who conceals her anger lest it blow the family apart.

But we *must* inquire after the body, touch it to believe, and beg God for forgiveness, knowing that each of us holds a little piece of the blame. Mike's departure may not be a death in the family, but a truth remains: he left us. We pray for him. We can reassure him that, in our hearts, we have not judged him or withdrawn our compassion. And we can still gather together in the collective strength of our faith, and tell stories of survival and hope and deliverance. I

hope to write Sister about returning to Belfast. Would she participate in a ceremony of healing and reconciliation and celebration? Would the Bishop come;
would Father Mike; would the parish? The Catholic Church has always believed
that rituals are more powerful than words, and St. Francis Parish can use whatever grace it can muster.

Habits of the morning. I rose today on time and ran the "Route 1 Bypass." It
escorts the Camden-to-Bar-Harbor crowd around our town, skirting the
chicken plants and shoe factories and the sole stoplight in Waldo County. Two
months ago that strategy was complicated by a county planning board decision
to put a second stoplight at the junction of the Bypass and Route 52. So preposterous was the idea that local motorists refused to heed it, and drove obliviously
through the red light. So the Maine D.O.T., recognizing the nature of the beast,
brought in a neon sign that blinked SLOW DOWN MOTORISTS . . . EXPECT TO
STOP AHEAD in marching green letters. The reminder is gone, but the message
seems to have stuck.

My rituals have changed. I found myself looking out the bathroom window
for snow falling in the streetlights and plowed high at the roadside. None was
there, only gravel and twigs left in winter's wake. After the run, I made coffee the
old Mellita way, not from the drip machine that broke two months ago, or the
plunger method that fell into disuse after I shattered the carafe. The cats now eat
off whatever plate I can find, after The Maine Grange Centennial Plate curiously
cracked and could not be replaced. But still I rise at 4:30 and ply these plastic
keys to an airy Mass by Charpentier and the weeping gray skies of spring. It is my
last day as the office doctor; an uncommitted Sunday lies before me, with only
Mass and a run on today's platter.

It was a glorious weekend, free of responsibility. But I awoke Saturday morning
nervous and irritable, single-minded in my determination to clean the attic, rake
the lawn, go running, tidy my desk at the office, and write two letters for the
church. But Lindsay had other designs; she had made arrangements to shop in
Camden with a friend, and Cris had called hoping her daughter might come over
while she was at a Quaker retreat and Tim was stuck at hospital. Outside, the
rain poured and I sank into a waterlogged mood.

As the day got going, it seemed possible to accomplish at least some of the
agenda, and my gray mood gradually lifted. Tim and Rozy came late, and agreed
to take Clare to the Quaker retreat. They were gone for two hours, during which
time I was able to clean the attic, rake leaves, and nap on the sofa during the
Game of the Week. Why can't I let these compulsions go? Scott had sadly commented to Lindsay on Friday, "Doesn't David ever gaze out the window?" No,

I do not, unless it promises to lead somewhere. I have one foot in the door of obsessive-compulsive disorder, I often fear, but fortunately without a constant sense of compulsion and with a feeling of satisfaction from the work.

Later in the day, Tim dropped off Rozy, and the three of us—Clare, Rozy, and I—played two frenetic rounds of The Monster Game (a sort of touch-tag) and Peter Pan (a version of hide and seek), racing about the house and eventually tipping over a large potted plant, which shattered on the living room rug. All the racket caused our smallest cat, "Dinky," to hole up in the bedroom, motionless under the covers. She stole out only once during the afternoon, long enough to poop in my shoe and crawl back in again.

Sunday was a horse of a different color. Blue, clear, warm, and filled with hope. I tidied the attic, bicycled to Mass, ran the short loop around town, helped Lindsay with the yard, and played with Clare. We went cycling to the steps of St. Francis, where we shared a Hershey's chocolate bar. Twice she tipped her bike over and released a blood-curdling "Daddeeeee." Nowhere near the scene of the crime, I still caught the brunt of her frustration. When asked why she blamed *me*, Clare explained matter-of-factly, "Well, Daddy, who else could I?" Lindsay spent the afternoon caressing her garden, fussing over it, working her arms through the leaves and twigs and clumps of gravel that had been hurled on the lawn by the winter plows. Her glorious vision of a summer garden is beginning to materialize.

Clare does not go to Mass yet, except on high holy days, Easter and Christmas, and the special feasts when Daddy sings. I do not mind. She is learning reverence and prayer. The other day, she and Lindsay found a decomposed squirrel under a melting snowbank in the front yard. Clare immediately crossed herself and murmured a prayer before executing a proper burial in Bird Land (the timber behind our house). That is an incredible beginning; it made her father proud.

I called Mom yesterday, just to say hello and report on Clare's birthday. She asked if she had sent a card. "No, but that's OK," I swallowed. Mom offered an excuse that "the Christmas check was meant for both" and admitted that her memory was failing. But she is looking forward to seeing us this summer. A short visit, one planned around other necessities, a ripple in her doldrummed sea, in which one day merges imperceptibly with the next and is distinguished only by the severity of her pain or the number of stools. Her habits are well entrenched: breakfast at 7:15, lunch at 11:15, supper at 5:15; smoking in the lounge or out on the back stoop, interspersed between her meals. She has "her stories" (the television soaps in which she shows diminishing interest) and her photographs, the osteoporotic pain in her back, and Crohn's diarrhea. Dementia is a mercy that submerges as much as it gives rise to the banality of her life.

It is now four days later, a Sunday at the end of my weekend off. I rose at 4:30 A.M. The eastern sky, already lit, heralded the dawn. I folded the laundry for nearly an hour and finished watching *A Passage to India*, with its curious portrayal of the Mirabar Caves. Adele Quested had gone to the caves looking for the authentic India and instead found herself agonizing over her betrothal to the city magistrate of Chandrapore. She had come to India with the magistrate's mother, Mrs. Moore, who would later experience, within the Mirabar Caves, a premonition of her own death.

The cave is an apt metaphor for the doctor's witness to the suffering of his patients. We are close enough to hear the echoing cries of our patients, see our reflection in the polished walls, and watch as they self-destruct or toughen from self-knowledge or despair. Patients do not ask that we join them in the caves, or suffer in their misery. They ask only that we guide them to the mouth and wait. Yet the intimacies of suffering can create confusion. Is it their experience or my own? Is it my father who is dying before we could say goodbye? Is it my childhood loneliness and the pain of my own past? It is in this capacity, as witnesses to suffering, that family doctors expose themselves to the greatest dangers and rewards in medicine.

I worry about the Mirabar Caves and my obsession with the memorial Mass. I feel the early loss of my father with each hospice death I attend. Am I now forcing that agenda on the parishioners of St. Francis? I must try to cling to Dr. Gadpole's words of Hindu wisdom in *A Passage to India:* "It makes no difference whether I worry or not [about the rape trial of Dr. Azziz], because the outcome has already been decided."

State of the state. The office has become harder with fewer OBs. Prenatal visits are often an oasis in the schedule where I can recover lost time. A routine OB visit requires five minutes of the doctor's time. We ask if there are any questions; is the baby moving; are you taking your vitamins; are your preparations complete? We review the chart, measure the uterine fundus, listen for fetal heartbeat, and check for edema. Five minutes. On some visits we must discuss the pros and cons of testing for birth defects, or avoiding drugs during pregnancy, or preparing siblings for the new arrival. We must address medical or social problems as they arise, and answer thorny questions that find their way to lists that are brought in every week. But . . . there is always the possibility of shifting our teaching chores to the next visit if we are running behind. Stealing from Peter to pay Paul. In our schedule now, as with our population as a whole, there are fewer Peters to pay for the Pauls.

Friday we received our first check as a rural health center. We have been wishing, working, waiting for that day for many months. The program offers us the hope of making a respectable profit, sharing it with the office staff, planning for a secure retirement, and recruiting a new partner. The government will reimburse us according to the "reasonable costs" of caring for Medicare and Medicaid patients, who comprise 70 percent of our practice. It is a well-aimed program. Most of the emphasis on increasing the supply of physicians in rural areas has focused on placement, not retention. Scholarship recipients in the National Health Service Corps and Indian Health Service left in droves after their obligation was satisfied—or even before, when buy-out options were still available. The RHC program takes a different slant: It emphasizes retention of health care personnel through wage supports and other benefits. It tries to reward those who have already chosen to live in areas designated as a government priority.

There are two patients on the Hospice Wing whom I know nothing about. Are they officially enrolled? The reins of the program are slipping from our hands, but I know it is for the best. We are full-time generalists who cannot hope to carry hospice. We are still exploring whatever it is we have to offer.

News from Father Mike. He has been placed in a treatment facility for troubled priests in the southwest and anticipates six months in rehabilitation. Mike writes with hope of returning to parish duty, perhaps even in Maine, and reveals to me his reason for leaving, but "not as a pastor writes a parishioner; rather as a patient confides in his doctor." His words seem so cryptic, fearful, and paranoid that I fear for his health.

Though I am sworn to secrecy, I cannot bear the burden alone. At Thursday morning group I seek the attention and advice of Tim, Mary Beth, and Scott. They encourage me to send Father Mike my support and prayers, but not respond directly to his claims or to the many wild rumors in circulation.*

Yesterday's news caught my attention. A Republican filibuster had thwarted passage of President Clinton's economic stimulus package, but the nation read only this: CLINTON HANDED DEFEAT. The FBI sifted through the charred remains of the Branch Davidian compound outside Waco, Texas, looking for the body of David Koresh and an estimated ninety-five others who perished with him on Monday. After seven weeks of waiting, why now, why this? Officials at the Southern Ohio Correctional Facility successfully negotiated the release of five guards who were taken hostage by four hundred inmates, and the headlines

---

* The charges finally became public eighteen months later when a local paper reported that a civil suit had been filed in Cumberland County Superior Court. It alleged that Father Mike had an affair with a parishioner who came to him seeking spiritual counsel on his homosexual feelings. The suit was later settled out of court; the plaintiff's attorney, C. Donald Wilkie, could only say that "the matter had been resolved."

blared: OHIO PRISON SIEGE ENDS. And just last week, two "guilty" verdicts were returned in the Rodney King police beating. With them, L.A. hopes to let the sleeping dog of racism lie.

After arriving home from a delivery at 3:00 A.M., I slept through until 7:00, then hauled my weary bones to the shower and scrubbed my eyes open for another day. It went smoothly. A wonderful session with Mary Beth, Tim, and Scott. The four of us span a decade ripe for the midlife crisis. We are aware that ailing parents are part of the equation, and that it is their taillights we have been following for all of our lives. Suddenly, rounding a hill, they are lost. And, momentarily, so are we. Who stands between us and death? Who protects us and our children? The road is silent and dark, save for our searching lamps, save for the lighted glove box where we fumble in vain for the road maps.

I made unimpeded rounds on my three hospitalized patients, offered greetings to my new mother and her darling baby, and by 10:00 was staring at some free time before my office hours started at 1:00. Then the beeper caught me halfway out the door. A patient of mine, Nancy Newcomb, had arrived in the ER looking *sick!*

Mrs. Newcomb is an active, vibrant sixty-seven-year-old woman who lives by herself in Montville. Yesterday she came to see me with "the flu going around." No fever, no phlegm, no shortness of breath, only a week of generalized aching and a pain in her chest when she coughed. There was nothing localized or alarming about her physical examination; the lungs, in particular, were crystal clear. I confessed to having no effective treatment against a virus, but suggested ibuprofen to soothe her aching muscles, and a cough syrup to nip the cough. She accepted that advice and went home to rest. During the night her breathing grew shallow and labored, and she found it impossible to lie down without gasping. She telephoned her daughter about the pain in her left shoulder and scapula, but the daughter—having just recovered from a similar flu—reassured her that the pain would disappear by morning.

It did not. Her breathing became increasingly rapid and shallow and painful through the night, precluding a satisfying sleep. By morning she was exhausted and afraid, and reluctantly called the neighbor for a ride to the emergency room. At 10:00 A.M., I found her in Bay 6, slouched and gasping. The vital signs signaled that something serious was wrong: blood pressure 80/45 in this normally hypertensive patient; pulse forty-eight. She remained afebrile, but her respiratory rate was rapid and oxygen saturation had fallen to 85 percent. Though the patient's white blood cell count was normal, the differential had shifted to the far left, with toxic granulations suggestive of an acute bacterial infection. The chest X-ray showed fluid halfway up the left lung. Blood gas studies confirmed the obvious: Nancy was hypoxic and acidotic, and now even high concentrations of oxygen could not maintain her saturation above 90 percent. The EKG was unchanged from previous tracings, and this, along with the chest X-ray and the clinical course, argued against a pulmonary embolus. An overwhelming pneumonia seemed the most likely cause of her precipitous decline: likely bacterial on the heels of an influenza-like illness. The cardiologist was away for the week, and, lacking a definitive diagnosis, I dared not risk managing a life-threatening illness without him. I called the pulmonary specialists in Bangor to arrange for Nancy's immediate transfer.

Before my eyes, Nancy's color and confusion deteriorated, and breathing became more of an effort. She fidgeted on the gurney, failed to find a comfortable position, looked furtively from side to side. I studied her digital read-out blood pressures: systolic of eighty despite the Lactated Ringer's solution that was flooding her veins. With a low serum sodium and a low blood pressure, Mrs. Newcomb was likely "third-spacing."* But without the reassurance of a central line, I hesitated to replace volume too quickly, no matter how badly she needed it, for fear of overshooting the mark and sending her into pulmonary edema.

I kept watching Nancy from the nurses' station, posted like the captain of a ship (or was I the ship and it the anchor?). From the helm I conferred with the pulmonologist Dr. Frey, consoled the good neighbor who brought Nancy in, and spoke to her daughter, who is a prenatal patient of ours. I ordered IM Toradol, studied the flow sheets, experimented with the oxygen masks until we found one (a non-rebreather) that kept the oxygen saturation above 90 percent. The ambulance still had not arrived! Breathing status and chest pain were growing worse, so I drew off fluid from the patient's lung before transfer. I aspirated over a pint of cloudy, greenish-yellow fluid from her left lung and sent a sample for gram stain, culture, and analysis. The laboratory quickly called with the report. They had found strings of gram-positive cocci and numerous white blood cells: presumptive diagnosis of streptococcal pneumonia.

I rode shotgun in the ambulance to Bangor, along with the ambulance crew, an emergency room nurse, and the respiratory technician. It was an uneventful journey except for a gradual but clear decline in the patient's condition. She saved her energy for breathing, making no sounds except for an occasional inquiry about her daughter or the next-door neighbor. Within an hour of her arrival in the ICU, Nancy was outfitted with a Swan-Ganz catheter, chest-tube, foley catheter, and endotracheal tube. Assisted ventilation would be required for the foreseeable future. Six liters of electrolyte solution were flooded through her subclavian vein. Dopamine was added to insure that a marginal blood pressure would perfuse her vital organs. Yet the outlook remained positive: she had a

* Leaking fluid into the diseased lung without replacing it in the circulation.

bacterial pneumonia (streptococcal pyogenes, we later learned) that should be responsive to surgical drainage and a host of antibiotics. And Nancy had entered the fight strong, vigorous, and well-nourished.

The circumstance of Nancy's unraveling was kind to me. I had examined her the day before, not brushed her off with a telephone reassurance. I *knew* that, just twenty-four hours earlier, her temperature had been normal, her cough nonproductive, her lungs clear, and her breathing relaxed. The following day, I had the good fortune of greeting her in the ER and witnessing the rapidity of her decline. She had fallen through no crack in the system, and I was thankful to be there when she needed me most. I had respected that inner voice of alarm: get her to Bangor if you are this worried about her ventilation, or there's a chance that she'll crash in the night.

It is difficult, I now realize, for me to recognize the severity of a patient's illness. I rely upon the experience and judgment of the experts, especially Dr. McCarren, who had been away on vacation. I've lost touch and interest in critical care medicine and its aggressive (albeit life-saving) ways. Seriously ill patients deserve a firmer hand. My skills are less suited to the juggling of fluid balances and blood gasses and serum chemistries than they are to surveying the broader goals of therapy and attending to the family's needs. Thank God I did not abort the transfer after making the diagnosis of "only" streptococcal pneumonia in her lungs; or waver until a transfer was impossible; or embark on the ambulance run only moments before the patient went into respiratory arrest.

I am humbled by the onslaught of this pedestrian bug. In the era of antibiotics, people still die of bacterial pneumonia, as did Jim Henson of Muppets fame—of a ß strep pneumonia in the wake of a run-of-the-mill viral illness. Rapidly, rapidly. Our clinical decisions must reflect the sure knowledge that most respiratory viruses do not cripple the immune system, most headaches are not ruptured aneurysms, and most breast lumps are not cancer. But let us not forget the Jim Hensons and Nancy Newcombs of the world.

It is so wonderful to sit before the computer in a rested state of mind. Last night I drifted through seven uninterrupted hours of sleep until four A.M. when my beeper went wild. A "low cell" ringing the false alarm. I disarmed it, climbed back into bed, and lay still and stiff for another half hour in a slow-pulsing state of awareness, like the beacon light in Belfast Bay.

Yesterday was a restful day, too. The air was surprisingly cold, dry, and dusty; the wind blew hard and steadily all day. Mary Beth, along with eight-year-old Evan and four-year-old Maria, came up for the morning to do "the Belfast thing." I guess that means hanging out at the creative playground, finding treasures on the beach (sea glass, jelly fish, and skipping stones), lunching at Th' Cup, and raiding the Belfast Food Co-op for granola and other organic staples.

Mary Beth lives in Camden and, after all these years, still apologizes for residing in that idyllic coastal town. There, the people are noteworthy, the boutiques are cute, the harbor is deep and blue and dotted with yachts and schooners. But Belfast residents have cultivated an attitude as strong as the Camdenites. We are self-righteousness about living "close to the land"; we take seriously our vows of poverty, abstinence, and a wariness toward outsiders, especially those who bring change. We resent Camden for what we cannot afford and must therefore reject. These two towns, twenty miles apart, serve each other well, reflecting the "other reality" that is hidden within.

In the afternoon, a friend and I went running. The wind riffled against our bodies and we struggled to maintain a pace, concentrating on stride and breath rather than words and ideas. I spoke briefly about my hard week, about Wednesday night's C-section and Thursday morning's ambulance ride to Bangor. "Do you mean with Mrs. Newcomb?" he inquired. "I'm friends with her daughter." A small town it is, I am forever reminded.

When we returned, one of our babysitters sat astride her bicycle in our driveway, speaking with Lindsay and Clare but waiting for me. She had come—I later learned from Lindsay—to extend a supper invitation for Thursday night. Just for me. She is both my patient and our occasional babysitter, a quiet, slightly built, happy, but (I now discover) lonely sixteen-year-old. She had bicycled over the night before "just to talk," ostensibly about her chances of needing back surgery, but mostly just to talk. She came as we were eating supper, and rather than send her away, I asked her to join us. Afterward, Lindsay and Clare retired to the living room for a video while we remained in the dining room to chat. She told me that her parents divorced when she was eight. Her father remarried and is now expecting a third child from his second marriage. Formerly "Daddy's little girl," she feels expelled from the center of his life. She cannot speak honestly to her father, share her true feelings (especially her dislike for the stepmother), because she lacks time with him and fears the stepmother will read all her correspondence.

And now her mother is dating, off to a concert tonight with her new boyfriend, dinner last night with friends. This is school vacation week, which is particularly hard because her friends are stranded on the island where she attends school. She has chosen a ferry ride over a ten-minute walk for reasons unknown. I worry about her loneliness, and her affection for me. She needs her father; she needs friends her own age. I'd like to help her but need to set limits. How to do this without pushing her away or embarrassing her? Perhaps I should talk to her mother or to her therapist.

The evening brought a stillness to the air; a warmth, finally, even though the day's high never topped fifty degrees. I grilled salmon on the barbecue, surrounded it on the dinner plate with broccoli and hash browns, and shared the better half of a bottle of chardonnay with Lindsay. Ah, weekends. Afterward, we retired to the living room for *The King and I* on video, and collapsed in a great heap by 9:00 P.M.

I spotted Yellow Eyes again at 4:30 A.M. By the time I had fed the cats and chosen the morning music, he was gone—around the corner from Condon to High, disappearing beyond the neighbor's stand of pine.

Last evening the babysitter's mother called Lindsay. It seems mother will be out of town for the weekend and needs a place for her daughter to stay. Daughter had thought of us. Would we mind terribly? After yesterday's letter and last week's overture, I felt we should decline. I am her doctor, first of all; her occasional employer, secondarily. I like her and do not resist becoming a friend in need, but I must avoid becoming a surrogate father. She is lonely. I must talk to mother today about my concerns.

I couldn't believe my eyes as the sky lightened and the ground became visible, blanketed with a lily-white coat of new snow. I raced to the thermometer. Thirty degrees and snow, and it is nearly May!

Last night's wine is clouding my head. Lindsay and I dined with friends who own a string of "camps" called the Wonder View Cottages. A friend and his father (both of them patients and fellow parishioners) had invited us for supper and asked us to bring dessert. They would supply the salmon, potatoes à la Julia Child, steamed snow peas, and a reserve Chardonnay from Monterey. It was really quite a delightful evening notwithstanding Lindsay's challenge to the chauvinism of the Church. After discussing the sorry plight of the American priesthood, she made the apt analogy: wouldn't you prefer a woman behind the wheel of the car instead of a drunk? We tiptoed around politics, but found common ground in English ale and conversational French.

Lindsay and I are trying, these recent days, to conceive another child. We both desire it, but wanting isn't enough. Have our procreative parts become obsolete? Has luck swung the other way? Has sex become too much of a goal or burden? I am loving my fatherhood now. Clare has increasingly showered me with affection (healthy oedipal feelings, Lindsay is quick to observe). I am not feeling too old for the job, although projecting one's health and well-being ten years hence is always a risky proposition. I know that a crying baby will put a crimp in my writing and delay our "freedom." But I remind myself that there is no perfect time to have a child. Now is good enough. I prayed yesterday—for the first time in years—that Lindsay and I might bear a child. And I pray again today. It has been a long five months trying.

We all came to Thursday meeting, Scott, Tim, Mary Beth, and I. We talked of time: its expansiveness and compressibility. Not the standard measure of time we clock and bill for, but the fleeting impressions, the lingering memories, the flow in which we live.

Tim is surprised to learn of our mutual regard for Mr. Lincoln. He tells me that years ago he read Carl Sandburg's biography. He was smitten then by the darker, veiled, enigmatic side of Lincoln, which survived despite his rise to fame and his life of public service. Lincoln was a passionate man, prone to depression, a lover of words. It is probably the latter quality that hooked me—his commitment to words, his belief that they can move us toward nobler ends.

And because he believed they could, they did. Or so Gary Wills proposes in *Lincoln at Gettysburg.* Lincoln's Address at Gettysburg, he says, transformed the nation's view of the Constitution. He "stole the game" by taking a single proposition about man's equality and turning it into a supreme national commitment. "The Gettysburg Address has become an authoritative expression of the American Spirit—as authoritative as the Declaration itself, and perhaps even more influential, since it determines how we read the Declaration. For most people now, the Declaration means what Lincoln said it means, as a way of correcting the Constitution without overthrowing it" (pp. 147–48). We are now a single people (a singular United States, not a set of fifty) united in one proposition. Through Lincoln's vision, we have been changed and live in a different America.

Scott was down at the mouth yesterday. He talked of the tomb, and of death stalking him in that last April snow. He talked of the dawdling spring, always a latecomer, more so here than in any other place in the world. And he talked of the terrible waste in the packaging practices of the drug companies, who plasticize their samples and gloss their advertising brochures. Someday he'll be forced to leave, Scott wagers; he'll flee this frigid wasteland, this cul-de-sac of squandered hopes and pruned possibilities. Debbie (his wife) could be happy anywhere, he admits, with practically nothing to do or wear or eat, but not so our curmudgeon comrade.

Scott swears his love to the animals and birds, simply for their beauty's sake, and for their freedom and their innocence. Man, if left to his own devices, would destroy the whole ball of wax. But I challenge Scott. Why must we pit the innocence of nature against the savagery of man? With whom do you stand, Scott Bailly? You have chosen this Maine; *you* cavort with the drug companies for their free samples. There are few among us who are not guilty or complicit. Yet among us, too, are seeds of redemption, of love, of passion, of yearning. I want to shake you, I say to him, shake you into acknowledging the brighter possibilities instead of staring blankly at the wall, down the cul-de-sac, into the depths. Choose love and life, my dear aging friend, instead of the rose's diadem only.

Later in the day, Scott tells me that he believes in the power of words, too. He feels better after that "good shakin' I commenced to lay on him" this morning. We power-walked at noon with our faithful nurse Bonnie; had ourselves a good chortle or two and a fresh, salt-misty saunter through Moose Point State Park. Tim and Scott and I are all closet depressives. I have waded into it only occasionally, never at serious risk of losing my footing or overstepping the bounds of sanity. Tim strokes through it, in and out in his even strokes, like the rhythm of his sculling oars. Scott hunkers down in the Swanville marsh, his beady eyes barely blinking, toadlike, at the water's edge. It is a part of our lives, whether we desire it or not.

It has been a week since I packed Nancy Newcomb off to Bangor. I keep in touch with the doctors and nurses on a daily basis and can report that she is still on the ventilator but weaned of medicines to maintain her blood pressure. A slow recovery, but not unexpectedly so for someone of her age. Yesterday, too, a young hemophiliac called complaining of a high fever, pain behind his eyes, flulike aches, and a stiff neck. It might be the flu, or viral meningitis, or an opportunistic infection in this young man infected with HIV. But three days ago I started him on a new medication (rifabutin) that we hope will prevent or delay the wasting disease called MAC, and there's a good chance that rifabutin and these new symptoms are connected, according to the manufacturer. Who knows, especially when his immune system is, by every measure, bereft of a cellular response? The infectious disease consultant in Portland advised me against launching into an exhaustive workup. See what tomorrow brings, he hedged, after you stop the rifabutin. Tim will be holding the reins by then. It always seems to work out this way: my sick AIDS patients get sicker on Tim's watch. We are both familiar with this spin, and it has solidified our partnership.

I have been learning a lot about parish life through the planning of Father Mike's Mass. Last evening I had talked to a coworker who is handling the "telephone end of things." She has invited two dozen parishioners to participate, as well as ministers from the Methodist, Episcopal, and Baptist churches; representatives from our mission church on Islesboro; leaders of the various groups and commissions within the parish; lectors and altar servers and Boy Scouts and Brownies. She is doing right to involve as many people as possible and to solicit as many suggestions and revisions in the plan as she can. One prominent parishioner was offended because he had not been asked to sing; he would pray for Father but could not bring himself to attend Saturday's Mass. I called him last night and apologized for the oversight, invited him to participate in any number of ways, asked him if he knew of others who had been inadvertently neglected.

The apology came easily because I felt less the cause of his injured feelings than a caretaker for them. But that is not the point. We stand together in our broken-ness before God.

It has overwhelmed me to realize how many parishioners cherished their "privileged" or "special" or "intimate" relationship with Father Mike. That was his gift, and the source of our deep loss. It should be a sparkling Mass with many facets: healing, thanksgiving, farewell, and the invocation of God's grace. What comes of it will come, for again, in the words of Dr. Gadpole, "the outcome is al-ready decided."

A day to remember. After two hours of pushing, little Marian Grace was born at the stroke of midnight, all five pounds and seven ounces of her. Mother apolo-gized about keeping me up all night. The delivery came between services—Fri-day evening's Hospice Memorial and Saturday morning's Mass for Father Mike. What a fine bit of timing it proved to be.

The Mass for Father Mike went wonderfully. The attendance did not disap-point me, even though I had hoped for an overflow crowd. Perhaps a hundred twenty-five people attended; all seemed to appreciate the effort, and maybe even enjoyed themselves. Said one elderly woman to me afterward, "Thank you for showing us how to say goodbye." It's true. We all need help with what might oth-erwise seem a "natural" process. As Lindsay has learned through her bereavement support groups, people have forgotten (or never learned) how to mourn; they need permission, guidance, and support to do what society has hidden away. I have learned this lesson coaching mothers in labor: though childbirth is a natural process, it nevertheless requires guidance and support. That's all I provide, but it can cut four hours of pushing into two, make for a less terrifying and agonizing ordeal, and sometimes spell the difference between perceived failure and unmis-takable success. The Mass was graced by Father Mike's parents, who drove up from Biddeford. And even Father Mike granted his blessing, calling the parish secretary Thursday night with a prepared message to be read at Saturday's Mass.

We may have set a parish record yesterday for most participants in a single Mass. If so, it was worth the effort. Our success lay in a people gathered; in seg-ments of our parish and the wider community coming together to read petitions on behalf of Father Mike; in the lectors and cantors, ushers and servers, eucharis-tic ministers and singers who gave up their Saturday morning to join us and to mingle afterward for refreshments in the parish hall. If only a handful had come to the Mass, I should have been happy. But, I admit it, my neck was on the line with the parish council after I spoke out so forcefully about the needs of the parish. I suddenly began to question, "Was it their needs or mine?"

I hope that our words and actions have honored Father Mike. We did not want a Requiem Mass, or a spectacle, or something grotesque in the name of religion, like the cult of saints where bodies (or fragments thereof) are exhumed and displayed to feed superstitious belief.

I spoke my piece yesterday, after Communion, after all the worry and misgivings of the last several weeks. It was not Mr. Lincoln's address at Gettysburg, nor did I pretend to have the power, through poetics, to restore our loss. I did not seek applause, or even posterity, for if it were not for the videotape of the Mass, these words would have sunk from my lips to oblivion. But I am thankful for the one comment I made before my reading, which may have been the only words that hit home. I thanked all who came to the Mass, especially those who came with heavy hearts, or mixed emotions, or doubts about whether this Mass was the right way to help Father. I admitted to doubts of my own but said that, in the end, our gathering seemed the Catholic thing to do, the instinctive and time-honored and sacramental action. We gather as a community of faithful to pray for God's blessing upon us all. Then I continued:

I would like to offer a few words on behalf of Father Mike. Not about the kind of person he is, nor about the good works for which is revered. Many of you knew him better or worked with him more closely and could write a far better tribute to the man we remember today. I should speak only about his leaving, which has affected us all, and all of us differently.

A priest is no mere interchangeable part, the "sparkplug" or "drive shaft" of parish life. Each is his own man, albeit a servant of God with special gifts and human limitations. Father Mike was such a man. Like many of you, I gradually came to know a personal side of him, a guarded and private side, one piece in a puzzle.

Many of my conversations with Father came at the end of an exhausting day, or in the deep part of the night, when I needed him urgently for Last Rites with a dying patient. He always came. I would come, too, on rare occasions, to morning Mass, as on the Feast of St. Blaise when he blessed us against afflictions of the throat, and joke with him about his "practicing medicine without a license." As his family doctor, I helped him uphold the Boy Scout motto "be prepared" by immunizing him before the Brazilian Jamboree. I appreciated his warm welcome for my singing friends, a Quaker and Episcopalian, though he admitted that he didn't follow the music that closely, anyway.

And I was shocked and saddened when, three Mondays ago, we learned that Father had left us and would not be returning. I searched for an explanation between the lines of the official announcement. I wanted to hear his goodbye, see him one last time, be reassured that he was alright, and that we would be, too. I felt abandoned, lost amid the fears and rumors, stranded in the stride of Holy Week with a Passion all of my own.

Yet, help came in the persons of Father Jim Goyer, Father Paul Pare, Sister Rita Mae from the Portland Chancery, but most importantly from each of us, as we became neighbors to one another. We pulled together, and pulled through these worst of times. Still, questions, concerns, and tears linger. How can we best mend our wounds before moving on?

I have been in family practice for nine years in Belfast. During that time I have felt a great sympathy for the work of the parish priest, similar to my own in its rewards and challenges, yet lacking any partner with whom to face them, or a family into which one can escape. Yet both the priest and the doctor have their "flock," upon whom we depend more than you will ever know.

In the last several weeks, I have been reminded of one former patient who first taught me the importance of saying goodbye. He was a jolly, plump, semi-retired Italian, impossible to dislike; it was inevitable that we should become friends. One day he came to see me with his skin and eye grounds as yellow as a squash. After a battery of tests, we arrived at the diagnosis of pancreatic cancer. He received the news in shock and utter despair. We spoke—haltingly—of his grim prospects, about the few treatments available, of my desire to stick by him until the last.

He asked for heroic treatments and got them, far away in a Boston hospital. After his return, the treatments were exchanged for the loving attention he had always deserved. My wife and I visited Tony and Kate often, shared marvelous meals together, listened to tales of the olden days, traded intimate conversations where labels disappeared, those of "doctor" and "patient,"and life's priorities became blindingly clear. During the final weeks Tony was surrounded by his siblings, tended tirelessly by his wife, and given peace in his long passage unto death, even as the bloating and nausea and pain accelerated. Then one Sunday morning, as he struggled to right himself in bed, Tony turned pale as a ghost, vomited violently . . . and was gone, eyes blank as stone. What happened, what did he die of, Kate would implore of me afterward? Did he feel any pain? Her nightmares of those last terrifying seconds have taken years to subside.

Shortly after the diagnosis, Tony availed himself of the latest weapons in the war on cancer. He underwent a promising operation by a famous surgeon and received adjunctive radiation therapy in a great teaching hospital. But after his homecoming, the supersubspecialist called to report that the mission had failed. Would I—the family doctor—pass along bad news? So the cancer was still there, and Tony would die of it. Nothing more now to offer him, other than my support. And my promise to be there until the end.

But, of course, even that promise would be broken. The European vacation that my wife and I had been planning was fast upon us. Tony was bad and would not likely survive until our return. We made our tentative, awkward, eye-averting goodbyes, still scheming for a rendezvous on the shores of his beloved Italy. The scene of our final parting haunted me for days. Finally, on the Spanish frontier, I wrote Tony a letter. Said goodbye. Said I loved him. Said I hoped that I would see him again, and listed those parts of his life that have survived in my own. I slept soundly for two weeks until we reached Rome, when a trans-Atlantic call informed me of his death. Tony had died the previous week, having never seen the letter, his wife reluctantly acknowledged. But I know now, knew then, that he had been listening as I wrote it, and listened every time Kate reread it in the months ahead.

It is hard to lose someone we care about under any circumstances. Especially when they leave us suddenly, miserably, or in our absence. We cling to all that we have left, the most immediate memories, often the most painful ones.

Now it is important for the parish to move on, to focus on the unfinished work before us, yet cherish the memories that bind us together. It is right that we should gather in this way. We owe Father Mike our thank-yous and goodbyes. Not as we might have wished: a reception in the parish hall, glowing testimonials, and hearty handshakes all around. But a closure nonetheless.

The good news is that Father Mike can still hear us, in our cards and in our prayers, and in words of appreciation and pain murmured as softly as a heartbeat. He needs our prayers. He would that our parish pull together and move on, with social action that bears his unmistakable stamp.

With God's grace, and with the blessings that flow in a supportive parish, we have survived. We offer this Mass, this prayer of the community, not to extinguish our sadness and pain (nor Father's), but in order to lift our hearts to God, under whose grace and guidance we might all emerge stronger in body and soul. That is our prayer of healing. Godspeed your return, Father Mike.

MAY

This is what Yahweh asks of you, only this: to act justly,
to love tenderly, and to walk humbly with your God.

Micah 6:8

Yesterday we reached a pinnacle for the new year: sixty-six degrees, nature's ideal temperature. Saturday was perfect in other respects: An offshore breeze blew away the black flies and mosquitoes. We enjoyed a long, sunny afternoon of gardening, running, shopping, raking, putting on the front door screens, and reorganizing my brick pile. In the morning, we distributed a dozen May baskets but received none in return. So while Clare and I did errands, Lindsay composed a lovely basket and placed it on the front steps. Clare squealed with delight as we pulled in the drive. Then, later in the day, she received an authentic May basket from her friend Lucy. That evening we barbecued a chicken with friends; the warm, sweet day pushed gently into evening to a chorus of peepers and crickets and other insects that rub in the night.

I am leaning hard into the home stretch of the journal. There is a restlessness about it, perhaps a yearning for the end and the hope that I might arrive with some satisfying conclusions about the joy and organic rhythm and mystical oneness that sustains this rural life. But I finally believe that I live here not because it is good for mankind in general, nor good for me alone, but because it has become home.

We talked in group yesterday about the two sides of nature. Scott spoke of an adorable, domesticated red squirrel who comes to munch at his bird feeder. Or at least he came until Scott squirrel-proofed the feeder last week. Now Red is looking longingly at birds, and has spotted one of Scott's favorite nests under the eave at the rear of the house. Sooner or later he will get it unless Scott intervenes. What is the appropriate action on behalf of the squirrel, the bird, and the balance of nature? Should Scott move the garden tools and barbecue stand away from the side of the house so that the squirrel cannot reach the nest; should he borrow a gun and destroy the squirrel (even though Scott abhors the thought of violence)? Red and his companions can be ruthless when it comes to sating their appetite. Perhaps *he's* the critter who has been gnawing at the substructure of their house; perhaps he will not stop until he has done violence to Scott's domicile, his dog, his wife.

Yet, what if the chewing sound persists after the squirrel is dead, or the baby birds are gobbled by a blue jay or fall helplessly to their death? Scott recalled the tragic episode of the doe in the woods, whose mournful cry behind the house awakened him one morning. Crashing through the forest, he and Debbie came upon the doe—only to discover a fisher clenched to its throat. Despite their rescue and a mad dash to the veterinarian, the doe died and the fisher went hungry. Eventually nature wins out, and man pays the price for his meddling. Death, suffering, ignominy are part of a natural order that tempers the will of man.

Mary Beth revealed that she is pregnant. Seven weeks, cautious but happy. I reluctantly brought up Lindsay's miscarriage, and the graphic, violent dreams that followed it. It was, in a crazy way, hard to look at Mary Beth as I spoke. Does my pain spoil her joy; is she thinking just the reverse? With my mixed emotion, I could not congratulate her. Perhaps later; perhaps in time.

An undercurrent of stress rippled through the workweek. I spoke with the daughter of Nancy Newcomb, who reports that Nancy received a tracheostomy to permit prolonged mechanical ventilation without damaging her windpipe. Today surgeons will crack her chest to release loculations of pus and fluid that surround her left lung. This may be her only chance. My prayers are with them both.

John Geyman, editor of the *JABFP,* also called. He wanted to know how my writing was going, how the practice was holding up. I took it as a collegial, perhaps fatherly, chat to which E-mail or an interoffice memo would not be adequate. Probably, too, he was fishing for more contributions to the journal, or at least keeping the door open. I saw it as trimmed with all the best intentions, a reaching out to one engaged in the solitary affair of writing.

Clare—it was announced yesterday—was chosen from among the applicants for a multi-age class at Peirce School. Next year she will start kindergarten with a third of her classmates similarly aged. The other two-thirds will be selected from first and second graders. Clare so much enjoys, imitates, and is challenged by older children. She will be in a cooperative day camp this summer and exposed to a whole new complement of kids, scenery, activities. She is growing, with opportunities and a safe environment that so *many* children in our country lack. I have chosen to live in a poor, rural community with at least this one tangible benefit.

Clare and Lindsay woke before 7:00 A.M. and we enjoyed a breakfast of glazed twists from Mr. Weaver's Bakery and chocolate croissants from 90 Main—customary fare for a Saturday morning. Then Clare and I set off on an adventure while Lindsay spent the morning with her gardening friends. We drove to the waterfall under the Doak Road bridge, as I had promised. The broiling waters had quieted, but the noise and spray were still very impressive. Clare was frightened and preferred to look at the wildflowers along the roadside and point to blossoms on the flowering trees. She spotted the osprey nest atop the utility pole, with its two residents circling the sky in great swathes and casting shadows like a low-flying air plane.

In the afternoon, when Clare and Lindsay left for a birthday party, I set off on the long run in sixty degrees of sunshine and an offshore breeze, in running shoes that have finally conformed to my feet. We all finished the day together with an early supper on the barbecue, and a movie in Camden with the Thomases.

The murder trial at which I am scheduled to testify is still selecting its jury. Yesterday the district attorney called me with an update, "Friday at the earliest." I am not looking forward to it. In 1985 there were two brazen, brutal drug-related murders in our tiny town. Both were allegedly the work of the same assassin. I had been the county medical examiner, and vividly recall that disturbing walk around the cordoned grounds with the state crime lab, interviewing police and eyewitnesses, preparing a seemingly insignificant report drawn from their accounts. Too close to the violence. Now, on yesterday morning's local news, I hear that the streets around the courthouse have been barricaded and all visitors must pass through a metal detector. I am a witness for the prosecution and will supply observations from that evening, July 2, 1985, 11:00 P.M. My testimony will show that the victim was dead and that the body lying in the blood-soaked grass was the same one autopsied by Henry Ryan, the state's chief medical examiner.

After the initial murder, the defendant was released on bail. During his release a second murder was committed. It was for the second murder that Joel Fuller was convicted and is now serving time. But why, after eight years, is the first murder case coming to trial? I don't know, but I'll be glad when this business is behind me.

Yesterday was a day of varied fortune. Gayle Stephens called with his regrets: he will not be in Birmingham when I make my visit. Father Will called to say he would. There were no interesting stories in the office until the last of the day. A patient whom I had delivered came to see me about "the bug going around," a stomach flu. It began four days ago and was already mending. Her son had suffered from it for a week. Grandmother had also crowded into the small exam room with the family.

"Oh, doctor," interjected the old lady, glancing at her daughter on the exam table. "Maybe there's something my daughter should tell you about my grandson." The patient reluctantly took over the narrative and reported on her son's odyssey from birth. I had managed the pregnancy until we discovered—at term, with ruptured membranes—that he was breech. After the C-section she chose to take her son to another doctor. He had been a poor breast feeder, eventually took the bottle, yet never seemed to thrive, and cried "three out of every four hours he was awake." A heart murmur was evaluated at six weeks of age with a chest X-ray and EKG. Something serious was wrong. An echocardiogram and heart catheterization eventually documented a congenital heart defect. Half the heart was unformed, veins connected to all the wrong places, and three operations would be necessary to correct it. The first was behind her. The baby still needed a feeding tube and special formula.

I listened patiently as she talked, affirming her struggle and pain as a parent, which flies in the face of the universal belief that our own children, if not all children, will be born healthy. "Have you been riding again?" I asked, remembering the joy that horses brought her before the pregnancy.

"No, but I've been thinking about it."

"Anne, you need not sacrifice your own life for your son. You'd be a better mother if you took time for yourself and your husband." Grandmother nodded approvingly, and likely will be a strong ally of mine during the hard times ahead.

The day ended with a hospital admission at 2:30 A.M., a young woman with elevated blood sugar: 1,371, to be exact. She appeared alert and lucid and complained only of a bellyache and bruises. This problem (diabetic hyperosmolar state) is a correctable one; it is also an area where I enjoy some expertise, as I had written a paper on it during my fellowship in San Francisco. She needed IV fluids more than insulin or buffers, and *liters* of it poured quickly through her veins. But the real crisis was her social situation: twenty years old with two kids, living next door to parents who are divorcing. Her boyfriend left two months ago, and the new boyfriend of her ex-boyfriend's girlfriend "knocked her around" last week. They had both been drinking, got into a tussle, and eventually began ramming cars together. She landed in the ER, was given anti-inflammatory drugs, took twice the prescribed dosage, and developed a severe gastritis that ended in protracted nausea and vomiting. All the preconditions for hyperosmolar hyperglycemia: stress, dehydration, and poor compliance. According to the nurses, the patient's blood sugar fell to 350 with just a liter of fluid and fifteen units of insulin.

I visited Nancy Newcomb yesterday at the Eastern Maine Medical Center. Two hours of driving in exchange for a half-hour visit, sandwiched between hospital admissions at Waldo County and my rehearsal with Jean and Scott for the weekend's memorial services. I had not seen Nancy since our ambulance ride, and it was disheartening. She lay limp and pale in her ICU bed, with blue plastic tubing jetting from her body, a rectal tube draining feces, a NG feeding tube meeting her nutritional needs, and eyes making feeble attempts to communicate. Because of the tracheostomy, no sound came from her trembling lips. But after several unsuccessful attempts to use the language board, I worried that the brain centers might be in disarray. She looked at me, squeezed both hands on command, cried when I mentioned the frustration she must feel with her imposed silence, and cried again when I expressed astonishment at the length of her hospital stay. At one point, when I remarked on the quivering of her lips, she squeezed her hand into a fist and shook it at me, angry and outraged by her desperate straits. She stares at the ceiling, listens to the blaring radio (her usual source of "stimulation"), and lies, thinking, of what?

Last evening, late, I called the daughter with a report of my visit. I did my best to express support for her faithful visits, dismay at her mother's condition, hope in the news of her mother's progress, and my own concerns about anoxic brain damage from the septic shock and hypoxemia she sustained in the first hours of her illness. Time will tell—and language, when it becomes available next week with her weaning from the ventilator. I cannot imagine what mental anguish her mother feels. Is it more Purgatory or Limbo, a place of suffering or benign separation? What does she perceive of the lapsed time, the beige walls and blaring music, the parade of attendants and nurses and technicians, the futile attempts to understand her (not just her complicated moods, but her most elementary needs), the flicker of hope that she will survive all of this to return home someday to her books and her cats and her precious garden? Or, equally plausible, that she will never recover and that this gray, groping existence will stretch on interminably. We have constructed, Nancy and I and the doctors, an anticipated timetable for her recovery; it keeps hope in stock. It allows us to persevere from day to day. I have promised her daughter that I will continue my phone calls to the pulmonologist and will encourage him to look after Nancy's needs and opportunities for stimulation: talking books, rehabilitation, periods of sitting at the ICU window overlooking the Penobscot River.

Yesterday morning at our business meeting, Tim announced his plans to cut back at the office to three or four half-days per week. He has accepted the director's offer to teach on Wednesdays at the Augusta (Maine-Dartmouth) Family Practice Residency Program. He is squeezing that time entirely from his office schedule. Might it not make more sense to give up the hospital, give up OB, and have Tim in the office five or six half-days a week? What does the future hold? How long will we lash together this Searsport Family Practice, with our good employees and the promising reimbursement program and the array of services we now provide? But I worry most about the waning of Tim's commitment, and the loss of an equal partner at my side.

I have been fretting it all week: this murder trial of Joel Fuller. He stands accused of the shotgun slaying of Scott LaCombe on July 2, 1985. And I was there. There, at least, two hours after the fact, wearing the coroner's badge. I observed a dead body, a lake of blood, a stained path where the decedent crawled to his death, the gaping hole in his face created by a twelve-gauge shotgun discharging at point-blank range. The violence jangled my nerves for weeks afterward. Drugs were behind it, they say, all drugs.

Now, eight years later, new evidence has surfaced and the case has been brought forward. Having exhausted a pool of one hundred eight potential jurors owing to the notoriety of the defendant and the impact his murder had on the community, today thirty-five more would be questioned. "Set aside an hour," the DA had told me, "even though you'll be on the stand less than five minutes." On Friday, as I assisted with an inguinal hernia repair, I got word that they needed me at 1:00 P.M.

All morning long people talked of the trial. Belfast was blanketed with state police, who parked their cruisers in rows around the courthouse and posted rifled troopers on every corner. Almost everyone had an opinion about the La-Combe murder ("a good kid mixed up with bad apples") and his alleged murderer ("the worst apple of them all"). The DA's office had asked the local papers to muzzle their coverage until after the jury had been selected. But stories buzzed anyway; and the whole of it had tied my stomach in a knot, struck fear into Lindsay's heart, and lingered in my thoughts as I drifted to sleep.

I arrived at the courthouse at 1:00 P.M., as directed; the assistant DA quickly found me and led me to a side room. There we reviewed my testimony. She asked only those questions that were of concern to the prosecution: What was my educational background? Was the victim dead? What did I observe that night, directly (rather than read or heard about in subsequent reports)? The trial, not unexpectedly, was running behind. The key witness (the victim's girlfriend, an eyewitness to the crime) had just completed her testimony and endured the cross-examination. "You'll be on by 2:00," I was assured. "Does that pose any problems?" I called my office to cancel more appointments, but they intuitively had cleared the slate until 3:00. So I paced and studied patterns in the walnut paneling of the courthouse lobby; peered out the window at the sunshine and steady flow of state police with their tight strut and display of arms; worried about the upcoming courtroom drama. Would Joel Fuller study the face of each witness; would the defense attorney find holes in my testimony or my credentials, or ask incredulously, "So you had been county coroner for how long? What constituted your formal training in forensic science? How did you establish Scott LaCombe as the decedent and determine his time of death? No further questions, your honor."

I reviewed my report over and over and over again. I said what I intended to say a hundred times. Then I paused on one detail that I had long forgotten but that was immeasurably important that night: the fog. The dense, dripping fog. Fog that forced my slow, careful crawl to the crime scene at Saturday Cove Antiques. The soft yellow haze of headlights piercing it, the glow of squad cars and darting of flashlights through a cordoned-off darkness. The smells that the mist intensifies, especially blood and flesh on your hands. All of that imparted an eerie otherworldliness to the evening, a timelessness and intimacy with the particulars and a melodrama that might have otherwise been lacking. Would I dare say any of this on the witness stand, or was I mistaken or romanticizing or simply feeling a surge of adrenalin in my blood?

At 3:00 the assistant DA found me in the lobby (luckily, for I may well have been on my tenth trip to the bathroom) and relayed the bad news. "They changed the order of witnesses, and the cross-examination took longer than expected, but we'll need your testimony in a half hour. Can you wait? Many apologies, but we're on trial-time. It's a little like waiting for a baby, isn't it?"

I called the office to cancel appointments until 4:00, but I definitely wanted to make my last four of the day. Definitely. By now fear and anxiety were mixed with anger. By stringing out the testimony, by reordering witnesses without regard to their prior commitments, the prosecution was turning a friendly witness into a hostile one. I was fuming, pacing, sputtering. What good would I be on their witness stand now? Time ticked. 3:25 . . . 3:38 . . . 3:52 . . . Then, at a minute before 4:00, the upstairs doors flung open and the jury filed out, recessed for the day. The assistant DA followed on their heals, sought me out, brought me privately aside to make amends, and dared not hope for my return on Monday. "Only," I discouraged her, "if it is absolutely necessary."

So there was my day in court. My exposure to the American system of justice. The trial may continue for another week, or so they say. But I will listen now without trepidation. I may even peer from the gallery on my Monday afternoon off just to experience it, say I was there.

Delays and disappointments. My new sidewalk lies bedded but unbricked for want of a compactor, a hack saw, and a masonry chisel. I need unfettered time to find them, and that means the weekend. Yesterday Robert Coles's secretary called to schedule my appointment for sometime in late July or early August—publishers' deadlines and graduation ceremonies and much too much on Dr. Coles's mind to make for a relaxed meeting now.

Our neighbors up the street miscarried yesterday. I had taken the call two nights ago when she began spotting; hadn't recognized the name; referred her to her family doctor without a second thought. Yesterday morning I saw the husband and wife in the lobby of the X-ray department as I breezed through. "Waiting for an ultrasound," they had volunteered, and I remembered hearing about their pregnancy a few weeks earlier from their six-year-old son, a friend of my daughter. "Well, I'm glad you're here for good news and not bad," I chirped.

Not until evening did I put two and two together, and called them on the telephone immediately. The husband answered and confirmed what I had correctly deduced: the ultrasound revealed an empty gestational sac, and a miscarriage followed. I had put a big foot in my mouth. But it was not so bad, he intimated. Now he will go through with the operation he had promised his wife, and they will both better appreciate the blessing of two healthy children. I commiserated with him and told him of our miscarriage last fall. It is comforting to think that neighbors with nothing more in common than an ill-fated pregnancy could share these kinds of thoughts and feelings.

It is Monday morning, and I have only a few hopes for the week. Run thrice, finish the yard work, struggle with an essay, and prepare for the retreat to Gethsemani. Lindsay has two hospice meetings this week, and then the bereavement groups will be over. Saturday, supper with the Baillys and the photographer Michael Simon. Quiet, so quiet that I have to think awhile before reporting the news in my life.

Perhaps that is a reason why I need a retreat. It is pretentious, I agree, to fly to a Trappist monastery in Kentucky when here, in my own back yard, there is plenty of peace and quiet. Yet I have wanted to visit Gethsemani for a decade, ever since reading Thomas Merton's *Seven Storey Mountain,* and meeting the Trappist monks near Dubuque, Iowa.

Only one storm cloud over the week. At 8:30 last night I received a telephone call from Leane Zainea, the assistant DA, who asked me back to testify. I would be the first witness, she quickly assured me, Monday morning at 9:00. Out by 9:30 at the latest. Probably. Well, she'd do her best, although "I don't control the proceedings."

I arrived early yesterday morning and retrieved my medical examiner papers (forgotten last Friday in a fit of disgust) from the Grand Jury room. Here the present jury gathers each day before filing into the courtroom. Over the weekend, I had gnawing fears that my papers would be discovered by "unauthorized persons" and that a mistrial would be declared on the basis of this irregularity. But I was delivered from this humiliation and could now sit patiently on a hallway bench, reviewing my eight-year-old notes.

I sat beneath an oversized oil painting of Justice David Nichols, a recent Superior Court Judge in Belfast, shown brooding in his flowing robes and resting a worn copy of the Revised Maine Statutes on his lap. My mind wandered; what questions would be asked in cross-examination? By what route would the baillifs lead Joel Fuller in and out of the courtroom, or back and forth between "Supermax," the maximum security prison in Warren? And why such intense security? To ease my mind, I had brought along William Styron's *A Darkness Visible* in order to skim for passages that I might include in a forthcoming essay.

Finally I was summoned to take the stand, swear to tell the truth, and face both the prosecution and the defense. The room was largely empty; I recognized only two local newspaper reporters from among the dozen who populated the gallery. To my left, and partially hidden by the stand, sat Joel Fuller, slumped in his chair and surrounded by a private investigator and his defense attorney, John Nale. He seemed too small a man to be charged with such a large crime, to garner so much press, to require so much security, and already to have shouldered one conviction for murder.

The room itself was ancient, paneled in the same dark walnut as the downstairs lobby, old and musty and in keeping with Perry Mason reruns. A large clock hung above the rear (main) entrance; I would study it carefully, refer to it frequently, as a diversion from the eyes of the courtroom.

My testimony lasted a few minutes, went smoothly, and followed the exact script of Leane's preview last Friday (although faster, I noted, and punctuated by more questions). Then Attorney Nale took over. He was particularly concerned about the size and shape of the wound to the decedent's face, and the exact location from which the lethal shot was fired.

"Is it not true that the weapon used to kill Scott LaCombe was a twelve-gauge shotgun, and that it was fired three to nine feet from the first bloodstain, where Scott LaCombe reportedly first fell? Does this bloodstain on the driveway—a single-vehicle driveway—lie in the only place where a car pulling up to the residence would park? Does the diagram in your report concur with the one on the blackboard?"

As the questions drummed toward me, I kept in mind Leane's words of caution: "You are only accountable for what you saw." And after eight years, what I can reliably recall has narrowed to what was included in my coroner's report. I declined to confirm or refute any information provided by the autopsy; I declined to comment on the driveway's dimensions, or whether it could hold one or two cars, or if it was the logical place a vehicle might park. Leane, by her repeated objections, reinforced these instincts. But the insistence of Nale's line of questioning confused me: was he trying to wedge some discrepancy between my account and Dr. Roy's autopsy findings, or was he simply trying to badger me and fill the jury's head with nonsense? I assumed only that he was leading me away from the prosecution's argument, and I resisted the leash, perhaps foolishly. He excused me from the witness stand thirty minutes after I took the oath.

Later that afternoon an alcoholic with booze on his breath came to the office. He is an old patient of ours, with high blood pressure and a smoking problem to boot, who today complained of blurred vision and a constant urge to pee. We have monitored him for diabetes in the past, and never has his sugar climbed above 158. Today it is 316 by fingerstick. Blood pressures were, on average, 180/116. I evaluated him for prostatism by digital exam, checking a PSA and measuring residual urine. His symptoms all seem related to his newly discovered diabetes. But he will not stop drinking; we have discussed it repeatedly and on this one point he is firm. Will he take his medication? Will he keep his appointments? George has been unfaithful in the past, and so I draw the line: if you don't make an effort to help yourself, then I won't either, and you will need to find yourself another physician. I have not made abstinence a condition of my care, nor have I been firm about his smoking—hoping, I suppose, naively, that he would come around in a trusting relationship. But I also want to be there when his fragile world shatters, after the stroke or heart attack or pneumonia, and help him to pick up the pieces. Glyburide and diltiazem, I order, and back in a week. If not, George, the boot. The boot.

The days are warming. This weekend, with clear skies and a Canadian high, temperatures may climb into the mid-seventies. Just what the doctor ordered for our basil and rosemary, which look pathetically brown and droopy in the herb garden. But yesterday was an indoors day: overcast and misty, cool and enclosing. Around noontime I went downtown to the cleaners with a pile of shirts. There, I learned from sources close to the trial (Embee Cleaners is just down the block from the courthouse) that Joel Fuller had been convicted of murder. The jury deliberated fourteen hours before reaching their verdict. I am glad it's over, assume that justice was served, and feel relieved that the principal witness (the victim's girlfriend, now married and a mother of two) can safely resume her new life.

Today, mad planning for National Nurse's Day and an eye to Mother's Day on Sunday. I wrote a brief card to my mom this morning; now to find something for Lindsay, and help Clare prepare a special card.

At group, I could see it in her eyes—or at least thought so—a look of distress and sadness. And so I invited her to speak first. "Mary Beth," I said, "what's going on?" She began with a catch in her voice, "I'm spotting. As you said a few weeks ago, I had put this embryo through college. What we take for granted . . . is all at risk."

Mary Beth is nine weeks pregnant, I discover; she has no cramping, just spotting. No sense in calling Clara, her midwife, she has concluded, because nothing can be done. I offer my prayers and regrets, then gently suggest that Clara would like to know. She might order an ultrasound, or request an examination, or simply offer some support.

I talked about my upcoming pilgrimage, the retreat to Gethsemani (where I am heading in my mind, high in flight over Atlanta). As I unveiled my plans, Tim squirmed in his seat until he could contain himself no longer. "Travel light," he advised. "Leave the camera home, and the computer, and your strap of books. A pad and pencil is all you'll need. How do you expect to find what you're looking for with your head buried in a map?"

If it is God we are seeking, there are many ways to find Him. Through faith, through reason, through love. Through journal-keeping and secular reading. Over the last few years, I have observed my professional life following a creative lead, as it did when our office T-shirt (sporting a skeleton) preceded our involvement in hospice. As it did when the scallop shell emblem on our office sign preceded my attraction to pilgrimage. And now my creative energy is flowing into words, ushering me to some undeclared destiny. Perception lays the groundwork for discovery. Faith finds what it's looking for.

Yesterday's work was overwhelming. After group, I treated a serious aspirin overdose in the ER and assumed care for two gravely ill patients, one with unstable angina and the other with Guillain-Barré Syndrome. This trio nearly filled our four-bed ICU. In the office, Bonnie (the head nurse) required special attention for her gimpy knee. She has been hobbling on a torn meniscus and needs orthopedic referral. Then came a walk-in with shortness of breath and weight gain, whom I will whisk to the ER, suspicious of pulmonary edema.

Yesterday was troubled by events of the preceding night. Lindsay felt the pangs of ovulation, and our newly purchased ovulation kit (which detects the surge in luteinizing hormone) confirmed it. Now there was an impetus to act.

Sex has never been our strong suit. In the beginning, of course, the appetite was hearty and natural and a wonderful preoccupation. But soon we had to "talk about it" as the spontaneity began to ebb. At first it seemed all Lindsay; she was depressed and inhibited and troubled by issues of conception. Therapy helped to ready us for a family but not to overcome all of the "obstacles." These seem to be written in the wiring, not something to be expunged from a traumatized past or fixable in an unhappy marriage.

But it was not just Lindsay. I recall a similar pattern in my first marriage as interest waned. Now it is easier to blame Lindsay than face my own ambivalence: have I lost my attraction or the desire for sex? Will we ever make love again?

Now the thought of performing on command seemed beyond our limited capacity. After crawling into bed, Lindsay's first words to me were, "So, are we going to act on the luteal surge?" We lay on our backs, not touching or speaking but rather brooding on our sad state of affairs and the duty we faced. We were immobilized. I drifted off to sleep, then awoke with a start and lay trancelike, waiting for Lindsay to make a reconciliatory move. Was she asleep? Was she angry or frustrated; did she care about our unborn child and the future of our marriage? I rose from bed, sat on Clare's small stool in the bathroom, stepped lightly downstairs, fumed and scowled and pitied myself, and finally, about 1:00 A.M., came to realize that the resolution lay in my hands, in my climbing back into bed, cradling my wife, and giving the opportunity another chance. We succeeded.

All of this is tied to another project simultaneously conceived: finishing the attic over the kitchen-ell. It would be our master bedroom and a necessary addition for a growing family. The plans were drawn, the contractor's estimate approved, a bank loan negotiated. We have no pregnancy, only aspirations. What if God decides otherwise? How will I feel about an empty guest room? Will it be a stinging reminder of our failure to bear?

We were pushed here as well. Micky, our contractor, starts a large project in July that will consume the rest of his summer. Now is the time if we want him. And friends will be visiting from New York and California in August, for whom the addition would provide necessary living space. Another nudge.

Exercise caution or plow ahead? Cast fear aside, toss logic to the wind, or plant them in the ground of faith and await the harvest? We seemed ready for the motto from the movie *Field of Dreams,* "build it and they will come."

At last night's dinner party, we were joined by a Hungarian-born friend of ours and found ourselves discussing suffering and Slavic cosmology. He says that Judeo-Christians place heaven above, hell below, and creation somewhere in the middle. Slavs put heaven on top and hell in the middle. His daughter, a recent college graduate, had joined us for supper; someone worried aloud that "all this talk of suffering deprives the younger generation of hope." The comment lay like a pall upon our lively babble. Does the awareness of suffering and evil in the world drain our capacity to dream?

America, like every nation, bears a legacy of unrealized hopes. We remember the Franklin Expedition to the North Pole, the unsinkable Titanic, and The War to End All Wars; we remember how the national mood sank successively with The Great Depression, The Bomb, Civil Rights, Vietnam, and Watergate. Hollywood and Madison Avenue could no longer distract us from the knotty truth, from seeing the human condition as a jungle, and evolution as a natural decline. We no longer doubt that we have the most to fear from our fellow man. We embrace suffering as the human lot and are resolved to the Gospel news that the poor (and all things wretched) will forever be among us.

But I do not find these thoughts depressing. We are constantly reassured by the miracle of birth, the renewal of love, and the celebration of life in the midst of suffering. We need only a context for coping with the pain, and a community to help absorb it.

We invent a cosmology, as did the early peoples, the Judeo-Christians and Slavs. We fabricate and cling to stories that give life meaning. This journal is one such collection of stories. It is written with an end in mind. It is predicated on a faith that the ordinary can become heroic, that odds can be beaten, that simple lives can be consecrated to great causes. In this sense it is "devotional" literature of the highest order.

The last entry before leaving for Gethsemani. I know that my first ten days back will be devoured by family practice call. The chaos of leaving deprives me of the focus to write, or the free time to pack or to tie up loose ends. My hemorrhoids are flaring, due in part to garden work, but also to stress. The hospital pace has been furious. I discharged three patients yesterday, but one returned overnight.

I have high hopes for the journal while I'm gone, but they are false and grand. Even if my writing is productive, I know that true success will hinge upon participation in the Daily Offices, on entering into the presence of God, on inspiration, on chance. My first aim is to be Alone with the Alone, as the Desert Fathers say, in a place and time set apart.

Standing in the garden in my red pajamas, pitching compost with my new fork, I watched steam rise in the crisp morning air. It is easy to draw an analogy between this labor and the doctor's sleight of hand: we attempt to create a valued commodity out of something worthless, joy from suffering, like the ancient alchemists. The strong stench of decomposition is God's cologne, which he wears on the occasion of such miracles. Hope springs eternal, that from death shall come life.

The hospital remains in overdrive this week. On Monday morning I inherited seven patients, all troublesome in some respect, none ready to budge from their hospital beds. We have two patients in the Hospice Wing who require "only" time and energy; another worries me with her recalcitrant diverticulitis. Isabelle Rooney is whiney and demanding, and Richard Talbot is a menace to the foot traffic outside his door; both have brittle diabetes that has whittled them down to a couple of limbs each. One elderly lady is dying from stroke, another will find a home at Tallpines, and a proud old man—a gentleman in every respect—will return home after surviving yet another bout of dyspnea. I saw two patients in the ER, one with acute urinary retention, the other with polymyositis, and both needing immediate referral to a specialist. Not surprisingly, the office was a beehive. Add to this my own needs, and it makes for a stressful week. I had a period—around midnight or 1:00 A.M.—when I could not lie down, but instead returned to the bathroom and gazed out the window and listened to the rustle of trees in the night breeze.

Last evening, I saw a darling three-year-old who had swallowed (and passed) a nickel, penny, and dime. She sat on mother's lap and stared me squarely in the face, while her third and fourth fingers popped playfully in and out of her mouth. This sight, this story, is all too familiar. Two years ago in Santa Clara, while returning by interstate to San Francisco, Clare suddenly sat bolt upright in her seat, became bug-eyed and still, and moaned. I wheeled to the side of the road, raced to the passenger side, and realized that the coins Clare had been fingering were now nowhere in sight. After a few sips of juice, she vomited a nickel with projectile force, followed in turn by a penny and a dime. How odd that another little girl, sucking these same two fingers, had swallowed an identical sixteen cents at the identical age. Fortunately, nothing more than that was wrong and we could smile at the coincidence rather than anguish over it.

I am grateful to be here in Birmingham, Alabama, spending a few days with my good friend Will before the Gethsemani retreat. It is a place of strange sounds, odd opportunity, dormant memories. I am grateful, too, for my connection to Maine. I miss the whit-ter of the cardinal, the forlorn ee-oh of the morning dove, the twittering of the rose-breasted house finch at 5:00 A.M. I miss my kitchen window and making coffee and feeding our cats (who must be, at this moment, prancing about Lindsay's bed, wild with hunger and whining over the poor service they have received in my absence). But here in Birmingham I have—on this floor alone—a tiny chapel, a Jacuzzi, a swimming pool, a hot tub, and a retreat house, which I can see through the trees below the crest of the hill. I have silence, solitude, and unfettered time. I have religious conversation, prayer, and a challenge to faith. I have a thread of history that connects me to a time when my first marriage was crumbling, my residency program was in turmoil, and a friend (the monk, William, the very symbol of Christian holiness) began seeking God apart from his cenobitic vows and his Catholic faith. I was twenty-eight and living in a cataclysmic time.

I have finally arrived at my retreat in Trappist, Kentucky. The only excitement in the drive to Bardstown was spotting signs for Lincoln's boyhood home and birthplace, just before my turnoff to Gethsemani. There's a real chance that Mr. Lincoln will meld into my pilgrimage plans.

It has been ninety degrees since leaving Maine, and I began to worry that the oppressive heat might disrupt my sleep. But Brother Raphael changed the room assignments; he booked me in Room 309 of the air-conditioned retreat house instead of the sweltering South Wing. I do not conceal my elation. The change was made—it is rumored—after a terrible windstorm on June 4th deposited 150 feet of the South Wing roof into the courtyard. No one was hurt, but many trees were toppled and roofs demolished. The wind rose and fell within a span of ten minutes.

I have lost most of the romance that once drew me to the monastery. What was it then? Father Will, Thomas Merton, or some inexplicable lure to the interior of the Catholic faith? To order, to perfection, to the most excellent praise of God through the exercise of the Daily Offices? What remains for me is time and solitude and silence. The main chapel reflects Cistercian simplicity: white brick walls, pebbled concrete floors, wooden beams supporting the roof, slabs of yard-thick stone forming an altar. The only adornment is the icon of the "Theotokos" (Mother of God) painted by brother Lavrans Nielson of Gethsemani. At Vigils, I note seventy choir stalls divided among four rows, two on either side of the center aisle. At Lauds, I count forty-nine seated monks below ten rows of windows from entrance to apse. The organ's pure pitch diffuses by quarter tones through the uneven voices of the monastery choir, prismlike. After all these observations, I still have time to listen and wait. And to bow, singing the doxology after the psalms, "Praise the Father, the Son, and Holy Spirit, both now and forever. The God who is, who was, and who is to come, at the end of the ages."

I tried to pray today, a few simple words of thanksgiving for my safe arrival, and for the joys of a life I left behind. But within moments my head clouded, and I felt an inescapable desire for sleep. Some twenty minutes later I awoke, but not in dispair, for I remembered the good counsel of the guestmaster at New Melleray Abbey, who once told me: "God looks after your physical as well as your spiritual well-being."

After Compline, Father Matthew Kelty read the poetry of D. H. Lawrence, Ezra Pound, and John Donne to the retreatants gathered in the guest chapel. Later, a heavy rain soaked the land. It will clear the air, we wanted to believe. Father Matthew has the appearance and demeanor of an aged Humphrey Bogart, with a long face, cropped white hair, and a low, gravelly voice. But this morning, he was celebrant at Mass, and his voice rang like steeple bells.

The next morning, after Lauds and Compline, I made the compulsory trip to the grave of Father Louis (Thomas Merton). It was marked by a plain white Celtic cross, knee high, lettered in black with the date of his death and glory, December 10, 1968. It lay on the west side of the abbey church, outside the monastic enclosure in a cluster of forty-two identical markers. He was flanked on either side by monks; immediately to his left lay his abbott, Father James Fox, who followed him in death.

I walked to Gethsemani Garden in the afternoon, under trees felled by the June fourth winds, to view two statues and an inscription, "May we always remember that the church exists to lead men to Christ in many and varied ways. But it is always the same Christ." I idled a few hours in the retreat house library, reading *Commonweal* (the book reviews, and essays by John Garvey and John Shea) and a biography of William of St. Thierry, friend and contemporary of St. Bernard of Clairvaux. I poked around on the computer, wrote letters to Lindsay, postcards to Clare, a note to the office. Then spent a long-overdue hour reading a manuscript sent to me by a friend. He is a writer with abandonment issues (like myself); it has been months since his materials arrived, and I now owe him the favor of an immediate and worthy reply.

The best part of a retreatant's day is entering cloister. This happens twice: during Mass at 6:15 A.M., and following Compline at 7:50 P.M., when the whole community is blessed to dispel the fears and dangers of the night. It is a great privilege to walk on the pebbled floor of the cloister, join the monks in their life of unending prayer, and sit motionless in that resounding chamber.

Again tonight, I sat alone in the guesthouse garden and opened my mind to God. This is a beginner's prayer, my own muddled attempt. But I am heartened to know that He is making no demands, except that I desire Him, face Him, and reflect His love in my relations with others. I am grateful for this monastery, these walls and this solitude, for helping me to see (though I fear, and at every turn evade) what the animals know, what the desert monks understood, what peoples who have never heard the word of God have found in their daily life: that we are all one in our dependence on God.

The beginning of my third day at the monastery. It is 3:00 A.M., and in a few moments I will leave for Vigils. I have showered, made my bed, and outlined the day's schedule. I hope that I can relax more, enjoy the Offices, have time for meditation, but there is so much to do in this place that exists solely for the praise of God.

Yesterday I embarked on a two-hour excursion to the birthplace and boyhood home of Mr. Lincoln. They seemed, to the untrained eye, nothing more than tiny, decrepit log cabins. It is my duty to report that the Lincoln Temple is an impostor. A plaque acknowledges the error, announcing that, after reviewing "extensive new research," historians have concluded that the cabin was not *exactly* Lincoln's, just a facsimile of the original. When I casually asked the Park Service attendant about this, she snapped, "What do you mean we've got the wrong one? Don't you think people a little closer to the time of Lincoln's birth might know better which cabin was the real McCoy? We can't *prove* that this was his cabin— we don't have his fingerprints or the deed or anything—but think about it: why would the Lincoln Farm Association or the National Park Service or your average taxpaying American go to all this trouble for a *replica?*" Her rebuff served me right for asking.

After the assassination, the Lincoln Farm Association sponsored a nationwide tour of the "birthplace" cabin. I wonder if the idea for "Lincoln Logs" came from the countless disassemblies and reassemblies of the cabin during this period.

A curious fact about Mr. Lincoln: he had no progeny. Within three generations of his assassination, the seed had died out. His children, and their children's children, had either died in infancy, never married, or bore no offspring. I also note that the state of Kentucky preserves that wonderful custom of marking highway fatalities with roadside crosses. This practice was prevalent in Iowa during my youth but is now abandoned. Perhaps issues separating church and state forced its extinction. Would the painting or replacing of a cross constitute a misuse of tax dollars? What should be planted if the victim were a lapsed Catholic, or no Christian at all?

I have made no new acquaintances since coming to the monastery. The vow of silence inhibits that, but on the other hand, I am thankful for a respite from social obligation. Only two guests are in any way memorable. At breakfast on the first day, a man sitting next to me smacked, chomped, slurped, sniffled, and hacked his way through the "silent" meal. I confess that I harbored some uncharitable thoughts about him. And yesterday at Mass, a small man with white hair, balding and bearded, refused to shake my hand at the kiss of peace. "Refused" may be too judgmental a word, but at least he ignored, and awkwardly so, my outstretched hand. He may have his reasons. But silent communal life would be difficult for me if I could not redress these insults to the ear and soul.

What good will come of my trip to the monastery? A well-deserved rest? A satisfied curiosity? A payment of respect to Thomas Merton? Or the opportunity to dwell on the fact of suffering? I try not to forget Elena Moulton, who dies a slow death, and Nancy Newcomb, who was given a reprieve. I try to recall those patients who suffer innocently without relief and without end, those who suffer outside the reach of love, or those who submit to the severe demands and sharp instruments of the merciful doctor and come away further harmed.

Every day, and during most of my free time outside the abbey church, I have worked on an essay. It is about the doctor's devotion to suffering.* The monastery is an ideal place to consider it: here, there is a rhythm, a receptivity, and the time for writing; here, suffering rains upon us in the chanted psalms that swing between anguish and hope, in the shrines that depict Christ's crucifixion (inscribed with the words, "I have suffered this for you. What have you done for me?)," and in the solitude that bares our deepest wounds.

On this Feast of St. Brandon, I realize that I am a pilgrim also, not simply to Gethsemani but in my life. I am on a sacred journey, more in the tradition of those Celtic monks than in that of the wandering penitents of the Middle Ages or the great *peregrinatios* that were the Crusades. The Irish monk set out upon his sojourn not to visit a sacred shrine but to discover his rightful place before God. His *peregrinatio* was undertaken purely for the love of Christ and in imitation of Him, an "exercise in ascetic homelessness and wandering."† His destination would be revealed by the God of the Elements, not by social dictates. Thus, the monk's journey was mysterious, his destination unknown, but it always led him to a divinely appointed place where he would be united ultimately with God.

Says Merton, "the geographical pilgrimage is the symbolic acting out of an inner journey. The inner journey is the interpolation of the meanings and signs of the outer pilgrimage . . . For man's pilgrimage to make sense, it must represent a complete integration of inner and outer life, of his relation to himself and other men." For Merton, pilgrimage is an indispensable structure and program for man. The fruitful pilgrimage is one where—after coming to the end of a long journey—the pilgrim sees himself as the stranger, and also *in* the stranger, the aborigine, or native. It is another way for us to see Christ in our neighbor.

The last five years have seen a gradual integration of my private and professional lives. The parallels have hit me now like a thunderclap, as when Saul was thrown from his steed. Our house on Salmond Street and the office on Route One were both bright yellow when we purchased them. The office, too, has a domestic feel; it is merely a remodeled bungalow with classic architectural lines. When I was looking for an emblem to adorn our new office sign, I unwittingly chose the scallop shell, which once marked pilgrims along their great routes in the Middle Ages, especially toward the shrine of the apostle James at Santiago de Compostela in northwestern Spain. These congruences are meaningless except to the person of faith who is already searching for symbols of integration.

---

* The essay remains unfinished, and lies in waiting for answers that I am unable to provide. There is no resolution to the problem of suffering and the doctor's inability to solve it, or justify it, or bear it each moment in the lives of his patients.

† Merton, *Mystics and Zen Masters.*

There is something else important about the theme of pilgrimage. Historically, Merton notes, pilgrimage became increasingly internalized, so that monastic literature eventually portrayed the monk's *peregrinatio* in entirely spiritual terms. It became synonymous with his vow of stability, a vow to stay with one monastic community forever. My commitment to Belfast has been lately recast in thoughts of where I will be buried. In Belfast's Grove Cemetery, of all places? Why, there is no ocean view, and who will come find me in such a far removed place? And what of my temptations to travel farther, to a more perfect place, where my maker must surely reside?

I have come here to contemplate the gnawing discontent, the restlessness—for new projects, for an accelerated pace, for endless variety—that moves me off center in my life, where otherwise I must face the wants and fears and loneliness I harbor there. The monastery contracts the struggle for happiness to these four walls, in clear terms, through plain ritual in the immediacy of the here and now. It teaches me to find self-fulfillment in my emptiness. To see it for what it is: a hunger for God.

Being here, paradoxically, turns my longing homeward, to the place and people I have come to cherish above all others—my wife and daughter, my partner and practice, my parish and community. Love ripples in a widening arc. But it is one and the same love, which, for me, begins and ends in the intimacy and trust of marriage.

Noontime, following Sext. It is the best of days, breezy, clear, and sunny. The closing prayer perfects my intention for the day: "God of mercy, this midday moment of rest is your welcome gift. Bless the work we have begun, make good its defects, and let us finish it in a way that pleases you."

We have come to the monastery—the twenty or so of us bedded in the guest house—with Benedict's blessing. He reminded his followers that all guests should be welcomed as Christ, because He will say, "I was a stranger, and you took me in" (Matt. 24:35). "Show them every courtesy . . . for it is Christ who is really being received."*

We have not earned the right to be here. We are welcomed not on account of our station in life, nor for the purity of our faith, but rather because we come in Christ's name. Here, it is the "stranger" in all of us that is embraced—a wonder that, in Patricia Hampl's words, supplies religion with its profound reassurance: one is loved, not personally, but because one is (p. 146). But I should forewarn potential pilgrims to call ahead. It can take six months to reserve a better room in a popular house. Nevertheless, a bed is always there for the wayward traveler. We are here—all of us—on account of the hospitality.

---

* *The Rule of St. Benedict,* pp. 89–90.

We have also come to realize our unmet, unformulated, desire for God. If, as Henri Nouwen says, God dwells where man makes room, we stand a fair chance of finding him here. For all monastic activity—the liturgy, the silence, and the simplicity of the meals, the clothing, the order of the day—converges to minimize distractions and differences and elevate our attention to the one God.

This is why the first monks fled to the deserts in fifth-century Egypt and Syria and the Sinai; they were "simple men who lived their lives to a good old age among the rocks and sands [in order to] be themselves, their *ordinary* selves, and to forget a world that divided them from themselves."* They knew that a man "who has attained to true prayer and love has no sense of the differences between things: he does not distinguish the righteous from the sinner, but loves them all equally and judges no man, as God causes His sun to shine and His rain to fall on the just and unjust."† They welcomed the lowliest daily task or sinner as a gift from God and the ground of common worship. They came quickly to the realization—which the "little muddler" Bernanos's *Diary of a Country Priest* took his whole life to grasp—that "What I had believed was so far away, beyond imaginary seas, stood out before me. My death is here. A death like any other, and I shall enter into it with the feelings of a very commonplace, very ordinary man" (p. 279).

In a world of distraction, where false reflections of our better selves are peddled in the shopping centers, social circles, playing fields, and classrooms, we lose an appreciation for the ordinary. We know that it can be retrieved by returning to the place where the words *fuge, tace, et quiesce*—solitude, silence, and inner peace—are lived each day. But just going to the monastery is not enough. There, too, the challenge awaits us, as we read in Father Nouwen's account of his extended retreat:

> When the monastic life does not hold anything new any more, when people do not pay special attention to you any more, when nothing "interesting" is distracting you any more, then the monastic life becomes difficult. Then room opens up for prayer and ascesis . . . The monastery slowly makes you aware of a powerful sameness that transcends time and place and unifies you with the one God who is the Father of all people, all places, all times, and who is the same through the ages unending . . . When we have given up our desire to be different and experienced ourselves as sinners without any right to special attention, only then is there space to encounter our God who calls us by our own name and invites us into his intimacy.‡

---

* Merton, *The Wisdom of the Desert Fathers*, p. 23.
† *The Way of a Pilgrim*, p. 85.
‡ *The Genessee Diary*, pp. 60, 67, 81.

During his retreat, Father Nouwen received counsel from the abbot John Eudes, who urged him to explore the feelings of loneliness, boredom, jealousy, and pride that followed him to the monastery. He needed—we *all* need—a place where we can find the time, support, and courage to face painful self-truths. To recognize the many and fundamental ways in which we are petty, imperfect, and merely "average," and in this way share something in common with our neighbor.

Back home in my practice, life brims with feelings of self-importance and urgency. My days are preoccupied with "saving the sick." Yet I seldom question what it is I am saving them from: risk factors? abnormal test results? fear of a "natural" death? Or, more importantly, what I am saving them *for*.

The Feast of St. Joan of Arc. It is my last day, and a holiday at Gethsemani, but thankfully we found Brother Anselm in the farm building after Lauds. He wrapped a "three-pack" of Gethsemani cheese for me to bring back to Lindsay. Of the varieties, only the aged cheese (they also make mild and smoked) has been served in the retreat house. It stands squarely in the the tradition of "stinky French cheeses": strong but good, and better when cut with cream cheese. The solemnity has doubled our time in the abbey church: an hour at Vigils; 2 at Lauds and Mass. Father Matthew provided some ecclesiastical trivia at conference today: the names of the notes in the musical scale (Do, Re, Mi, etc.) derive from the first letters of the Latin hymn sung at Vespers on St. John's Feast Day. Each line of the hymn was sung on successively higher notes through the octave.

Praise God that I am leaving. It has been a full four days of *Ora et Labora*, with prayer at the Offices and toil on the computer. Now I am returning to Lindsay and Clare, six days of mail, five days of work on our new addition, two weeks' growth of grass, and a ten-day stretch of call to test my clinical skills. Back into the thick of things, starting tonight with bedtime stories at my daughter's side.

She is an amazing kid. Lindsay reported in our Sunday telephone call that, after stubbing her toe and screaming bloody murder, she crossed herself to regain composure. She has been dealing with my absence by making gifts, endlessly, and counting down the days until my return. She has wonderful instincts for self-preservation and leaves little doubt that she is spiritually alive even if not yet accountable in the Catholic fold.

Last night I suffered misgivings about spending so much time and money on a monastic retreat. Why travel to rural Kentucky in sweltering June, for God's sake? Well, it is only money, and about the same as Lindsay spent on her jaunt to Paris. I needed to see the land and the community where Thomas Merton lived, and from which he cast his spiritual spell.

I did not know about Merton until well after his death, probably (I recall it now) in 1973, during my second year of residency. His writings were then very much in vogue among young, radical Catholics. And it was during a visit with my young, radical Catholic friends in New York City that I heard his poetry read by Daniel Berrigan at the lower Manhattan Catholic Worker House. My interest was piqued further when I learned he was Trappist, an order I had become familiar with two years earlier. Soon I was reading his books voraciously. *Thoughts in Solitude, The Sign of Jonas,* and a biography by Michael Mott called *The Seven Mountains of Thomas Merton* have became my favorites.

I have read his poetry, quoted him in my essays, copied his habit of wearing a black watch cap, and fancied him as my alter ego. Merton's life was contemplative; mine is of the world. But his struggles have seemed my own. He made a vow of stability to his religious community that would forever tempt and try him. He squeezed time for writing between his regular duties. He professed humility yet sought public recognition and pursued a voluminous correspondence with his friends. As an intellect, a convert, a mystic, he has represented for me the triumph of faith over reason, of free thinking above the rigidity of doctrines and vows. We share March 19, 1953—the day of my birth and his Ordination, a coincidence of great significance to me.

To pause before his common grave, to see a new barn standing where the old had majestically blazed, to talk and pray with his brethren, to imagine his night watch through the bell tower and silent corridors of that rambling stone structure, to drive the same winding miles to the monastery where so many have driven in pursuit of Merton's message . . . and drive now, in search of what? Through his writings, Merton became my spiritual advisor when—because of my divorce—the Church could not comfort me. His personal journals served as an inspiration for my own. He taught me about the reality of the great mysteries, including intimacy with God and the workings of universal love. I owe him too much to resist the visit. My last bow at the Abbey Church door is for you, Father Louis, with embraces and farewells for the mystic monk.

The simplest treasure of homecoming is the 4:45 A.M. cup of coffee. In the monastery, I would go from Vigils (3:15 A.M.) to breakfast (7:15 A.M.) without a drop of caffeine or a hint of its addictive aroma. The rest is more complicated: within an hour of my return the neglected demands of family, community, and work are already upon me.

My sister called several times in my absence. She needed money to buy a new trailer by tomorrow because her landlords banned her cats from the apartment complex. I managed to squeeze two hours out of yesterday's cramped schedule to help her secure a loan from our family bank in Iowa.

Clare has been clingy, moody, and desperate for attention ever since I returned. It's understandable but a darned nuisance when I want to talk to Lindsay or leave home in the morning. Yesterday, I couldn't peel a sobbing little girl off my leg, so I toted her along for the 8:15 meeting. An extra half hour on Daddy's lap set a bad precedent but soothed my daughter's worries.

The lawn is overgrown, compost needs turning, laundry is in piles, Cathy is depressed, our savings account has been bled dry by the workmen, and Bonnie has almost certainly torn a meniscus in her knee. It disturbs me that her doctor ordered a $1,000 MRI "just to be sure." I know that he knows that he will perform a laparoscopy no matter what the scan shows, so why waste the money? Because that's the way he likes it. I feel badly for Bonnie, who, despite having "good" insurance, will still pay a hefty deductible and a 20 percent copayment.

After vacation, I found myself eager to receive the list of hospitalized patients from my partner. Topping it was Isabelle Rooney, our chisel-toothed, gravelly voiced, leather-skinned patient with brittle diabetes, now in her third hospital week. At fifty-eight, she nears the end of her life—and of our rope. Isabelle is legendary for having worn through the roster of Waldo County physicians before landing—intractably, it now seems—on our doorstep. The difficulties lie in her self-destructive bent, her passive-aggressive behavior, her bold-faced lying and thievery. I also knew that her medical problems—brittle diabetes, pancytopenia, primary biliary cirrhosis, kidney stones—deserved whatever care we could muster.

Already running behind, I nudged open the door to Room 212 and gazed at the curled ball in the far bed, which stirred at the sound of my voice. Isabelle rose up like a lopsided inchworm on the stump of her left arm. "Morning, Dr. Hughes. Boy, am I glad to see you. I didn't know how I was going to get to see Dr. Patch, the kidney man, in Bangor, being holed up in the hospital like I am, yah. He's going to help me because I don't know who else can."

Then a tone of resignation muted her voice, and tears ran in streams from her eyes. "I'm not much use any more, Doctor Hughes-I-mean-Lobstercam. I try to keep a weight on by shoveling the groceries to me, but it's no use. Maybe I could go to the nursing home for a spell and give my hubby a rest. He's been awfully good to me, awfully good, but there's only so much a body can do, yah."

"Isabelle," I interrupted, "what is it that you hope Dr. Patch will do for you?"

"Tests, dear, tests," she replied pointedly. "He'll run some special tests, and I don't want to miss them on account of being parked in the hospital."

Tests and treatments are, of course, what doctors do, when we are puzzled, insecure, overrun, falling behind. "Let me listen to you," we say as we plug our ears with a stethoscope and press it hard against the whistling ribs. True, our testing demonstrates that we have taken the complaint seriously. It offers hope of understanding and cure. But it has become a poor substitute for the doctor at the bedside. No technological advance, no unrestrained expense, can fill the needs of a wounded soul.

I remember standing that morning beside her door with my fine notions of suffering culled in a monastery cell. The essay that I had worked on so diligently will not conclude. It could not prepare me for Isabelle's grating voice, her mutilated form, her pathetic groping, or the revulsion gnawing inside me. In the afternoon, and much to Isabelle's delight, I would perform the bone marrow biopsy that her consultant had recommended. But that morning we sat quietly in her darkened room, beside the moaning air conditioner, tending to her questions and worries and fears.

In those fifteen minutes Isabelle and I tied the sacred knot between physician and patient. We talked and attended to her pain. *Pati* is the Latin word for "suffer" and forms the basis of words like "patient" and "patience." In the derivation we sense, again, the temporal side to suffering. Ecclesiastes tells us that there is a time for every purpose. A time to hurry and a time to cast stones. Time to perform procedures and tend to common colds. A time to judge and to withhold judgment. A time to spend with those who accept their woundedness or still struggle against the fear and pain.

I recall my thoughts in the monastery, and the liberating desire to be average. It creates room in one's heart for humility; it brings balance; and it offers a sustainable pace for a professional life. It helps us to overcome our pride and preoccupation, and to slow down for the needs of the suffering. It brings us back to the mission of our profession, which is to prolong life, cure disease, and (when these ends escape us) to share with our patients whatever meaning and love has blessed our lives. To treat with hope, and our enduring presence.

Telephone calls interrupted me all of yesterday. There were three long conversations about the possible transfer of Nancy Newcomb back to Belfast. She is now off the ventilator, without a tracheostomy cuff, needing no oxygen, and beginning to sip clear liquids, but still very weak, terribly confused, communicating poorly, and a long way from home. She may be too healthy to be transferred to an acute care hospital such as ours. For Medicare to pay, we must document a need for services beyond those commonly provided by skilled nursing facilities. What Nancy needs, more than anything else, is physical therapy. But she also needs "watching," close observation for signs of relapse; and she needs a gradual advance in her activity level, dietary intake, and stimulation. We must write her H&P persuasively. But Waldo County General Hospital is not enthusiastic about the risk or hassle. We'll see how it goes.

I hesitate to assume all the responsibility for Mrs. Newcomb, but I am willing to gather up the loose ends, anyway. I know that Nancy's daughter is exhausted and bewildered; the transfer back to Belfast will offer her a shorter commute, a less imposing face of technology, and fewer nurses to contend with. I am still the daughter's obstetrician and her family's physician, and I find her in my thoughts daily. It is not that we know best in Belfast, but nursing and ethical issues are now foremost in her care, not the life-threatening infection that had necessitated her transfer.

Clare is up for her five-year-old shots at 10:30 A.M. today; I have agreed to be there if I can, and hospital duty seems light enough to allow it. We wouldn't worry except for Clare's ordeal with the pilomatrixoma; special attention now seems appropriate.

Happy Anniversary. Eight years ago Lindsay and I were married on a sunny Memorial Day weekend in Belfast. Lindsay's family, my mom, and a few friends gathered on the back porch of our home at 96 Union Street, lilacs blooming and the rhubarb ripe for pie. A Methodist minister performed the ceremony, and afterward we served our guests boiled lobster and champagne. Half of the guests are gone now, not dead but simply out of our lives; my mom has "gone by," too. But we are still happy to be here (in the words of another Midwesterner come east, Garrison Keillor), just up the block and around the corner on Salmond Street, with a more handsome lawn and a better view, stronger than we might ever have imagined, with beautiful Clare and the golden hopes of pregnancy.

I saw the flicker today for the first time this spring, studied him with the Bushnell binoculars as he preened himself in the neighbor's birch tree. Spotted breast, swathes of black beneath his eyes (looking for all the world like Will Clark in the batter's box), and a red chevron on the back of his head, the signature sign of a woodpecker. Occasionally he would stop, twist his tiny head, and let loose a shrieking call from his mechanical beak. Before flying way, he strutted his feathers so that I could observe his yellow undermarkings. When I reported my findings to Scott, he shouted animatedly "the yellow-shafted flicker! On the west coast, those very same markings would be red." The cardinals are now back in great numbers, all about the neighborhood, along with the northern (Baltimore) orioles and catbirds and blue jays and goldfinches. And, three days ago, a *heron* flew over with its long legs trailing like a kite tail.

Mamie returned to the office yesterday, repeating every few minutes that "I'm not sick" and "I only came because my daughter made me." She is terrified of being admitted to the hospital after her ordeal two years ago, when a small stroke led to unremitting seizures and several days of mechanical ventilation. She denies abdominal pain, reports a healthy appetite, and is still "putting on a face" every morning. I listened to her heart and lungs, drew blood, but mainly wanted to see her again, this incredible lady, weathered and worn but hallowed in her role as family matriarch.

Clare accepted her immunizations bravely ("it's part of going to school," we told her) and sat on the exam table big as you please. We were worried; would she be terrified of the needle after the trauma of her surgery? Fortunately, Clare accepted our explanation about the difference between the two needles and made her parents proud. She was proud, too, and wore her bandage like a badge all day.

A glorious Memorial Day weekend. Cold winds buffeted the coast, but I barely noticed them in the exhilaration of a holiday weekend. I ran every day, taking a longer eight-mile circuit on the first and last. Between runs we journeyed to Schoodic Point, on the eastern edge of Acadia National Park, just beyond Mt. Desert Island. Here the rocks jut precipitously into the ocean, and I had to struggle against fears for my daughter's safety. I am acrophobic, and Clare's youthful daring only magnified my anxiety, and triggered, no doubt, last night's avalanche of violent dreams. On the far side of the peninsula were beaches more delightful than the dramatic cliffs. Here lay strewn perfectly round granite stones as large as cantaloupe. We brought two home as souvenirs.

Tim's current project is a pebbled walk to his boathouse. He has been gathering stones from the shore and embedding them in a walkway for weeks now. Several hours of foraging for stones harvest only enough to lay a foot of path. But the task is redeemed by the love and patience he brings to it. Much as this journal is, or so I hope.

Sleep is a strange activity that brings the household into synchrony. Lindsay and I often awaken together, intertwined in each other's limbs, anticipating Clare's cry from the other room. Or both of us will rise half-consciously to use the bathroom or fetch a drink or toss sleeplessly in the stillness before dawn.

Yesterday was a kinder, gentler day. Early that morning I spotted a familiar yellow-orange bird dart to the top of neighbor's maple tree. With binoculars, I studied him carefully: black head and wings, splashes of yellow-orange along the sides, and a clarion call that sounded like "do-ri-to, do-ri-to." I couldn't wait to discuss my findings with Scott at the office. He pondered it for a while, furrowed his brow, and then guessed aloud, "drink your tea, drink your tea. Sounds like a rufus-sided towhee, which I haven't seen inland for years, but is probably still plentiful along the coast. You get such a different offering than we do inland." Unbelievable! I raced home to the Audubon Field Guide and looked up the towhee. There he was, just as I had seen him in the binoculars, save for the white breast that I will study hard to find next sighting.

Good news. Nancy Newcomb will be transferred to Waldo County General Hospital today or tomorrow for another week of physical rehabilitation. She has been totally free of the ventilator for nearly a week, and her only difficulty now (save for weakness) is the tendency to choke on her secretions. Tom Frey, the pulmonary attending, has no concerns about anoxic brain damage. He believes that she is only weak and disoriented from her extended stay in the ICU. The daughter was delighted with the news, and I am anxious to see Nancy again, now on the road to recovery.

I ran seven miles again yesterday, the old run, and my mind reworked the essay on suffering. This distraction took me effortlessly out High Street Extended, through the canopied descent along the river, past the wide breech of the Passy at Head of Tide and the falls at Doak Road bridge, then up the mile-long incline until I coasted clear. Fifty minutes. After arriving home, I showered, succumbed to a fifteen-minute nap, and enjoyed another two hours at the computer before picking up Clare at day care.

Lindsay announced, upon crawling into bed last night, that she might be "preggers." Her period is a week late, and yesterday she developed breast tenderness and a "weird feeling all over." I suspect that a pregnancy test would turn positive, but will it *stay* positive? Will this pregnancy fare any better than the last? I dare not raise my hopes. There is the first trimester to survive, then the results of an amniocentesis, and only *then* will the reality sink home. It is tempting to count chickens. If the nest counts for anything, our marriage is in a far better place for receiving the news, good or bad. We are ready for a pregnancy if God will grant it.

Samples. We have long felt it worthwhile to have them around. We store them properly in a back room at our office, keep an "approved" list of those we will accept, and dispense them to our destitute patients, to our family and friends. We have always defended the policy by appealing to "the greater good," knowing full well that samples are only another form of advertising, that their cost is passed along to the consumer, and that there is never any free lunch. But they *seem* like something for nothing, and appeal to a gullible side of the human psyche.

And they generate their own set of problems. A young asthmatic's chart crossed my desk yesterday, with a request from Scott to review it. She is an obese ten-year-old who moved to the area two years ago and first came to our office with a diagnosis of "severe asthma that requires intermittent pulse treatments with prednisone." Her panoply of drugs includes theophylline and three different inhalers. She has been seen in the office sixteen times over the last two years, evaluated twice in the ER, once prescribed prednisone, ordered to have a home nebulizer machine "for emergencies," and certified to have "severe and disabling asthma" in a letter to some governmental agency. *Yet never once has anyone heard her wheeze!* The only evidence has been her mother's word over the telephone. Every pulmonary function test performed by her former physicians (probably six or seven) was normal; Scott has not repeated them, pushed for allergy testing, followed theophylline levels closely, or sought specialty consultation, because the mother has pleaded poverty.

Indeed, she *is* poor, has no insurance, and receives workman's compensation as a major portion of her income while her husband is looking for a job. The child's illness contributes to the family's poverty—except for the samples Scott provides her, a tidy bagful at each visit. It would seem that we have become "enablers" in some strange family dynamic whereby the daughter must be disabled, too. I have seen her only twice. During the last visit, now over a year ago, I was struck by how passive, pliant, doughy she was, this only child who sat quietly on the exam table and let mother run the show—possibly to the child's detriment, if the concerns about the overuse of theophylline in children are valid.

But more importantly, we have sanctioned an illness, made a diagnosis, and forever altered Nicole's outlook on life and the way her mother and her teachers and her classmates will regard her in the future—even the way other doctors will come to consider and manager her symptoms. She has asthma, first of all, because we say so, whether or not (and for whatever reasons) reactive airway disease impinges upon her life. Is there a way to back off a bit, to give her breathing room, to spare the medicines and the medicalization that have created an invalid, and invalidated her life? Scott and I spoke last night after office hours. He vows to take the bull by the horns. He will recommend tapering back her medication, limiting the dispensation of samples, offering pulmonary consultation if mother is unconvinced by his arguments. I know mother better than daughter, and know that it will not be easy. "Do your best, Scott," I encourage; "let me know if you are stymied."

With this strategy, we risk being proven wrong, in full view of a controlling mother whose daughter's health is at stake. But there are risks to staying the course; greater ones, we perceive. Science is on our side, and the social "authority" of medicine. We must exercise it wisely, with wisdom and courage.

JUNE

The doctor is the familiar of death. When we call a doctor,

we are asking him to relieve our suffering, but,

if he cannot cure us, we are asking him to witness our dying.

✺

JOHN BERGER

A Fortunate Man

Elena Moulton is back in the Hospice Wing. She entered three days ago on a Sunday afternoon during my weekend off. I happened to be at home when the telephone rang, and I could find no good excuse to spare me from the responsibilities. She was feverish, unable to swallow, and so weak and emaciated that she could barely lift her eyes, those last remaining vehicles of expression. Did she wish intravenous fluids or antibiotics?

I met Harry outside, hunched on the hood of his car in front of the emergency room entrance. He was smoking a cigarette, or rather allowing it to smoulder unnoticed in his thick, arthritic hands. When he saw me, he motioned me over to speak with him before I saw Elena. "Doc," he began with eyes scanning the ground, "she's tired. She wants to be here . . . and I can't take it anymore ta' home. I've tried. I know where she belongs. But I haven't slept, haven't showered, haven't tended to anything but Elena for the last three days and I can't go on no farther." He stopped short, his gravelly voice breaking beneath the burden, sobbing now with long stretches of silence that I finally broke off, after taking in the full measure of his pain and exhaustion and personal failure.

289

"Harry," I nodded, "you've done the right thing, the best you could, more than most men with two good ears and working hands. This is where Elena belongs for the time being. Once you are rested and we see how she's doing, we might decide that she can go back home. But not now." Harry followed inside to Bay 3 of the emergency ward where his wife lay curled on the gurney, faintly smiling and groaning her greetings. I explained our decision and she nodded. Elena would remain on the Hospice Wing until Harry was rested, but without intravenous fluids or antibiotics, even if they could forestall her death.

Death seemed, still, not part of the immediate picture. With the message board, we ploddingly clarified her condition. "I can swallow. I am starving. More than jello. Sit up to eat." I made some nursing suggestions to the family doctor on call, but left him with the busywork of the admission and hurried home to join my family.

It has been so incredibly beautiful this past week that few patients have bothered with their ills. Many more "no-shows" than usual; virtually no hospital admissions or deliveries. I'm not complaining, just a little anxious. There is an insecurity that attends underemployment, even for the doctor. How do you measure up? How can you feel satisfied by pulling a lightened load? But how much worse for the sardine packer or shoe factory worker who has lost his job permanently, along with his income and benefits and self-respect? But, with the beautiful weather, I'll not go begging for business.

God has sent me a major penance: I have been asked to sing "Kumbaya" during Communion at the Children's Mass this morning.

It was a glorious weekend, the first of the summer. Temperatures in the low seventies, blue skies, ocean breezes, and freedom from Friday to Sunday. After Communion at 10:45 Mass, I thanked God for having plucked me from St. Joseph's Orphanage in Sioux City, Iowa, and delivered me here. Here with a wife and daughter, home and garden, partner and practice, friends and neighbors, and a safe and handsome community. Tears fell from my eyes, and I felt wholly connected to this place. While waiting for Communion, a patient of mine whispered her concerns about her husband. After Mass, I spoke at length with Tim's rowing partner, David Simmons, about Elite shells and our Catholic upbringing, and I invited him to join RENEW. Another patient waited ten minutes to report, happily, that her husband's sinuses improved on the antihistamine I had prescribed.

I had two long runs, mowed the lawn, pitched compost, laid a stone walk, emptied the attic for the workmen (who begin today), organized the garage, and repositioned Clare's tree swing. There was still plenty of time for Clare and Lindsay: a row on the ocean in Tim's skiff, a trip to the park with Clare and Justin, a family bicycle ride to Th' Cup for cones. There we met the Bakers, who have sealed their decision to move to Boone, North Carolina, where Bernie will accept a faculty appointment in the American Studies Department.

Last evening, I talked to Clare about sleeping in the big guest bed for awhile, maybe a month, while the workmen remodel the attic. Then she could return to her own little bed. But as I laid out the plans and considered the labor involved in breaking down the guest bed, reassembling it, breaking it down again, moving it to the new guest room (our current bedroom), it all seemed too much bother. "I've changed my mind, Clare. How about staying in your own bed until we can buy you a new twin?"

She burst into tears and sobbed uncontrollably. Was this fatigue, or were there deeper issues tied to the larger bed? Should I hold my ground or give way? If my daughter's happiness hinges on something so small (a little work a little later) then why not do it? OK, I said. A big bed it is. She immediately hugged my leg, shrieked "thank you, Daddy, thank you," gleefully helped with the assembly, proudly climbed aboard her new bed, and awarded me with the reading of tonight's bedtime stories, which she *never* does. Coming at the tailend of a long day, this was less of an honor than I let on. Of the many items on Clare's wish list—a hammock, a swing set, a pet goldfish—I have provided so few that this one concession seemed the least I could do.

Lindsay is sounding more and more pregnant. No period yet, but breast tenderness, queaziness, and profound fatigue. Lindsay *is* pregnant, I hesitate to say, hoping not to court disappointment or arouse notice among the gods of miscarriage. Clare and I picked up some prenatal vitamins for Lindsay at the pharmacy yesterday, but we hesitate to crawl any further out on the limb. For now, anyway. I have higher hopes than last fall, and dread the thought of another failure. Lindsay and I talked at supper last night about how things might change with a new baby. I will help more and am willing to contribute my three afternoons off (every other week) to spend with the baby, at least for the first year. After we finish the back room over the kitchen-ell and turn our attic into a master bedroom . . . but here I go making grandiose plans before the pregnancy has declared itself.

We have had exquisite weather for the last two weeks. Clear skies, warm days, thirty-six degree nights, and enough ocean breeze to clear the black flies. Our sugar snap peas, asparagus, and sweet basil are thriving in the garden, having escaped the killing frost that haunts the gardener who plants before Memorial Day.

At group yesterday I talked about a patient I had seen the day before. I knew her from the early years of the Pen Bay Singers when we sang together, and before I left for San Francisco she saw me infrequently as her doctor. She was twenty minutes late, but I saw her anyway for a scheduled physical, knowing that she had left work early to drive an hour to see me. No, a *complete* physical would not be necessary, she offered; the obstetrician had done that in February, including a pap smear, blood tests, and hormone prescription. Could I simply listen to her problems (on a list quickly retrieved from her purse) and fix a few?

My patient was much heavier than at her last visit three years ago, but neatly dressed and not unattractive in a blouse, skirt, and "mannequin legs" (her husband's term for industrial-strength panty hose). She inquired about a tiny mole on her skin, irregular periods, low back pains and facial hair. The obstetrician had given her a clean bill of health four months ago after ordering a battery of blood tests and an abdominal ultrasound. She had recently seen a chiropractor for what sounded like (in allopathic terms) a facet joint syndrome; these do (and did) respond quickly to manipulation. But now she was seeing him weekly for the low back pain, the result of "hip slippage" from a leg-length discrepancy. The pain is no better, and I presumed (correctly) that she had come to see me for a second opinion.

After a brief examination of the spine, I determined that her legs were nearly equal in length, reassured her about the benign appearance of her nevi, and read aloud the pelvic ultrasound report. Impression: normal study.

I could feel my resentment mounting: toward a patient whose tardiness left me only ten minutes for an examination and no time to ponder the "real" agenda behind her visit; and toward the other doctors who chose to ignore the obvious problem of obesity, even though it complicates everything else. I resented being the doctor of last resort, the one who charges the least and bears the greatest burden. For now I must mention the weight, and exercise, and the grim facts of aging. What did her mother look like? When did her facial hair grow? Are you willing to see a dietician or try a daily exercise program? Do you want to change or be reassured? Today I even resent the appellation "family doctor," which denies me any claim to expertise, earns me but a fraction of a *real* doctor's wage, and leaves as my only ally common sense. What is my role here? Why did her visit provoke such bitterness?

Tim put his finger on it instantly: respect. My patient had arrived late, chosen me last among her doctors, and left our forty-five-minute appointment without the exercise sheet I had selected for her. I mailed it to her the next day, attaching a brief note of encouragement.

Respect provides the leverage in a doctor-patient relationship; it allows the wary patient and weary doctor to move off dead center. Doctors too often destroy it by our tardiness, paternalism, inattention, or rush to judgment. Without a bond, the patient feels relegated to the sidelines so clearly described by Leo Tolstoy in *The Death of Ivan Ilych:* "To [the patient], only one question was important: was his case serious or not? But the doctor ignored that inappropriate question. From his point of view it was not the one under consideration; the real question was to decide between a floating kidney, chronic catarrh, or appendicitis. It was not a question of Ivan Ilych's life or death, but whether the floating kidney or appendicitis were to blame. And that question the doctor solved brilliantly, as it seemed to Ivan Ilych, in favor of the appendicitis."

Doctors show their respect simply by listening, by cherishing the intimate details or petty concerns that others might disregard. We do not flee the disfigured face, the stench of incontinence, the spasmodic sobbing of a jilted lover, or the litanies of complaints by those in chronic pain. We stand by. We are there. We may limit but not refuse. Sometimes, perhaps most of the time, patients are grateful for our services. They appreciate not only the results of treatment but every effort made on their behalf. Only the "difficult patients" deny us their gratitude, punish us with veiled insults or open hostility, cling to us desperately or refuse to get better no matter how petty the complaint. Some say "thank you" only by an episodic return sandwiched between broken appointments and collection threats. Some leave abruptly after a troubling interaction or unmet need, offering not a word of explanation. These cases test our commitment to medicine. They must be shared with our colleagues, explored to their roots, and let go.

After drenching rains all of yesterday, the morning is distilling to a hazy-clear day redolent with the smell of soaked earth.

An old drunk returned for his scheduled appointment yesterday, but without the usual stench of alcohol. I was stunned. He greeted me with a loud, cheerful "Hello, Loxterkamp," and in the privacy of our cubicle boasted that he had been dry a fortnight and weaned to a pack of cigarettes a day. "I needed a kick in the pants," he confided. "What good does it do to cry for help and not meet the person halfway?" Hey, that's *my* line, but it doesn't matter. What matters is how long the conversion lasts. I hold out little hope, but will see him back often enough to support his sobriety.

His blood pressure and diabetes have responded modestly to medication, and the urinary symptoms have all but disappeared. He feels like a new man, and I give him all the credit. Today I will adjust his medication and schedule a return appointment in two weeks.

Yesterday morning at check-in, Tim brought up a remark that I had made the week before at our hospice ITD meeting. Discussion had centered on which doctor should speak at the hospice volunteer training session. The coordinators had considered a list of four internists (all of whom politely declined) before choosing a colleague who had never once made a hospice referral and seemed the least likely candidate to expound a hospice philosophy. Why were Tim and

I overlooked? Perhaps, I teased, because of my partner's sullied reputation. It hit a nerve. Tim harbors a wedge of professional insecurity; unpleasant interactions or outright rejections cast a long shadow over his ego, as they do mine. But because Tim is so competent and able, I sometimes forget how deeply the wedge penetrates.

Why *were* we overlooked? A matter of speculation, but my comment was callous. That morning I avoided the main reason why Tim had mentioned the remark: his feelings were hurt. But I could not apologize even though I wanted to, and even though Tim was not pressing me to do so. Later I wrote him a short note of apology and deposited it unsigned on his desk. He thanked me; I felt absolved. These tiny acts of kindness, clumsy and veiled, are the pillars of our relationship.

I rue the days when I don't see enough of Clare. Yesterday she slept past my morning departure time, and I worked until nearly her bedtime. I had forty-five minutes to parcel between my daughter, my wife, the mail, the news, and the food trough. When bedtime rolled around, Clare's tug-of-war convinced me that she needed a bigger share of her father.

It was a weekend of overdoing. Too much sun, too much toil for my poor back, too hard a run, too many loads of laundry. But what beautiful weather for the doing of it!

I see the Mass with ever-changing eyes: eyes that trace the interconnecting strands among the parishioners of St. Francis, those who join me in worship and those whose names are read in the rollcall of the sick; eyes of a hospice doctor who bears witness to the inevitability that all of this shall pass away and every slate shall be wiped clean. Many on bended knee today are my patients and neighbors whom I met through RENEW, or acquaintances I recognize through my work. At Mass today there is no cantor, and the organist whispers a greeting into the microphone. In front of her, ahead and to the right of the first pew, I notice a man slouched in his wheelchair. He is mentally retarded, smiles broadly, waves his palsied limbs. He is ready for every rhetorical question posed from the pulpit, ready to wail the Kyrie and other responsorials he has memorized, appreciative of the shoulder pats of parishioners who pass him by. At one time, two years ago, he was situated in the pews, close to the front and next to the center aisle. From here he could reel around and offer his hand to those in the Communion line. Some gladly accepted it in the spirit of Communion, the very symbol and salvation of our community; others would study their folded hands as they bobbled obliviously by; a few even crossed the center aisle to avoid him.

As a welcome respite, the readings today are delivered in a thick, passionate Brooklyn accent. I realize at the Kiss of Peace that I am sitting next to the man

JUNE

who called me on the carpet for using the feminine gender throughout the Bobby McFerrin arrangement of the 23rd Psalm. A patient of mine is the eucharistic minister, looking gaunt but cheery after his chemotherapy and radiation treatments for lung cancer. I notice a neighbor in her flowery, wide-brimmed hat and a friend of Tim's whom I trail to Communion. We are an oddball lot, linked by faith, a pickup team chosen by some invisible hand. Small parishes, small practices, small towns make visible this element of community, stitched together by the challenge and blessing of sharing a common ground.

I ran into one of Tim's rocks yesterday, working on a new flower bed for Lindsay's dahlias. I kept hitting its crown with my shovel but could not get under it, around it, or budge it in the least. Rather than break my back on it, I'll accept it where it lies.

At the office yesterday I found a hand-scribbled note on the nurses' counter: "Should I restart Pravachol, now that I'm back home? Nancy Newcomb." *Unbelievable! Nancy Newcomb is back home.* She had improved so rapidly that the medical center decided to send her home rather than transfer her to Belfast for more rehabilitation. I called her back immediately and was greeted by a wisp of a voice, but one that enunciated her thoughts clearly. She admitted feeling tired "down to her corpuscles." Her memory of the hospitalization is threadbare; of the ICU, gone entirely; only filmy images, scenes from a bad dream, the touch of my hand on the ambulance run, the gradual focus on faces and voices through her recent recovery. A physical therapist comes to her home daily, but she needs no oxygen, antibiotics, pain or anxiety pills. Should she restart the heart medicine, the cholesterol pill, her vitamins? Just come to my office whenever you can, I blurted, and we'll talk. We'll see. How joyful it was to hear her voice!

It was a pleasant, efficient afternoon in the office, full of patients who were improving and old faces with no new complaints. Time enough to joke with Cathy and Scott and the nurses, to have lunch with Lindsay and Clare when they surprised me at noon. We went to Dexter's Dogs, which opened on May Day for the summer. But I fear that too many comfortable days undermine the doctor. Once we get used to the routine, we tend to settle into it and even to believe in it. A healthy, necessary self-scrutiny is more than I can muster on a day of waning energy.

Clare was yawning and curling into a ball by the time I picked her up at the high school pool. Tonight was a daddy-night, as Lindsay was gone to meetings. Though the hour was only 5:30, the day had been long and exhausting. Clare and I barreled through the grocery store for supper items, but quarreled at the checkout counter. Clare, in her hunger and fatigue, wanted three candy bars instead of an allowable one. I won the argument but lost my temper. We survived our ride home, scrambled together a meal, ate, and collapsed together on the sofa.

I stroked Clare's beautifully domed forehead as she sprawled, unconscious, across my lap. This evening alone with Clare was opportunity lost, I realized afterward. I had lost my composure and now my priorities, choosing the evening news over a bedtime story for my daughter. Our chances are not unlimited. I should well remember this, after my father's early death and my experience in hospice, where so many families come to the lesson late.

Yesterday began and ended with Roberta Wilson: shortness of breath at dawn and a family meeting at dusk. She had been found that morning drenched in sweat and gasping for breath. Heart rate in the one-fifties, respiration in the forties, and blood oxygen saturation below the seventieth percentile and falling. I instructed the nurse to string an oxygen cannula, raise the head of her bed, and allow me five minutes to dress. Roberta had likely thrown a pulmonary embolism, a life-threatening complication of prolonged bedrest. We had not thinned her blood for fear of excessive bleeding into her badly fractured leg. Now that decision plagued me as I raced to the hospital.

When I arrived, Roberta lay flat in bed, lungs noisily drawing air, eyes glazed, arms cool and wet, right leg strung in traction to prevent her strong thigh muscles from contracting around her fractured femur. I immediately set the nurses in motion. We needed an EKG, portable chest X-ray, heart enzymes, blood gasses, and someone to keep a log of the proceedings. I called the son-in-law and asked him to notify the others. Did they want their mother resuscitated or let go, I needed to know. Roberta was frothing at the mouth, her lungs soaked, so I ordered diuretics in successive boluses until urine began to pour from her foley catheter. Then I paused to study the available data. The EKG and chest X-ray confirmed what had become clinically apparent: Roberta was in pulmonary edema (fluid on the lungs) as the result of an acute heart attack. I called the consulting cardiologist to seek his counsel, and the orthopedic surgeon to cancel surgery.

Throughout the day, we added higher flows of nasal oxygen to offset diminishing saturations in the blood; morphine was discontinued because it aggravated Roberta's falling blood pressure; the IV rate was slowed to prevent fluid from accumulating in her lungs; dopamine was added to raise the blood pressure and kidney perfusion. By midmorning, Roberta was conscious and gaining color. Ten hours later she still held her ground, though I cautioned the family against optimism. The next several days would reveal the outcome, not these few hours.

Lindsay and Clare had spent the previous night on Vinalhaven, visiting friends whose parents own a summer cottage there. The island is an hour by ferry from Rockland. It is still largely a fishermen's community despite the many summer visitors who come "from away." I had hoped for a pleasant evening and morning by myself, reading quietly, but it was not to be. I had arrived home late the night before and spent the last rays of the day running. Then Roberta's emergency exhausted my morning.

Roberta is a tough old bird. But the mortality rate from heart attacks complicated by pulmonary edema and low blood pressure is exceedingly high. She is not out of the woods yet, and I worry about our choices and their consequences in the days ahead.

These have been incomparable mornings, exquisite days. Yesterday, while crossing Memorial Bridge, I glanced out across Belfast Bay. She was swollen at high tide, full-figured in her indigo gown with sequins glittering in the spotlight of the morning sun. Today the clear, warm air is redolent with summer smells, chattery flicker calls, the green and kaleidoscopic splash of Lindsay's exploding garden. We worked together for an hour yesterday morning (around six o'clock) transplanting basil plants, sprinkling pine needle mulch around the blueberry bushes, and expanding a garden bed behind the garage. Office hours are no more satisfying than this good labor. Lindsay, who deserves all the credit for the garden's success, has assigned me the brute tasks of preparing the beds, fertilizing the soil, watering seedlings, cultivating weeds, and praying for good weather.

This week depleted me, wore me down and scattered my bones (as the psalmists say). But I couldn't put my finger on why. Too much hospice, too frenetic a pace, too little cheer. All I know is that I had nothing left to offer Lindsay and Clare last night other than blank stares and grunts of annoyance.

A review of the charge: Roberta is still alive, to no one's surprise. Yesterday her blood pressure rose, oxygen saturation hovered near the ninetieth percentile, urine flowed freely, and no morphine was needed throughout the day. But what of Roberta? She seemed all the more depressed for having muffed her departure, deferred the battle to another day. In the meantime she is tethered to her bed by the cast on her leg, as she is tethered to life. She motioned to speak with me and her hospice volunteer yesterday, and I saw in her eyes a mixture of frustration, confusion, desperation. Here lies a *useful* woman who worked hard and loved every minute of her life. She did for others without a second thought. Now she lies strapped to a bed, waiting, for what? Death? Declare yourself, then, and get on with it. Roberta is no coward, but she is tiring of your tactics, the stalking and the feinting and blows below the belt. She spoke, once when we were quite alone and her family had retreated to the sun porch, of the essay her granddaughter wrote about her. "Won a prize," Roberta whispered proudly, "and right on the mark. What truth children speak at the age of ten." Then she asked of me, with emphasis on every word, "Why didn't I die?"

What was I to say? "Here is the evidence, Roberta, your heart would not quit."

"That's a pretty lousy reason for living," she replied angrily.

"It's a fact, Roberta. Now *you* have to supply the reasons."

And she will, given time; given solitude and a chance to think things through. I spoke to her family and gave them permission to return to their regular lives. And I gave Roberta permission to mope and stew about this distressing turn of events. She has nothing left to give. She disdains the spotlight. She seeks the shadows, seclusion, a chance to sit with her unfamiliar self, a self full of fears and loneliness and the need of others (she asked last night, for the first time, if the family could sit in vigil). Good things are happening in the Wilson family, and there are reasons, I suspect, that she remains among us.

After I explained to the family how important it was for Roberta to rest, to draw back, and for the family to resume their lives, Roberta remarked, typically contrary, "Oh, I enjoy having them around." How to figure that woman!

Isabelle Rooney is awaiting placement and awaiting her kidney tests in Bangor. She, too, is tired of living. She would not let go of me yesterday, explaining it all to me and going over a list of questions. But what she really wanted was the company. She is broken down, she tells me, in ways the doctors cannot mend.

Two home visits, a couple of ship's physicals, lunch at Dexter's Dogs. And twelve patients scattered across the afternoon hours. Oldtimers, many of them, patients with whom I have a history of six or eight years, stories to share, familiar ruts we travel together. But that old friend depression, dressed in his shopworn suit, found me as I circled home. Was it the full face of the moon? Or the new prenatal patient who canceled her appointment, giving me one less opportunity (among a dwindling pool) to deliver? More probably it is the journal's end, after a year of comfort and security, and the infusion of purpose it has brought to this lowly practitioner. The journal has become more than a ritual; it is the underpinning of my day.

OB is the symbol of my medical prowess, the feather in my cap. If I gave it up, would I be less a doctor? Would I begin the slow slide toward the rocker? Am I ready to grow old with my patients, cut a deal with the debilities of age, follow my own advice to the octogenarian crowd, "simplify, simplify"? At forty, life is changing around me. When I grow old, I hope not to find myself in the same condition as Roberta, unable to adjust to a dying time when utility is gone, and when a few kind words and companionship and your whittled down hopes are all you have left to live for. Will I do it better than she? That is one of the beauties of my work: it lays out these questions in advance. Life is an open-book exam. I read it daily in the lives of my patients, find it in their struggles, their tentative conclusions, their errors and corrections. I have done well to stay attentive. And I look forward to the cast of thousands (including Roberta) whom I will meet again on Judgment Day.

Yesterday's group offered some refreshing honesty and a little pain, a sense of playing with knives. Scott related his conversation at a neighbor's house last night; they asked if he had ever considered writing about birds and nature. He couldn't, he confessed; it would change his experience, transform his beloved nature into something captive and marketable. Besides, he claims, his talents are too meager. Scott repeated his old saw about benevolent nature and malevolent man, throwing up his hands in despair. Maybe he should chuck it all, volunteer a month or two for Greenpeace, work toward the salvation of the world instead of tossing donuts to the seagulls. But will he ever do it? Not without Debbie, who is attached to her home, friends, and new job.

Tim challenged him. "Scott, here we go again with your dichotomies, man versus nature, us versus them. Don't belittle yourself, just take a risk."

There are risks even in writing. It has required me to turn my cloth inside out and expose what matters most. It has demanded of me a commitment. Writing is a relationship as serious as any other, lived often in secrecy and nourished by the simple pleasures of turning a phrase, or finding a metaphor, or bringing some niggling doubt to a tentative resolution. Whether we write to friends or for a commercial audience or with a college of peers in mind, the process sinks or sails on our relationships, on our commitment to friendship, to conversation, to truth.

Once, it was my most fervent wish that Lindsay should to convert Catholicism. Did I secretly hope that *her* faith would save mine? That her attendance at Mass might bolster my own, shore up my doubts, confirm those tenets of faith that have worn, in places, to mere habit and repetition? If she really loved me, wouldn't she wish to share in something so central to my life? But it doesn't work that way. It is my faith. It is my commitment and not Lindsay's. I cannot hold her hostage, but must allow freedom on this matter, and trust that our independence and self-fulfillment will strengthen our bond.

Amazingly, I have reached my computer before sunrise all week. A hospital week, no less, but a calm one owing to sheer luck. Only one admission to the floor, a repeat C-section yesterday, and sidetracks to the nursing home. I have moved efficiently from office to home, allowing Lindsay time to wing to her evening obligations. Our routine has found Clare asleep by 9:00 P.M. and lights out by 9:30. Last night was the only close shave, when Lindsay burst upon me at 9:45, all chatty and buoyant and charged with energy after a hospice bereavement support group. This morning my puffy eyes blinked reluctantly until a stiff cup o' jo and a Geminiani concerto revived my drooping spirit.

Our group yesterday morning provided a safe and fertile ground. I wanted (but failed) to tell Scott how much he is loved, as evidenced by the birthday cards, salutations, and awards that are plastered above his office desk; I wanted (but failed) to tell Tim that I salute and cheer his high adventure in the Maine-Dartmouth Residency Program (where he will teach one day a week), and as he takes his seat in another support group. Rather, we talked, each in our own way, about suffering.

I am tired and stiff after a weekend in the garden. My duties were menial; Lindsay requested only that I scatter a dump truck load of blended manure* over the various garden beds, and leave a small portion for the compost heap. I love it, this compost and manure; they are incontrovertible proof that from death comes new life. Each steaming forkfull reminds me of my native Iowa; it has the color of topsoil and the smell of silage. Lindsay exhausted her Mother's Day gift certificate at the garden store so that we would not run low on weekend projects.

What beautiful weather! Temperatures in the mid-sixties, seagulls screeching from the rooftop, blue skies and balmy sea breezes where low tide fills your nose with the smell of moss and mud brine and clams. Walking down Condon street toward the sparkling bay—Lindsay at my side, Clare in the wheelbarrow—I burst with joy at *living* here (not simply vacationing). It is very nearly paradise.

The walk on the shore beneath Tim and Cris's home produced less sea glass than our usual harvest at City Wharf. There, exactly a century ago, The Dana Sarsaparilla Company bottled tons of the famous root extract and distributed it nationally. Shards from the translucent green Dana bottles are still abundant in the gravel, and a cache of fragments, with the letters DA . . . or . . . PARILLA still distinct, line our bathroom window sill. A friend recently offered us a shipping crate with Dana's boast burned into it, "The only sarsaparilla guaranteed to *absolutely cure disease. Remember it! Remember it! Remember it!"* In its time, Dana was the largest of the sarsaparilla manufacturers in Belfast, but not the only one; there was Dalton and Leon, Skoda Discovery, Compound Rheumatic Oil, Rodolph, R. H. Moody, the Nutriola Company, and others who vied for a market that mushroomed and collapsed in the last decade of the nineteenth century.

A long run in the afternoon. I strode by the nearly completed Pitcher House, where restoration crews are scrambling for a Memorial Day open house. The owner is keenly aware of the esteem in which old homes are held in the community; over the holidays she will allow the curious and sentimental of Belfast one long, inside look.

The waterfall under Doak Road bridge is still roaring. Someday I will take Clare back there. While padding along the back roads, I realized the wisdom in

---

* Fritz Tisdale claims that chicken, sheep, and cow droppings are mixed together, but after it has composted, who can tell?

transferring some of my productive needs from work to home. Healthy work and a balanced life require it. How much harder it will be when the vagaries of age and infirmity deny me the opportunity to run, or lug manure, or chase my daughter on her bicycle.

All of these things are remembered on a Tuesday morning instead of Monday. Clare's cry of "Daddy" at 5 A.M. yesterday, wide-eyed and expectant, ended my brief solitude. I truly rejoice at my daughter's newfound affection, even if she demonstrates it by anchoring herself to my leg as I slink out the door to surgery or the office or a breakfast meeting. I am not being ignored, which is a better fate than I deserve.

Yesterday was another glorious day, but it was held to a mild sixty degrees by a steady offshore breeze. The big surprise was an occasional cheep . . . cheep . . . cheep of a cardinal, back in the neighborhood. She was browsing for nesting materials. I had worried that we (our cats) had made them feel unwelcome somehow, what with Dinky's alarming habit of shinning the tree trunks, and last year's discovery of a dead baby bird in the matted grass. Its identity was unknown, but all summer long I worried that it had been a fallen cardinal.

A strange and complicated day in the office. I noticed in the hospital mail that my alcoholic friend had been admitted over the weekend. He will receive close observation and testing for homonymous hemianopia, a one-sided loss of vision that suggests a stroke. George has not touched a drop of booze since that first visit three weeks ago. Will he blame his condition on abstinence? Do I hear him muttering already, "Doc, I'd be better off drinking." Tim, who is covering the hospital this week, will have to answer.

Then a plumber presented with a complaint of hearing loss, but as the story unfolded, it twisted into the bizarre. He is a man in his mid-forties; we sidestepped his past except for the passing remark that he was "raised Catholic, but I'm searching for a synthesis, East and West." The hearing loss began as a ringing in his right ear, and since has involved both ears progressively. He has seen two specialists (one of whom was convinced he had Meniere's; the other said definitely not); he has been treated by an acupuncturist and a chiropractor, and so concludes that the problem is likely "an energy thing." He reports the sensation of electrical shocks traveling the length of his spine and around his body; bouts of nausea (without whirling) that occur twice daily; strange visual manifestations of lights, patterns, shadows. He is now seeing an analyst and describes much of his three-year journey through the health sector—both alternative and allopathic—as a spiritual quest. His favorite poem, he confesses, is the ecstatic "Hounds of Heaven" by Frances Thompson.

Are the problems entirely emotional, or is he filtering organic disease through his symbolic imagery? Does he have multiple sclerosis or another degenerative process? And why in God's name has he come to see *me*? Partly, the patient now admits, because the second specialist recommended extensive testing that he, as an uninsured consumer, can scarcely afford. Yet he senses that "things are coming to a head"; he appears worn by the constant ringing, the incapacitating nausea, and the left-sided ear pain. I see an opening here: the ear pain can be attributed to grinding his teeth at night; and my physical exam confirms a tender jaw joint. But nothing else. And so we part with a treatment for his jaw, a referral to a good neurologist, and advice that he contact Medicaid for application guidelines should his medical bills pile too high. We agreed to reconvene after the neurological evaluation.

One of our prenatal patients has all the signs of pre-eclampsia: sudden weight gain, puffiness of the face and hands and feet, rise in blood pressure, and marked protein in her urine. I marshaled her off to the hospital, but the prognosis is not good, not this early (27 weeks) or severe. A couple requested diet pills. Another prenatal patient is near term but not ready yet to deliver; her last baby was large and developed shoulder dystocia, and she has gained 55 pounds this pregnancy. I read her the riot act about dieting, which she has ignored. Another patient is at the end of her rope since her daughter ran away for the umpteenth time. She has not been taking her thyroid supplement, despite a TSH of 90 and a goiter the size of an orange. She cannot afford it, or remember it, or even care about it when her life is disintegrating around her.

And then I was startled by Lindsay, who brushed beside me at the doctor's station and whispered "I'm bleeding." It had just begun, but it was as heavy as a period, more than a little spotting. So it was over already, this possibility, this chance, and I slipped into a glum mood until day's end. We had just collected her urine that morning for a pregnancy test. I had taken the kit home last night and tested her urine anyway: faintly positive, consistent with today's miscarriage, our second within a year.

The rains poured heavily through the late afternoon, so that by early evening, when Lindsay and Clare and I took our walk, the fog and mist rose in wisps ahead of us. We walked by the Pitcher House, which is still getting primped and painted for the open house. We angled over to St. Francis to inspect the perennials I had helped plant the day before. I could not shake the mood, as heavy and obfuscating and damp as the night air. And all through my dreams, I experienced the violence and terror of living in the worst residential neighborhoods of L.A.; breaking and entering, stolen property, threats against our lives with knives and guns, scene after horrid scene. One vivid scene with Tim: a body lay in the middle of the room and was certified dead, cold to the touch, yet began to twitch as I observed her, then she breathed and rose up and approached me, exhaling warm sweet breath in my face. I was relieved when the alarm provided an escape, even though I am still troubled by the violence, fear, and death that was conjured in my dreams.

It was a bad day in the office. I don't know if the cause was fatigue, or my allergy-swollen sinuses, or depression plain and simple. But it was a day for trudging, an interminable, cool, gray, misty day that pinched to a close with an absolutely lethal medical staff meeting, where I was again reminded of how little I know my colleagues.

It did not help (except for clarification) that I had seen three depressed patients that morning. The first complained of a burning numbness in the skin over her right iliac crest. The complaint was unchanged over two prior visits. It might stem from early shingles or myralgia paresthetica, I explained again, but why does it matter so much?

"Why do you always say I'm depressed?" she challenged me.

"Because, first of all, you *are* depressed. Depressed patients eat too much, which your weight gain suggests, and dwell on their ailments. You have been thoroughly evaluated by the experts. To the best of our knowledge, nothing serious is the matter. My diagnosis may be mistaken, but before we discard it, can we work with it together?" There is always, I mutter to myself, the possibility that I may be wrong. But she agrees to a support group, a dietary referral, and daily exercise. She also agrees to return if necessary, but I doubt she will: I have named the spade.

My next patient was someone whom I had delivered several months ago. Shortly thereafter, her husband was laid off, which led to money woes and the added irritation of his constant presence. She took up Tupperware for extra cash, and to have a project outside the house. But the burden and demands became overwhelming. She is now crying at whim, fitful in her sleep, forgetful and careless at work and in her mothering, and preoccupied by dark thoughts (suicide, she confesses, like all five of her siblings). Father was an abusive alcoholic; mother was often absent to support the family. She was horrified at the thought of repeating the nightmare, but saw her life being "sucked down the same drain." The stream of conversation flowed unobstructed; I let it pour, the tears washing away time and memory. She carries a medical card, so that many doors for counseling are closed. In the end, we agreed to weekly meetings, antidepressant medication to jump-start her recovery, counseling with Mary Beth when an opening develops, and a pledge to call if thoughts turn suicidal.

The last depressive of the day was a successful, attractive woman with a list of complaints: fatigue, recurrent canker sores, chest tightness, fitful sleep. Symptoms of anxiety run in wolfpacks, I explain to her. Any pressures at work, any reason to feel depressed? She admitted to thoughts of a career change. The catering business is too much; cooking has become void of all charm. Personalities, the pressures of business, the tiring routine have sapped her of the satisfactions she once derived. There is a door behind which more secrets lie, but it is closed to me now. Yes, she has two good friends with whom she talks things over; no, she has not seen a therapist. She accepts my explanations, and the caution to avoid anything rash. I offer to test for "organic explanations"—diabetes, anemia, hypothyroidism—if she wishes. No, not now. And she will chew on the idea of a therapist.

I wanted to shake these women, shout at them "I am the one who needs help now." But instead trudged through it all, stifling yawns, sniffing loudly, and feeling dull and vacuous and uncertain at every turn. It is a two-edged sword, this wound of depression. It provides a sensitive ear for hearing the sad ring of a story. But when the doctor is slumping, he loses that necessary shield, lacks the energy to defend himself against the great stampede of human suffering, cannot throw off the bodies as quickly as they stack at his feet.

A good day for hospice. I met Elizabeth, one of Elena's favorite nurses, on my way to the Hospice Wing. She relayed Elena's request for the priest, "not now, but before it is too late." The Church has revamped the last of her sacraments. The names "Extreme Unction" or "Last Rites" were shed in favor of the less declamatory "anointing of the sick." The priest's arrival no longer signals the death knell. Elizabeth also sang high praise for bedtime Demerol, which helped Elena achieve ten hours of welcome rest. At home, she had been sleeping a dozen hours at night in addition to a three- or four-hours nap in the afternoon, after the home health aides departed. The aides, the home health nurses, Harry and Billy (Elena's nearest brother) all visited in turns, amicably and with a sense of common purpose and approaching end.

I found Harry at the end of the long hallway outside his wife's door. He was sitting alone, steeped in shadow, head in hands. She's asleep, he gestured with the flat of his hand against his cocked head, and motioned me closer. We talked at length about their twenty-two-year-old marriage, and their adopted son, John. Harry was thirty-nine, Elena thirty-seven, when they tied the knot before the justice of the peace. After changing the date three times, they finally eloped. Only afterward did they pass the news to Elena's dour and disapproving parents. Harry recounts that, while they were dating, Elena still sought their permission to extend an afternoon visit into a dinner date. Elena appreciated Harry's "coming down on her stern," which was a "rare but necessary" event when Elena became too silly or superfluous. Her greatest flaw, he allowed, was the spoiling and sheltering of John, not unlike the way that Elena's parents had spoiled her brother Billy. They had adopted John over the strident objections of Elena's sister-in-law, Hildy, a Germanic, matronly woman twenty years her husband's senior. John had not cried since the day they brought him home from foster care at age fourteen months. Nor did he so much as shed a tear when, as an infant, he fell on his front teeth and split his gums. Unable to cry, he would laugh instead, which only incurred his parent's annoyance and wrath as they tried to comfort or discipline him. But he was a loving boy, especially to Elena, and provided her with her greatest joys and memories.

Upon hearing the voice of the nurse as she fed and fussed over my patient in the next room, I rose to visit Elena. She was propped by an array of pillows, smiling as always, and snugly bibbed. I crouched beside her asked if she would like the priest to come. Her eyes blinked approvingly. I asked if she would like to be remembered in the roll call of the sick at Mass, and again her eyes flashed. All the while generic pink liquid oozed from between her teeth and dribbled onto her bib and nightgown as she smiled. No matter how hard Elena tried, she was unable to swallow or support her head. To signal "no," she had only to wag her head laterally. But nodding a "yes" had become impossible, and so a blink was substituted for the affirmative.

I inquired again about IV fluids and antibiotics, but Elena shook these off as emphatically as before. We returned to the language board. With Irene's help, the first few messages went smoothly: "pillow up. I am still hungry. Shot helped." Then a confusing line, one that required me to backtrack and decipher more carefully. Finally we eked it out, guessing the completion as Elena squeezed her eyes "yes." "I want a shot to put me into oblivion."

I was prepared for her request even though, oddly, it had not been raised by Elena or any other patient. I had discussed it academically, expressed my opinion on doctor-assisted suicide and the media-mongering of Jack Kevorkian, on all the permutations and what-ifs that might justify doctor-assisted suicide. I crouched low before Elena's face in order to reduce the distance between us, the potential for error, and possibility of doubt in the limited range of her expression. "Elena, I can do no more than I am doing. I will give Demerol to relax you and help you sleep, but I cannot knowingly give a dose that would put you away forever. I am not judging you by your request; I cannot climb inside you, experience what you are feeling, know the extent of your suffering. Perhaps you see my hesitation as cruel. But my pledge remains: I will do my best to keep you comfortable, to be honest and forthright in our discussions, and to go the distance with you."

I rubbed her emaciated arm, which had withered to bone and drooping skin, and squeezed the nubbly fingers lying limp on her lap. Just then, a twinge of remorse. Had I overreacted to her request? Was she merely asking for a few hours more of sleep, a longer respite from the grim reality of her disease? But I put aside these doubts and I spoke unhurriedly into her eyes, "You almost certainly will not choke to death. You may starve if you stop eating and drinking. Or, more likely, you will die peacefully in your sleep, kept comfortable by the Demerol that I will gladly provide. The time is coming soon. You might pray that God will take away your fears and frustrations and sorrow, and bring you close to Him in peace at His appointed hour. I want you to know that, although I hate seeing you suffer, I will miss you terribly when you're gone. I like you very much, Elena. And I will promise to look after John and Harry, especially during the immediate months ahead."

I had said enough, could no longer watch the tears as they welled in Elena's fixed and sparkling eyes. I could not bring myself to imagine what she might be thinking or feeling, or what trials she would face in the hours and days ahead. I called the interim priest, Father Paul, before leaving the hospital, and learned later that he had stopped by around noontime to administer the holy oils.

When I visited Elena yesterday she was sleeping, having just received another bolus of Demerol. Harry and John waited outside the room, anxious for me to confirm a slight deterioration in her condition that might herald the end. Harry was exhausted, prayed for the ordeal to close, begged me to keep Elena "rested" in a twilight sleep where she might wait without misery. But Elena was still running the gauntlet, attempting painstaking speech through the message board, requesting puree and thickened liquids that found their way back onto her saturated bib. I reminded Harry that Elena had chosen this ending. She might give up all together, lay down her fears of choking, her restless thoughts trapped inside a useless body, the discomforts of odd and unrelieved positioning, the humiliation and frustration of her total dependency.

Despite this, she has found reasons to live, if in nothing else than the pain of parting from her family and the fear of losing even this thin thread that has become her life. We, the unafflicted, can only imagine what it must be like, and that is painful enough. I reassured Harry we would all rather avoid those eyes, visit her only while she sleeps, and sigh in her presence instead of wrestle with complicated feelings, or fumble with the message board, or meet those wanting eyes, or squirm at the sounds of her moaning and gagging and feeble cough. Harry told me that John would be going to the dentist in a few minutes, so I wished him luck. As I turned to leave, something clicked in John's brain, and he wheeled to capture me with his dancing eyes. "Good luck to you, too, Dr. Loxterkamp," he shouted back.

A journal runs the risk of becoming a crude and disjointed affair, coarse and chaotic compared to the refinement with which a novel pursues the story line, or an essay the truth. But in its defense, the diary can show the connection between words and events. It is the vapor plume of an author's life, fresh and obvious in the making. It affords an intimacy with the author, a familiarity with his circumstance, and some sense of how he arrives at knowledge. I have often confessed to my patients that if you want to observe the doctor's reasoning in action, watch how he shops for groceries or assembles a Christmas toy "in five easy steps" or solves the Sunday crossword.

Knowledge in the wild is not your mounted steed, but a gamey, tick-infested, crop-crunching pest. Family doctors make a thousand clinical decisions a day, often ignorant of which will become the serious, pivotal, or irrevocable ones. We stumble across self-knowledge, or the most piercing clinical truth, as if it were roadkill, startling and vile with the guts hanging out. Truth that matters is often a scary sight.

A diary can show you this truth-in-action, a knowledge born not so much *from* experience as *through* it. It is in the here and now that doctors can make a difference, before the opportunity escapes. Sometimes we embark on a treatment plan in fog so dense you cannot see a hand before your face. On lagging days we are pushed along by the money and duty and need; on better days, when the top-sails billow, by curiosity and suspense and the sheer terror of it all. This is how a diary travels with the actual practice of medicine.

And what shores up the doctor as he stands solitary at the helm? Not only science, or good breeding, or the pearls of his clinical training, but something called common sense, which Dr. John Sassall roundly warns against: "Common sense has been a dirty word for me . . . It tempts me to accept the obvious, the easiest, the most readily available answer. It has failed me on almost every occasion I have used it—and God knows how often I have fallen and still fall for the trap."* There must also be intuition, caution, criticism, and support of the severest kind, much of which will be branded as heretical by the pure scientist, little of which could be defended in court.

But the doctor must also bring love to his work, without which all becomes drudgery.

Yesterday I ran into Tim on Condon Street, bicycling home, and we talked briefly about his interaction with a colleague that morning. Several nights ago, Tim had been in the ER when a youngster was brought in with ulcerative colitis. The child had not been previously diagnosed, though his doctor had seen him several times for persistent stomach cramps and fever. The doctor prescribed antidiarrheals, ordered stool samples for parasites, restricted his diet, and watched while the boy grew more wasted and wan. It was Tim's good fortune to find the child with a bloated abdomen. Upright roentgenogram of the abdomen disclosed an ominous and telltale toxic megacolon. Now treatment began in earnest: IV fluids were hung, steroids administered, and groundwork laid for his evaluation at the medical center.

* John Berger and Jean Mohr, *A Fortunate Man* (New York: Holt, Rinehart and Winston, 1967, p. 56.

Though our colleague had missed the call, no harm was done. It was a lapse any of us might make, and all of us have in our own fashion. But how do you broach it with your peers; how will they respond? With trepidation, Tim broke the silence at his next opportunity. Though he wished only to convey a snapshot of his evaluation, the interaction was awkward and unproductive. The next morning, the doctor challenged Tim on his management of the transfer: a little more Solu-Medrol, a little less electrolyte might have served the child better. But why, Tim thought, this accusatory tone? Why was Tim being blamed for having stumbled upon his colleague's error? If we cannot face our mistakes and acknowledge them, what lesson is learned: that, for fear of exposure, our patients should never be allowed to fall into the hands of another doctor?

When is the doctor let off the hook? When does he get the help, reassurance, and support he needs? Continuity of care—which is nothing more than the practice of medicine in one place over time—is a doubled-edged sword. It can be brandished over our heads as a duty, and we can use it to cover our tracks. But it also allows us to lend out our patients and accept them back, even when the exchange uncovers a mistake; it allows us to become intimate with the fact that we live, suffer, die, and err; and it provides us with one of the deepest satisfactions in medicine: a patient's gratitude for our "being there" and treating them with every good intention.

So I go back now, review my handling of Nancy Newcomb's illness, wonder if a clinical clue or telltale remark would have prompted an earlier, more aggressive intervention—an X-ray, perhaps, or a swifter transport to the medical center, or more immediate attention to her impending shock. That I was available in the ER on the morning she arrived was sheer luck, but somehow it dissipated the spectre of blame. I feared less the judgment of my colleagues than my own self-scrutiny and sense of responsibility. I had access to every point along the course of her decline. This is what we live with, especially family doctors who, more than anyone else, work in the shadow of the experts. Like FAA investigators, the specialists are always there to poke through the wreckage when things go bad.

Two bright spots in the day: The first, a telephone call from *Medical Economics* magazine wanting to schedule a photographer to take my picture for an article on rural health centers. I had the staff going. "It's for their swimsuit issue," I insisted. And upon my arrival home, Clare hugged me with such enthusiasm and charm that I could not help but relinquish some of the gloom that I had been storing up for a great sulk later that night.

It rained all day yesterday, spritzing at times but mostly falling in a steady, relentless, downpour. Unfortunately, I was forced out into it for an hour. After laying the brick walk, two large piles of earth, processed gravel, and washed sand remained in the driveway. And I was sick of looking at them. I pitched the excess gravel beneath the back porch and piled the remainder (one wheelbarrow full at a time) next to the compost. Transplanting the blueberry bushes could wait; filling a hole and sodding it could wait; turning the compost and returning Tim's wheelbarrow could easily wait. But the gravel and sand had to go. Now I feel jittery this morning, with pressure in my temples and a cold chill down my spine, the kind of chill that warmer clothing or resetting the thermostat will not touch.

Lindsay and Clare and I drove down to Camden in the rain and joined the Thomases for my first taste of beer at the Sea Dog Brewery, a micro-operation that just opened in the old Knox Woolen Mill. Fancy schmancy, heavy on pub decor and the sailing motif, but hardly a view of the vats or a whiff of malted barley. The waterfall that once powered Knox Mill had center stage and has become the pub's signature. But the beer itself will not. The "special extra bitter" ale that I sampled was warm and flat in the British tradition, but not the least bit "special" or "extra." Other beers are listed on the menu, and I'll reserve judgment at least until I've tried a wheat beer, Scottish ale, doppelbach, or barley wine.

Four o'clock in the morning. The hospital calls with word that Elena has died. The emergency room physician will pronounce her, but what now? No funeral home has been listed; Harry is deaf and cannot be telephoned; it is too early to request that a home health aide arouse him with the news. I take a number (the director of home health) and agree to call at 7:00 A.M. and make arrangements. Elena is finally at peace.

I hadn't communicated with her in two days. She slept more and more, especially in the mornings when I rounded, staying "comfortable" on Demerol and Phenergan. Her sleep was also merciful for the caregivers. Most of us found it excruciating to be near her, even for brief periods. Communication had been reduced to the basics at a time when so much swam in our heads. I felt taxed by the language board and those exasperated stares. Feedings had become an exercise in futility, as thick pink liquid oozed from her mouth faster than the syringe could replace it. It became increasingly difficult to prop and reposition her toothpick-like limbs and bobbing head, or to keep them restful in any position. And all of us felt the anguish of her predicament. I needed daily reassurance that the medication was treating Elena and not the rest of us.

As I write, Harry, who has stood by Elena steadfastly over these grueling two years, sleeps unaware.

I first called the visiting nurse and the director of home health, but reached only their answering machines. Next I called the Village of Liberty, hoping to enlist the services of their police department, but I had forgotten that they lacked one. I dialed the Waldo County Sheriff's Department in Belfast, but the deputy was off duty until 8:00 A.M., and even then we would have to "wait and see" if he had the time. By then, Harry and John could well be on their way to the hospital. So I dressed and headed to Liberty, grumbling all the way about the lack of foresight surrounding Elena's death.

Fluffy barked ferociously at the side door but was silenced by John's appearance in striped pajamas, and I entered to a cacophony of bird song. "She doesn't like the color of your car; she thinks it's red," John said, speaking for Fluffy, as he motioned to my teal green Jetta. Harry hastily dressed in the back bedroom and joined us in the dining room, where I had often come to visit Elena as she sat in her brown overstuffed rocker. The cloth restraints were still attached. The computer paraphernalia was nested in a box beside it.

"She's gone, isn't she?" Harry stammered. "Did she go in her sleep?" But without needing an answer, he continued, "I just thank God she didn't suffer any more than she already has. Sit down, won't you? Can you stay a moment?"

Harry ushered me into a chair and slumped next to me. He drew slow, deliberate breaths and spoke of the last few days and the long, tiring haul of the illness.

"She wanted me to destroy all her clothes. Once, when she was living in New Jersey, a friend of hers died young, and the family thought Elena should have her ring. It was a beautiful thing, fancy and jewelled, but when Elena wore it, misfortune followed her around—car wrecks, bad luck, things like that. She eventually took the ring to the Searsport dump and smashed it with a hammer. She didn't want any trouble to come from her clothes, even the things she never wore."

Harry studied the floor, stroked the arms of his chair, and continued, "I got her earrings for Christmas that are still in the box. She always asked for earrings every holiday and Christmas; oh, how she loved them. But this year she never put them on. I think she knew she was dying and wanted to be laid out in them."

John interrupted, and I turned to give him a share of my attention. "I feel so sorry for her, Dr. Loxterkamp, I just feel sorry. But I have my memories, my memories of places we've been together . . . to market for pizza, or the craft shop, or Sandy Point Beach. We don't know when she's coming home from the hospital. But I still have my dad."

"Yes you do, John," I replied, "and Fluffy and the birds and the garden and all those wonderful memories."

"I feel so sorry for her," he continued, oblivious to the news. "Once in school, I was eating a piece of candy and it slid too far back and I began to choke on it. It was too big to go down, so I spit it out, but by that time it had scratched my throat."

"That must have been scary, John," I said. And, groping for the connection, suggested, "Does it make you think of your mother and her choking?"

But before he could answer, Harry drew another breath. "It's so empty here. I just don't know how we'll go on, but we will. I'm sure we will. I'll summon up a stubborn streak and push ahead for John's sake. It's good to have that boy. We've been talking a lot lately. John told his mother, just after they made the diagnosis of ALS, 'Not to worry, Momma, Daddy and I will be OK.' I'll keep up with everything like Elena would have wanted, the garden and all."

"She loved this old house, though I don't know why, preferred it to anything I could have built for her. I'm partial to it myself, but I've lived here since I was a year old, and don't know any better. I never could have placed Elena in the nursing home, knowing how she felt about things. Mom wasted in one and I wish I'd never put her there. Dad withered away at home, like Elena, though faster, with a real bad case of hardened arteries, what the doctor said. At the end he couldn't move or swallow, just like Elena."

We exchanged words of appreciation for our mutual support over the final days. Harry thanked me for "all that ya done; you're more than a doctor, you're a caring person." And I praised him in return. "You couldn't have done more for your wife, Harry, providing her with happiness and love and a home to live in until the week of her death. It was an ordeal for all of us; many good people helped make the road a little easier. It should not end here. We will get together, we will stay in touch, and, if possible, I'd love to say goodbye to Elena at the memorial service."

I made telephone calls to the undertaker and hospital, apprising them of the recent events. Harry helped me package the computer, the headset, blink detector, and loudspeakers for MacInTalk, the printer and cords and all the paraphernalia that he had eyed warily from the start but allowed Elena to keep anyway. Because she wanted it. In the end she seldom used it; it was more symbolic than a useful extension of her arms or voice. Symbolic of what? Ed Regan's and my love for Elena, perhaps; or our desperate desire to do something in face of the overwhelming odds. In the end it accomplished little more than a referral to the specialists in Boston, as brother Roger had requested. Elena, in fact, negotiated her language board extremely well, once we got the knack of it and accepted the practice and patience and perseverance it required. Still, the language board communicated only a fragment of Elena's basic needs—no ordinary conversation, no sentiment, no ambivalence or deep longing, no love or forgiveness or last goodbyes. Only a drop in the ocean of her thoughts nodded and blinked onto the blank screen.

And that was that. I rolled out of the driveway and headed toward town, melding into the thickening traffic of the waking day. With Elena's departure from center stage of my routines, her memory will surely fade. All the attention and worry once accorded to her will fall to the next in line. I protest; it should be otherwise! But my regrets and best intentions, like seeds sown among thorns, will be swallowed up by the cares of the world (Mark 4:18–19).

I have returned to the computer each of the last three mornings, to my glowing green light and the print of St. Dominic, to the comforting rows of books that rise on either side of me and the strains of Brahms's *Requiem* lofting gently and with great solemnity past my living room door. At first I could only sit on these once-useful hands. I would listen to the rustle of cat feet and the groans of the furnace, and watch the first bluish hint of dawn as it peered in my eastern window and stirred a chorus of bird song and wind chime through the open back door.

Catatonia has given way to erranding; I have made list upon list, requiring my constant revision; I have found dishes to be dried, laundry to be folded, a cat box weeks beyond the possibility of restitution. Now I will attend to a long-neglected correspondence with my geographically challenged friends. But it is clear that the journal is in limbo; and that here, at this instant in the twelfth month, it should finally end.

Elena's funeral service was yesterday at 2:00 P.M. I could not, did not, attend as I had hoped; with Tim's upcoming vacation, there is no room in the schedule to reallocate the six appointments I would forfeit. Between patients, I penned a sympathy card to Harry and dropped it in the mail before leaving last night.

In my meditations this morning, I pause to remember Elena and Roberta Wilson, Mabel Towey and Greg Maguire, and the nine others who have died during the course of this journal. By the grace of God, the rest of us yet live for a time.

Ending the journal brings a sense of relief, a letdown, and a strong taste of humble pie. I realize now how ordinary a year (in an ordinary life) it has turned out to be. It does not claim to be heroic or grand. It has accomplished nothing of hard or lasting value in society's cynical eyes. But it has shown—if one can know such things by any means other than personal experience—how a certain people loved and labored and laid down their dead on this bare and rocky coast of Maine.

The journal's end is only a false alarm: I am one of the lucky ones. My life goes on. Good work stretches out before me without end in sight. I have a wife and daughter who invent me in their dreams as they toss in the cool sea breezes of a New England morning. And I have learned this: that life is not judged by our accomplishments, but by the love we have shared with our friends and with strangers.

Through my writing, I have tried to stay close to my patients. How can I forget Elena Moulton, who bore with Job-like patience her diminutive stature, a domineering mother, the retardation of her son, and an ignominious death from ALS. Her story joins that cacophonous debate over "doctor-assisted suicide." She taught us all—family and providers alike—that it is more often *our* pride and indignation that are put to the test.

The journal began as an accounting of the life of a country doctor. But it would not remain so. Nor is it, primarily, about growing older, coming of age, walking in my father's footsteps, or tasting the simple pleasures of a bucolic life. It is mostly about living in a small town, abiding by the conditions, and staking a spiritual claim. I can confirm in my own life what author Kathleen Norris discovered on the South Dakota plains: living in community is the only asceticism you need.

In the slow turn of the journal, I have grown more and more thankful for this measure of my days. Through it, and in the lives of my patients, I can imagine my own eventual decline. But I have been smitten, too, by a courageous spirit. And I have come to believe in something affirmed by every doctor who has found happiness in his work: that in the midst of death, we are in life.

Afterword

TAKING THE GRAVEL

It is Friday evening, two years hence. I hear the door latch behind the last nurse leaving. In the still of the deserted office, steeped now in its six o'clock shadows, I slump before my cluttered desk and brood on the comforts of a chosen life. Diplomas dot the east wall like a constellation, singing their laudates of daily devotion. On the opposite wall are mounted snapshots of my wife and daughter, grinning, from our sabbatical year. Japanese prints bow from the corners. They belonged to an AIDS victim whose mother came to me three years ago wearing society's shame upon her face, and they express, in ways we never could, the need for human companionship in the face of inexorable grief.

But I feel a burden in my breathing, like a boa wrapped around my chest. My partner of nine years has left on sabbatical. I know that while Tim has debated his decision to leave, I stew in mine to stay. Both of us demand answers: Can we be happy here? Will we survive?

I have reached the stride of my career. Because of my "efficiencies" (or level of competence, as they say), I rarely dip into the intimacies that once blessed my eyes and lips like holy water. Days peel off, patients whir through the schedule, tens of patient-care encounters are "generated" before I am forced to abandon the groove of the clinical routine.

Now the clinic has abandoned *me*. The day's din has dampened and the unconscious comes alive: Our faithful furnace clicks and groans, the telephone tinkles with calls rerouted to the answering service, and traffic drones on its merry way home. Angels shudder in the stygian darkness.

I have come to a dubious age. The specialty of family practice, like all of medicine, finds itself on sandy soil in a time of seismic change. The old pillars are falling; our leaders have left. And I feel not so much abandoned as vulnerable, like a hermit crab caught outside his shell. I have outgrown my old ambitions,

315

satisfied parental expectations, repaid my student loans, and earned that elusive right to self-respect. And I must now stake out the future on my own.

In school, you are valued for what you know; in practice, for what you can do. But who you are is another matter, something drawn in the lines of duty and given flesh through the relationships you forge over time. I am coming, thankfully, to that moment in my career, yet I still glance backward over the stages of formation: First, those frenzied years after graduation, of "proving myself" to patients and colleagues alike. Then, in my thirties, I began to notice how far the authority granted to me had outstripped my powers to use it wisely. There were moments of moral weakness, temptation and snap judgment, laziness and plain indifference at every turn. These added up, looming larger than the good I could ever have dreamed of accomplishing in my youthful striving.

The practice of medicine seems a hard life, harder than I imagined. I know now the sting of missed birthdays, the depths of exhaustion, the guilt of every mistake, the pressures of performance, the rigid limits of one's role, and the personal costs of treating pain too closely and death too often.

Sometimes I doubt if I can keep step with the march of medicine. It is a quest that fewer long for, and in which fewer last. I share cafeteria meals with colleagues who have turned their careers into marriages of convenience, a means to an end for paying off home mortgage loans and college trusts. I feel my tired eyes wander to newer, more seductive passions: writing, perhaps, or an assistant professorship. I listen for the distant hoofbeats of history that signaled my father's ambush by heart attack at age forty-nine.

From the chatter in the doctors' lounge, I can reel off names of colleagues who see their future through the filmy lens of a fiberoptic scope, or from the catbird seat of managed care. Others feel pinned at the Alamo of medicine, outnumbered by the circling crowd of malingerers and litigators and drug seekers, the hopeless masses with their hopeless wounds. Yet, even for the dispirited, I believe that idealism has not died. So again the words of Osler challenge us, "Ideals mean much, but that they are realizable means more.*

The doctor, to be sure, has an enviable life. I have lacked neither for work nor its reward. I am blessed with financial security, the trust of my patients, and a growing facility in the affairs of medicine. I could assure you that vocation's flame, with its warm and illuminating sense of purpose, still burns in my heart. My ears prick to the clarion call of duty; I have neither slowed to the chase nor long doubted the charge.

* W. Osler, *Aequanimitus with Other Addresses to Medical Students, Nurses, and Practitioners,* quoted by Charles S. Bryan, "What Is the Oslerian Tradition?" *Annals of Internal Medicine* 120, no. 8: 684.

I know something of what William Osler suggests in his line, "nothing will sustain you more potently than the power to recognize in our hum-drum routine . . . the true poetry of life—the poetry of the commonplace."* These are the same sentiments found in the poems and stories of William Carlos Williams, or John Berger's classic tale of *A Fortunate Man,* or in almost every writing that probes the genuine, sustaining, regenerative qualities of medical practice.

But poetry may not be sufficient to survive a career in medicine. I have been blessed with a love for literature, and have felt the love of my wife and daughter and friends, have reveled in the natural beauty of this land along the Penobscot. Yet even these are sometimes not enough.

I believe that the remainder is satisfied, perhaps completed, by a vow of stability: to my marriage, my vocation, my adopted community. It is a curious pledge, this vow, borrowed from the Rule of St. Benedict. In Benedict's time, Christian ascetics were often vagabonds, whose roving ways undermined the formation of community and distracted them from their search for God. Under the Rule, monks to this day vow to remain within a single community for a lifetime. St. Benedict saw mobility as the physical expression of a man's pride, independence, and free will, and believed that it should be brought under "the healing influence of obedience" to an abbot.

I have no abbot in Belfast, only my wife (who is lenient), my family, and a modest mortgage to repay. Yet I have stayed. And in so doing I have witnessed scores of patients close out their lives. That process draws you near to a person and earns you a setting, however briefly, at their family table. In staying I have watched my marriage change, my daughter grow, and a new son (at last!) spring miraculously into our lives. I live alongside my mistakes; habits and weaknesses have settled to a livable level; stories merge into other stories in which I play an increasingly central but less pivotal role.

At forty-three, I have crossed the Rubicon of my career. Patients and community alike know that I will not leave them. I have been hooked by the dependable rewards of patient care, with the same bait that lured William Carlos Williams, in whose poetry you'll find the exhilaration that many of us feel in the day-to-day care of our patients:

> It's the humdrum, day-in, day-out, everyday work that is the real satisfaction of the practice of medicine; the million and a half patients a man has seen on his daily visits over a forty-year period of weekdays and Sundays that make up his life. I have never had a money practice; it would have been impossible for me. But the actual calling on people, at all times and under all conditions, the coming to grips with the intimate conditions of their lives,

* Ibid.

when they were being born, when they were dying, watching them die, watching them get well when they were ill, has always absorbed me. (p. 119)

After a few years under these conditions, it is possible to believe that the wish for happiness and the wish for survival are two sides of a common coin. That in seeking one you find the other.

I reach to smooth the lump in my right hip pocket. It is a crumpled envelope, the letter I had stuffed there before leaving home this morning. I tear it open. A newspaper clipping catches on the ratty edges of my mother's notebook paper and tumbles out. I pick it up and carefully unfold it, working the creases like a Rubik's cube, until my eyes rest upon the bold lettering:

Dr. J. M. Hinds Dead at 74

This news pierces me in a strange, unexpected way; I freeze in my chair and funnel back through time. After my father's death in 1966, Dr. Hinds became our family physician. Gradually he grew into much more: the personification of the Ideal Physician. When I was a student in the College of Medicine, J.M. counted me among his colleagues. His signature topped the distinguished list on my first medical license, and his career broke ground for my own decision, years later, to swap the academic ladder for the level playing field of general practice. Now, in a stroke, he was gone.

Dr. Hinds practiced in the shire town, twelve miles over. He seemed cut from the same cloth as Watergate prosecutor Sam Erwin, "just a country doctor" who was also salutatorian of his medical class, chair of the state board of medical examiners, perennial delegate to the AMA. J.M. played musical chairs on the municipal committees, kept his busy practice at an even boil, chased after five children, and dodged a divorce from his neglected wife. It would take a movement disorder, Parkinson's disease, to finally hobble him into retirement.

It is true that the procedures of his day, breech deliveries and tonsillectomies and exchange transfusions, were out of vogue or beyond the pale of the new family physician. He was too busy to bother with educational objectives, decision trees, or the prevention protocols that tethered me in training. In skill and temperament, he was closer to a general surgeon than to his heirs-apparent in family practice. And though he might demur, I consider him my teacher. He executed, with poise and precision, the simple work of the general practitioner, whom Sir William Osler extolled as "the hope of the profession" and the "flower of our calling." Something of that life has become my own.

Although much of my memory of J.M. has faded, one image from a rural preceptorship in 1982 burns brightly. J.M. would perch on the exam stool and cradle his jowls in a leathery hand, then lean toward his patient and sop up her sadness like bread in gravy. Listening, with steely eyes cast, he seemed to gaze beyond, perhaps to puzzle after the hidden agenda or a pattern formed by the patient's recent visits. Or to drift to unrelated concerns gathering on his conscience like thunderheads over a parched prairie.

I'll not forget the sound of his laughter, a boisterous, unrestrained, bellowing laugh that he shared with friends. He could laugh with his patients and laugh at himself, and through it divide their differences while preserving a precious ground for honesty and frankness and savage self-scrutiny. He hung harmonies on a whole genre of sappy, sentimental tunes like "I've Been Working on the Railroad" or "Tell Me Why" and orchestrated shenanigans at the annual Society Barbecue in a preposterous chef's bonnet and apron. He loved his patients, though not all dearly; loved his job in an unfettered way that has became obsolete in the age of addiction theory; loved the spotlight, the lead role, the well-rehearsed line that so often began on the telephone at midnight, "Mmm, Doctor's residence."

There was something familiar about J.M. I first saw it in the mannerisms that resembled my father's; I saw it in the old stories, corny photographs, and favorite melodies of the Sagadahoc County Medical Society, where each played a principal role. In those days, before CME and the promise of "information highways," county physicians met monthly in a member's home for the noble purpose of "upholding the ethical and scientific standards of medicine." After the formal program they would revel in the fellowship born of a common struggle. There were highballs, often too many, that led to the inevitable cursing of the city specialists and admonitions to "take the gravel" home. Here, on these unpaved and deserted roads, they found safety in their journey. Perhaps, too, they found comfort in that same solitude that cloaked their practices. And forgiveness, in the still, open, starlit reaches.

The news of J.M.'s passing is magnified by the sight of my partner's vacant desk. Again, the questions stare back at me, the ones that have dogged me from the start: Can I be fulfilled by my work? Can I do it here in Belfast, and practice without regrets? Live with my mistakes? Accept my limitations? Settle for the portion of good mixed with the bad, the crumbs of joy mixed with the gravel? Or would I fling them to the wind, certain that I deserve better, like the million hopeful "finalists" in the Publisher's Clearinghouse Sweepstakes?

Nothing lasts forever. That is the one inescapable conclusion of a life in medicine. You discover how lucky you are to be captivated by your work, by a purpose, and by the people who surround you. You realize what a privilege it is to be invited into their lives, counted among family, enriched by their stories, and quickened by the certain knowledge of what becomes of all flesh. Our steady, important, respected careers will shudder to a halt before we know it. We will be left with a few cherished memories, scattered over the years, when pride or humility, grief or gratitude, or naked love shattered the sterile shield of our clinical experience.

My life here, and the keeping of this journal, have given me a glimpse of what J.M. Hinds and others of his generation learned in their lifetime. He taught me how to listen, how to quiet the voice of my own authority and so honor those who suffer in silence. His good humor blessed my own life with laughter, with great mouthfuls of sacrilege and frustration, tears and thanksgiving that I can now offer up to a Greater Glory. He believed that when you love your practice as a steward loves, you can expect to have love returned.

He left me with one final lesson: that true happiness, for which a man would gladly risk all, is won over the long haul. Through finding the necessary means to survive. Through accepting the bad that comes with all good. Through the long habit of taking the gravel.

Selected References

Anderson, Sherwood. "Death in the Woods." In *The Portable Sherwood Anderson*. New York: Viking Press, 1949.

Anon. *The Way of the Pilgrim*. Trans. R. M. French. San Francisco: HarperCollins, 1991.

Attwater, Donald. *Saints*. Middlesex, England: Penguin Books, 1979.

Berger, John. *A Fortunate Man*. London: Penguin Books, 1968.

Bernanos, Georges. *The Diary of a Country Priest*. New York: Carroll and Graf, 1989.

Brown, Raymond. *Crises Facing the Church*. New York: Paulist Press, 1975.

Colcord, Lincoln. *Sea Stories from Searsport to Singapore*. Unity, Maine: North Country Press, 1990.

Coles, Robert. *The Call of Stories*. New York: Houghton Mifflin, 1989.

Conrad, Joseph. *Heart of Darkness*. London: Penguin Press, 1973.

Dillard, Annie. *Teaching a Stone to Talk*. New York: Harper & Row, 1982.

Hampl, Patricia. *Virgin Time*. New York: Ballantine Books, 1992.

Hauerwas, Stanley. *Naming the Silences*. Grand Rapids, Mich.: William B. Eerdmans, 1990.

Kafka, Franz. "A Country Doctor," in *Selected Stories of Franz Kafka*. New York: Random House, 1952.

Merton, Thomas. *Mystics and Zen Masters*. New York: Noonday Press, 1989.

———. *Selected Poems*. New York: New Directions, 1963.

———. *The Sign of Jonas*. New York: Harcourt, Brace and Company, 1953.

———. *The Wisdom of the Desert*. New York: New Directions, 1970.

Norris, Kathleen. *Dakota: A Spiritual Geography*. New York: Ticknor and Fields, 1993.

Nouwen, Henri J. M. *Behold the Beauty of the Lord: Praying with Icons*. Notre Dame, Ind.: Ave Maria Press, 1991.

———. *The Genessee Diary: Report from a Trappist Monastery*. New York: Image books, 1976.

O'Connor, Flannery. *A Good Man Is Hard to Find and Other Stories*. New York and London: Harcourt Brace Jovanovich, 1976.

Pope-Hennessy, John. *Angelico*. Florence: Scala Books, 1981.

The Rule of Saint Benedict. Trans. Anthony Meisel and M. L. del Mastro. New York: Image Books, 1975.

Sillitoe, Alan. *Loneliness of the Long-Distance Runner*. New York: New American Library, 1987.

Tolstoy, Leo. *The Death of Ivan Illych*. New York: New American Library, 1960.

Williams, William Carlos. *The Doctor Stories*. New York: New Directions, 1984.

Wills, Gary. *Lincoln at Gettysburg*. New York: Simon & Schuster, 1992.

UNIVERSITY PRESS OF NEW ENGLAND publishes books under its own imprint and is
the publisher for Brandeis University Press, Dartmouth College, Middlebury College Press,
University of New Hampshire, Tufts University, and Wesleyan University Press.

LIBRARY OF CONGRESS CATALOGING-IN-PUBLICATION DATA
Loxterkamp, David.
    A measure of my days : the journal of a country doctor / David
Loxterkamp.
      p.   cm.
    Includes bibliographical references.
    ISBN 0–87451–799–0 (alk. paper)
      1. Medicine—Maine—Belfast—Anecdotes.   2. Loxterkamp, David.
3. Medicine, Rural—Maine—Belfast—Anecdotes.   I. Title.
R705.L69   1997
610'.92—dc21   96–54704